EDUCATION, AND WELFARE
1968

OFFICE OF PUBLIC INFORMATION

ASSISTANT SECRETARY (Planning and Evaluation)	GENERAL COUNSEL	ASSISTANT SECRETARY FOR ADMINISTRATION	ASSISTANT SECRETARY, COMPTROLLER

SOCIAL AND REHABILITATION SERVICE

Office of the Administrator

Rehabilitation Services Administration

Children's Bureau

Administration on Aging

Medical Services Administration

Assistance Payments Administration

SOCIAL SECURITY ADMINISTRATION

Office of the Commissioner

Bureau of Data Processing and Accounts

Bureau of Disability Insurance

Bureau of District Office Operations

Bureau of Federal Credit Unions

Bureau of Health Insurance

Bureau of Hearings and Appeals

Bureau of Retirement and Survivors Insurance

OFFICE OF EDUCATION

Office of the Commissioner

Bureau of Elementary and Secondary Education

Bureau of Adult, Vocational and Library Programs

Bureau of Higher Education

Bureau of Research

Bureau of Education for the Handicapped

Bureau of Educational Personnel Development

Institute of International Studies

Regional Commissioners	Regional Commissioners	Regional Assistant Commissioners

FIFTH EDITION

MUSTARD'S INTRODUCTION TO PUBLIC HEALTH

LENOR S. GOERKE, M.D., M.S.P.H.

Dean, School of Public Health
Chairman, Department of Preventive Medicine
School of Medicine
University of California, Los Angeles

ERNEST L. STEBBINS, M.D., M.P.H., Dr. Med. Sc.

Dean Emeritus and
Professor of Public Health Administration,
School of Hygiene and Public Health
Johns Hopkins University, Baltimore

With the Assistance of Rosabelle Price Walkley
School of Public Health, University of California, Los Angeles

THE MACMILLAN COMPANY
COLLIER-MACMILLAN LIMITED, LONDON

DEDICATED TO THE MEMORY OF

HARRY STOLL MUSTARD, M.D., LL.D.
October 10, 1888–August 4, 1966

epidemiologist, health officer,
dean, professor, scholar, and
outstanding leader in his profession,
who initiated and demonstrated
new and imaginative approaches
to the problems of public
health and preventive medicine

PRINTING   5678910   YEAR   23456789

Earlier editions entitled *An Introduction to Public Health*, by Harry S. Mustard, copyright 1935, 1944, and 1953 by The Macmillan Company. Earlier edition entitled *An Introduction to Public Health*, by Harry S. Mustard and Ernest L. Stebbins, © 1959 by The Macmillan Company.

Library of Congress catalog card number: 68–11858

THE MACMILLAN COMPANY
866 THIRD AVENUE, NEW YORK, NEW YORK 10022
COLLIER-MACMILLAN CANADA, LTD., TORONTO, ONTARIO

PRINTED IN THE UNITED STATES OF AMERICA

PREFACE
TO THE FIFTH EDITION

Tremendous changes have taken place in both scope and content of public health programs since the publication, in 1935, of the first edition of *Introduction to Public Health*, by the late Dr. Harry S. Mustard. These changes have been particularly accelerated in recent years, and for this reason the present edition has been completely revised and reoriented to the modern concepts of public health practice.

At the turn of the century, public health efforts in the United States were influenced largely by the need to control morbidity and mortality from communicable diseases. Remarkable progress was made in this direction in ensuing years, through advances in scientific knowledge of the causes of many communicable diseases and the systematic application of control measures. Environmental sanitation, as one of the significant measures, became a prominent part of public health programs. Today these efforts continue, but the nature of modern life has added new dimensions to public health and has greatly increased the complexity of health and welfare problems.

The scientific explosion, the vast quantity of federal and state legislation related to health and welfare, and the changing patterns of organization of health services are only a few of the numerous developments that are influencing contemporary public health. The community is assuming new and important roles in health planning, health facilities are expanding markedly, and new methods for the economic support of health services are being sought. Various social forces are also playing an important role in this dynamic process. These forces are manifested, for example, in the struggle to apply the results of science for the general welfare. They are also revealed in increasing public expectations regarding health services—expectations that have accelerated the demands for more and new kinds of health manpower throughout the world. Changes in population size and distribution are still other types of social forces that are creating new problems, the impact of which is likely to extend far into the future.

The purpose of this book is to introduce students to the concepts and principles that serve as the broad underpinnings of public health, and to

provide an orientation to contemporary modes of community health organization and practice. The current status of public health programs and
services is described in order to provide a view of present adequacies and
inadequacies and to communicate a sense of the challenge of unsolved
problems. Historical background is included in order to provide perspective.
Factors in the social, physical, and biological environments that influence
the magnitude and character of public health problems, goals, and the search
for solutions are considered, and the continuous changes occurring in these
factors are emphasized. The multidisciplinary nature of public health is
pointed out and viewed as an essential characteristic of the field. International health considerations are included in order to provide breadth of
understanding and an awareness of the magnitude of health problems in the
world today.

Traditionally, the advancement of health and welfare has resulted from
the interest, concern, and contribution of individuals from many disciplines
and backgrounds. Most professional schools concerned with the preparation
of health personnel require their students to take introductory courses in
public health. For still other categories of students, the hope is that this book
will stimulate them to consider their potential contributions to the health
field and to investigate the many career opportunities offered. The choice
of subject matter, references, and suggested reading has been influenced
by these considerations.

All subjects retained from previous editions of the book have been written
anew, with as much comprehensiveness and depth as are consistent with
the purpose of an introductory, manageable volume. A new chapter has been
added on the concepts and methods of investigation in epidemiology and of
research in other areas of community health. A chapter on the threat of
excessive population growth, and trends in solving the problems of overpopulation, has also been provided. A new chapter that reviews the health
manpower situation and describes professional services and careers in community health has been included in order to alert students to some of the
many professional and occupational opportunities in the health field.

L. S. G.
E. L. S.

ACKNOWLEDGMENTS

Special recognition and grateful acknowledgment are due the many individuals who have participated in the preparation of this volume. The primary collaborators, who are members of the faculty of the UCLA School of Public Health (unless indicated otherwise), are as follows:

Historical Development of Public Health	Arthur J. Viseltear, Ph.D., M.P.H.
Demographic Data and Vital Statistics	Jean L. Mickey, Ph.D.
	Virginia A. Clark, Ph.D.
Medical Care	Arnold I. Kisch, M.D., M.P.H.
Community Mental Health	J. Albert Torribio, M.S.W., M.S.S.W.*
Environmental Health	Charles L. Senn, M.S.†
Acute Communicable Diseases	Telford H. Work, M.D., M.P.H., D.T.M.&H.
Venereal Diseases	Walter H. Smartt, M.D., M.P.H.‡
Chronic Diseases	David P. Discher, M.D.
Maternal and Child Health	Audrey J. Naylor, M.D., M.P.H.§
	Marsden Wagner, M.D., M.S.P.H.
Health of the Child in School	Harriett B. Randall, M.D. ‖
Health Education	Guy W. Steuart, Ph.D., M.P.H.

Several other members of the faculties and staffs of the School of Hygiene and Public Health, Johns Hopkins University, and the UCLA School of Public Health have contributed to the book in a variety of ways. At UCLA, Dr. Charles E. Schoettlin and Dr. Jay W. Friedman provided valuable material on epidemiology and public health dentistry, respectively; Dr. Edward H. Forgotson contributed a comprehensive review of federal legislation pertaining to public health; Mrs. Elizabeth A. Hefferin provided

---

* Mr. Torribio is also chief of the Central Preventive Services Division, Los Angeles County Department of Mental Health.

† Mr. Senn is also environmental sanitation consultant, Los Angeles County Health Department.

‡ Dr. Smartt is chief of the Division of Venereal Disease Control, Los Angeles County Health Department.

§ Dr. Naylor was engaged in postdoctoral studies at the UCLA School of Public Health.

‖ Dr. Randall is also medical administrator, Health Services Branch, Los Angeles City School Districts.

material on public health nursing and assisted in the assembly of some of the illustrative material that appears in the book. Thanks are also due the following staff who typed the manuscript: Mrs. Helen Balch, Miss Margaret Weichel, Mrs. Barbara Brooks, and Mrs. Nancy Davenport.

CONTENTS

SECTION I

BACKGROUND
AND ORGANIZATION
OF PUBLIC HEALTH

HISTORICAL DEVELOPMENT OF PUBLIC HEALTH

The principal historical events that have marked the development of public health from antiquity to the present are described in this chapter. Throughout history, the nature of public health at a particular time and in a particular place has been influenced by the interaction of several basic phenomena; these are discussed briefly in the first section of the chapter. The second section describes early concepts of cleanliness and health and the public health developments of Greco-Roman times. The next three sections trace the nature of disease, theories and practices regarding disease, and significant social circumstances and developments from the Middle Ages through the nineteenth century. The revolutionary change in concepts of the cause, prevention, treatment, and control of disease that resulted from the emergence of scientific knowledge in the middle and late nineteenth century is described in the last section of the chapter. This section also discusses the influence of scientific knowledge on public health in the United States in the twentieth century, particularly in connection with the vast expansion of public health activities and the maturation of public health ideology.

PUBLIC HEALTH IN HISTORICAL PERSPECTIVE

The history of public health is an account of man's efforts to maintain himself and his community in a state of physical and mental well-being. By studying man's attempts to fulfill this purpose, the subject of public health unfolds as a continuum of events in time. A study of the history of public health has utility other than the intrinsic value of contemplating the past for its own sake. Thus, the ideas, attitudes, and institutions of present-day public health become more clearly defined when studied in a historical context. Moreover, connecting the past with the present in a continuous line of understanding provides valuable insight into what people of the past thought, felt, and intended; and a needed perspective and broadening of point of view are attained by examining the ultimate consequences of these actions and movements.[1, 2, 3] *

At any point in its history, public health has reflected the interaction of three basic phenomena: first, the nature and severity of disease; second, the theories as to the cause of disease and the practices regarding control and treatment; and third, the character of the prevailing social ideology and circumstances. In addition to manifesting a process of continuous inter-action at a particular time and place, these phenomena have also undergone marked alteration throughout history.

Over the centuries, the kinds of disease that have harassed mankind have changed, as has the severity of their effect on the population. The effects of the early, devastating epidemic diseases were mitigated as their true causes became known, and this knowledge in turn led to more effective control and treatment. Throughout this process, the kind and nature of the attention paid to health and disease were influenced by the ideologic concepts that dominated society at the time. The influencing ideologies were, variously, theologic, economic, political, and social. Situational factors also played a role and usually involved manifestations of the deprived and squalid circumstances in which the population lived, as well as the asso-ciated prevalence of disease. Throughout history, whether the promotion of health and the fight against disease lagged or progressed depended on the combination of dominant ideology, situational pressures, manifestations of disease, and status of knowledge.

It is apparent, then, that public health activity and thought, from antiquity to the present, have been intimately related to the nature of society at a specific time and place. From a historical perspective, the inter-action of disease, status of knowledge, and character of society is seen as a dynamic and continuous process, extending from the past to the present and into the future.

---

* Throughout the book, the superscript numbers pertain to References that appear at the end of each chapter.

THE ANCIENT WORLD

Early Concepts of Cleanliness and Health

Primitive man learned empirically to distinguish things that were good for him from those that were harmful. By observing animals he learned that bathing not only cooled and refreshed his body, but helped remove external parasites; he learned that application of mud assuaged insect bites; and by determining the actions of certain herbs, he learned their various medicinal or poisonous characteristics. To the primitive mind disease and infirmity were believed to be caused by the influence of magic or by malevolent spirits that inhabited streams, trees, animals, the earth, and the air. Purposively or accidentally provoking any of the spirits, it was thought, would result in dire consequences for the individual or his community unless propitiation was made to counteract the malignant influences of the offended spirit.[4]

As civilization advanced to a higher level and magical beliefs and animism were reduced to mere superstition, religion became the vehicle for hygienic thinking. All ancient religions demanded that a man who entered a place of worship be clean. This dictum implied spiritual cleanliness, but it was necessary for such cleanliness to have an outward expression. In ancient Egypt, for example, priests were robed in spotless garments and avoided touching unclean objects.

In no society of ancient times were the precepts of spiritual cleanliness and community responsibility more clearly formalized than among the Hebrews. The laws promulgated in the Book of Leviticus relate specifically to food, clothing, environmental sanitation, diseases, and personal hygiene. In the Talmud, which constitutes the body of civil and canonical law of the Jewish people, the hygienic code is discussed in great detail, as is the concept of contagion. Whosoever touched an unclean person or object himself became impure. The woman in labor was considered unclean from the moment her pains began until 40 days after delivery if her child were a boy, and 80 days if it were a girl. The menstruating woman was considered unclean for seven days.* Gonorrhea and zaraath (the latter being a loathsome skin disease that might or might not have been leprosy) were both highly prevalent in antiquity and also were discussed in terms of uncleanliness. Men who had discharges from their urethra were set apart from the community, whereas the man suspected of zaraath suffered an even harsher fate. He was examined by a temple priest who made his diagnosis on the basis of certain signs and symptoms recorded in Leviticus. If the signs were present and the disease diagnosed, the man was said to be "unclean" and compelled to leave the community. At some future date,

* Lev. 12:1–8.

when the man thought himself recovered and attempted to return to the community, he was examined again by the priest to ensure that recovery was complete.* In the Middle Ages when true leprosy became highly prevalent, the Church fought the disease by the rules found in the Book of Leviticus. The fact that the priests were responsible for the diagnosis of the disease indicates that the motivations for isolation, itself a public health measure, derived not from medical concepts, but from religious principles. As long as disease was considered to be caused by transgression or sin and inflicted by an all-powerful deity, the priest remained the physician of the body as well as of the soul.

The Greco-Roman World

Personal Hygiene. Whereas the Hebrews codified rules of hygiene for religious reasons, the Greeks created a system of personal hygiene which related to their attitude toward the human body. In the Greek world, the ideal man was perfectly balanced in mind and body and said to resonate with nature. Physical education, sports, and athletics were integrated into the educational system, and, with an emphasis on a simple regimen and vigorous physical exercise, the Greek youth approached an esthetic and hygienic ideal which remains unparalleled in history. Unfortunately, this refined personal hygiene was reserved for the upper social strata. The great mass of the common people—the slaves, farmers, and laborers—had no part in it.[5]

Environmental Sanitation. Although the Greek code of personal hygiene served as a model for all time, it remained for the Romans to develop public health. With respect to the human body and personal hygiene, the Romans differed little from the Greeks, but in the fields of engineering and administration the Romans far surpassed the Greeks. A notable development was the Roman water supply, an excellent history of which was given by Sextus Julius Frontinus, the Roman water commissioner in the first century A.D. Frontinus relates in his classic treatise on the aqueducts of Rome [6] that for over 400 years since the founding of the Empire, water was obtained in Rome from the Tiber or from private wells. In the fourth century B.C., however, the quantity and quality of the water increased markedly when the first large aqueduct, which transported water directly from the mountains to the city of Rome, was constructed. By Frontinus' time, nine aqueducts had been built which delivered many millions of gallons to the Empire (see Fig. 1-1).

As early as the sixth century B.C., Rome was provided with subterranean sewers called *cloacae*. Greece also had a sewage and drainage system which was maintained and supervised by *astynomi*, officials of the various city

* Lev. 13–15.

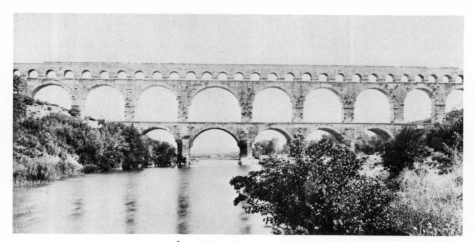

FIGURE 1-1. The aqueduct at Nîmes. Roman. (Courtesy of the Wellcome Trustees, London, England.)

states. In Rome, four municipal officials, called *aediles,* divided the city into police districts and were responsible for the maintenance and control of various municipal problems such as the construction and repair of public buildings; the cleaning and paving of streets; the control of nuisances of deteriorated buildings, dangerous animals, and foul smells; the destruction of unwholesome food; the suppression of false weights and measures; and the supervision of public baths, taverns, and brothels. The *aediles* also were responsible for the Roman sewage system, which included the Cloaca Maxima (see Fig. 1-2). Built in the late Republican period of Rome this

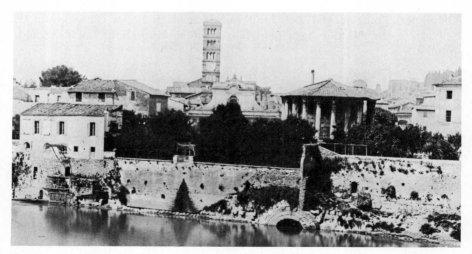

FIGURE 1-2. The Cloaca Maxima, a main drain of Rome. (Courtesy of the Wellcome Trustees, London, England.)

sewer drained the marshes at the base of the Capitoline Hill and emptied
into the Tiber. Today visitors to Rome may see this great sewer; it remains
a part of the drainage system of modern Rome, a testimony to the Roman
engineering genius of ancient times.[7, 8]

Medical Care and Hospitals.   In Greece, medical care was instituted
in *iatreia*, i.e., shops or offices in which the physician practiced medicine.
These *iatreia* were the private property of the medical men, and only in
the Asklepian temples was medicine practiced on an institutional level.
Other than the sanctuaries of the temples, the Greeks had no hospitals,
but they did have a primitive health service which was sponsored by the
individual city states. "Public surgeons and state physicians" were elected
by the citizens of the city states and existed side by side with private physicians. Once elected, the doctors entered into a contract with the city and
served in time of peace and war.[9]

In the Roman Empire, a significant contribution was the establishment
of hospitals. Suetonius, the second century A.D. Roman historian and biog-
rapher, has recorded the fact that an Asklepian temple was built on a small
island in the Tiber where sick and exhausted slaves were sent for nursing
and medical assistance. The Emperor Claudius (A.D. 41–54) decreed that
sick slaves became free if they recovered, and the island became a place of
refuge for the sick poor and may be considered an early form of public
hospital. Furthermore, Columella and Seneca both speak of *valetudinaria*
(infirmaries) which were used by slaves and freemen alike. Military ventures especially necessitated such infirmaries. As the Roman frontiers spread,
the wounded and diseased soldiers could no longer be sent back to Rome
and were placed in *valetudinaria* which were built at strategic points along
the frontier. *Valetudinaria* were also built in numerous frontier towns for
the imperial officials and their families. Many hospitals for the sick and the
outcast of the Middle Ages may be traced back to these Roman *valetudinaria.*

THE MIDDLE AGES

During the period of time known as the Renaissance, the practice arose
of dividing the history of the world into three major epochs: ancient,
medieval, and modern. For many centuries after this division, the word
"medieval" has connoted that period in time when civilization reached its
lowest ebb, a period of abysmal ignorance and superstition, when man's
concern was more for the "next world" than for this one. Even today "medieval" has become a synonym for reaction and lack of progress.

The Middle Ages, however, were not as stygian as has been thought.
It is true that the period immediately following the fall of Rome was characterized by a return to paganism, barbarism, anti-intellectualism, moral
asceticism, and political and economic decay. But with the Carolingian Re-

naissance in the West and the Arab ascendancy in the Near East, a renewed vitality flowed through the world. In the fields of literature, art, philosophy, and science, the human spirit soared to unprecedented heights. Public health and hygiene in this middle period between the ancient and modern worlds never attained the heights of a *renaissance*, but there were patches of illumination amid the political and economic chaos which characterized the early Middle Ages.

The Decline of Rome and Its Influence

Roman engineering and administrative genius reached its zenith between the second and fourth centuries. After this time the Roman civilization disintegrated owing to a number of external and internal factors which included the exhaustion of the soil, unfavorable balance of trade, epidemics of bubonic plague, and a persistent moral decrepitude. By the fifth and sixth centuries the impenetrable frontiers of the Roman Empire had been breached and Rome itself severely devastated and plundered. In A.D. 537, while Rome was under seige by the Goths, eleven principal aqueducts of Rome were destroyed, and without the financial means or the manpower necessary to repair them the water supply to the city after that time was perpetually disrupted.

Just as the barbarian invasions destroyed Rome physically, Christianity mitigated the hygienic precepts of the Greeks and Romans. The new religion found its disciples among the lower classes, where personal hygiene was not practiced, and as a consequence, an entirely different attitude toward the human body developed. Excessive care of the body, that is, man's earthly and mutable part, was unimportant in the Christian dualistic concept, which separated body from soul. For some Eastern churchmen and holy men, living in filth was regarded as evidence of sanctity: cleanliness was thought to betoken pride, and filthiness humility. Such an attitude was not favorable for the development of hygiene. Fortunately, the concept that the body was the perishable part of man matured in time until the body eventually was considered the abode of the soul while man was on earth, thereby permitting man to preserve and attend to its hygiene and cleanliness.

The Medieval City

Attendant upon the fall of Rome were the disintegration of the cities and the return of political anarchy. Large estates which were organized during the Roman supremacy were forced to band together in military and political units in order to withstand the attacks of the barbarians. A strong ruler conquered a district and immediately set about to defend his territory by building a fortress. Although the fortresses usually were founded for defense and military purposes, they soon became towns in the economic and social sense. Clergy and monks coerced those who came to the fortress for protection into adopting the teachings of the Church, and the traders who followed the soldiers and priests found a profitable occupation in exploiting the economic needs of the growing towns.

The physical appearances of the medieval towns were remarkably similar. The high walls were one of their most distinguishing characteristics as was the general plan of the town. The towns were plotted in squares with straight streets crossing each other at right angles. The main thoroughfares led directly from the main gates to the center of town where a town hall, market place, and church were built around the central piazza. As the town grew in size, the buildings and houses were packed closer together owing to the restrictions of the walls which encircled the city. As the populace spread outside the original wall, a new one was built, so that many towns eventually had two or three encircling walls.[10]

The rapid and haphazard growth of the towns soon made them unhealthy places in which to live. The buildings and houses were jammed close to-gether, thereby decreasing light and ventilation. Drainage was poor, latrines were connected to overflowing cesspools, and refuse was thrown into rat-infested streets. The houses had floors covered by straw or earth, and the people slept on tick mattresses which were usually infested by a host of insect pests. Municipal ordinances were issued by city councils in an at-tempt to control the health of the towns, but the towns grew too quickly for these to be effective. It is no wonder that epidemic diseases flourished in such a fertile environment.

The Wasteland: Epidemic Disease

Leprosy. The Middle Ages are characterized by the great epidemics. Leprosy was perhaps the cruelest in its manifestations. The disease spread from the Near East to Asia Minor, where it was contracted by crusaders who then brought it to the West. The terror of leprosy is related to the severe facial disfigurement of the leper, to the acute contagiousness and virulence of the disease, and to the biblical references to leprosy as a loath-some disease. All Western countries issued edicts against anyone suspected of having the disease and regulated every aspect of the sufferer's life. In some communities the leper was given the last rites of the Church and was compelled to wear identifying clothing and to warn of his presence by carrying a rod or sounding a bell. Such isolation usually brought about a speedy death from hunger and exposure, but some lepers found asylum in institutions created especially for their care and maintenance. The ma-jority of the lepers, however, never received this care and were especially susceptible to other diseases. When the bubonic plague of the fourteenth century passed through Europe, the lepers were all but eradicated, and thereafter leprosy decreased in prevalence and severity.

Bubonic Plague. The bubonic plague, known as the Black Death, may be considered the most severe epidemic in terms of mortality and disruption of society that the world has ever seen. Plague entered the Continent from Asia, and in three great thrusts moved westward into the areas of the Black Sea, Asia Minor and Greece, and Egypt and North Africa. Its progress was inexorable and in two years it had spread over all Europe.

Estimates of the casualties vary from 20 to 35 million, and it is very likely that Europe lost between a quarter and a third of its entire population. The effects of this great mortality were profound.[12] Many people reacted to the plague either by becoming licentious and hedonistic or by becoming severely ascetic, such as those who formed the sect known as the Flagellants. Jews were burned or exiled not so much because they were thought to have caused the epidemic, but rather because the nobles and communities were heavily indebted to them, and the deteriorated moral and ethical practices which accompanied the plague sanctioned escaping the debts in this way. The economic manifestations were also profound. As a result of the many casualties, a labor shortage developed with the consequence that prices rose. In 1350, the English Parliament was forced to pass a Statute of Laborers, which prohibited a laborer from seeking higher wages or going to another community where wages were higher than in his own. Many peasant revolts occurred in England and France at this time.[11]

Protection against the plague was all but impossible. Amulets were sold, magical formulas were recited, strange compounds were drunk, and prayers were offered to stay the epidemic. One apothegm dating from this period [13] was perhaps the only effective means to escape the plague:

> Three things by which each simple man
> From plague escape and sickness can,
> Start soon, flee far from town or land
> On which the plague has laid its hand,
> Return but late to such a place
> Where pestilence has stayed its pace.

In Avignon, where 60,000 people died, the pope was forced to consecrate the Rhone River in order that bodies might be thrown into it because the churchyards could no longer absorb the dead. Petrarch wrote of the great desolation in Avignon: "In what annals has one ever read that the houses were empty, the cities deserted, the farms untended, the fields full of corpses, and that everywhere a horrible loneliness prevailed." The famous fourteenth-century surgeon, Guy de Chauliac, who attended the citizens in this city, wrote in a similar pathetic vein: "The father did not visit his son, nor the son his father. Charity was dead and hope destroyed." [14]

Other Diseases. Plague and leprosy were not the only diseases which caused high mortality in the Middle Ages. The crusaders' ranks were seriously depleted time and again by outbreaks of typhus, dysentery, diarrhea, and scurvy. Jean, Sire de Joinville, author of a classic account of the Crusades, *The Life of St. Louis,* presented one of the first descriptions of scurvy: ". . . a disease spread through the army, of such a sort that the flesh on our legs dried up, and the skin became covered with black spots and turned a brown earthy colour like an old boot. With those who had this disease the flesh on the gums became gangrened; and no one who fell a victim to it could hope to recover, but was sure to die. . . ." *

Theories of Causes and the Control of Epidemic Diseases

Climate.   Joinville believed that the disease which caused the death of his comrades was due to the unhealthy Egyptian climate. The author of the Hippocratic treatise, *Airs, Waters and Places,* which dates to the fourth century B.C., was one of the first to express the fact that climate was one of the major factors to be considered in epidemic disease. However, the treatise informed the physician that not only was he to observe the meteorology and topography of an area but also that he should be cognizant of the soil, water, mode of life, and nutrition of the people. Such an enlightened and naturalistic approach to the disease of a community unfortunately did not become the standard guide for all physicians confronted by epidemics.

Divine or Demonic Wrath.   Diseases also were thought to be the expression of divine or demonic wrath. In the *Iliad,* for example, Apollo speeds down from Olympus loosing his arrows of pestilence upon the Greeks in punishment for Agamemnon's transgression, and in the Old Testament, it is written that the Lord smote the Philistines with a pestilence, characterized by small protuberances (emerods) in the region of the groin, for having stolen the sacred ark of the Jews.

The theory that demons and evil spirits were the cause of epidemic disease was always popular in history (see Fig. 1-3). In many sixteenth-century paintings, saints are represented as exorcising demons who emerge from the heads and mouths of diseased men and women. In a painting by Arnold Böcklin, plague is symbolized as a winged demon of horrific mien swooping down upon a terrified community.

Causes and Control of Plague.   Many treatises appeared in the fourteenth century in which the etiology and prevention of the plague were discussed. Jehan Jacme, the author of one treatise, wrote in 1348 that the disease was caused by five factors: by the wrath of God, by the corruption of dead bodies, by waters and vapors formed in the interior of the earth,

* Joinville and Villehardouin. *Chronicles of the Crusades,* translated by M. R. B. Shaw. Penguin Books, London, 1963, p. 237.

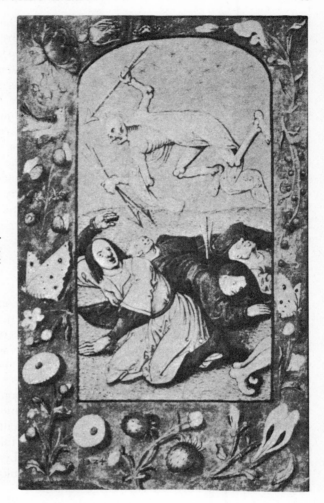

FIGURE 1-3. Symbolic representation of plague. (Courtesy of The New York Academy of Medicine.)

by unnatural hot and humid winds, and by the conjunction of stars and planets.[15]

Whatever views the authors of the treatises may have expressed regarding the ultimate cause of the plague, all agreed that it was contagious. The medical faculty at Paris, who also had published a plague treatise, warned that poisonous air might be exhaled by the sick. This concept of contagion dates back to ancient times. The contagious nature of many diseases was recorded in Hebrew scripture in the Books of Leviticus, Numbers, and Deuteronomy. Leprosy, of course, served as the paradigm of the contagious disease. The leper in biblical times was exiled and isolated, and this method of handling contagious disease again found vogue in the medieval period in connection with plague.

The plague usually spread along well-traveled land routes, and especially by sea. In the port city of Ragusa, along the Dalmatian coast, the city council in 1377 ordered that all travelers arriving from plague-ridden countries were to be barred from the city unless they spent one month on a nearby island where they could be observed. Venice followed Ragusa's example and also segregated travelers as well as imported merchandise. Cities kept their gates closed and placed guards along the highway; in some communities incoming mail was fumigated, and coins and other objects were dipped into vinegar as preventive measures. Those who were infected by the plague, or sick from other diseases, were removed to isolation hospitals located outside the town, where the disease was permitted to run its course. The period of isolation of travelers and of the sick was eventually extended from thirty (*trenta*) to forty (*quaranta*) days and hence the name "quarantine." Other than to escape an area where disease had erupted, quarantine was the only preventive measure of any success in treating epidemic disease in the Middle Ages.

The Cultural and Health Role of Monasteries

Monasticism had a strong influence on society and health in the early Middle Ages. The monks lived simple lives, often in a relatively enlightened and hygienic environment. They obeyed vows of poverty and humility, but their clerical responsibilities did not interfere with their secular interests. They wrote most of the books, copied the ancient manuscripts, and maintained the majority of schools and libraries. The monks also were excellent farmers, builders, and craftsmen. Drainage, sewerage, and water systems have been found in many monasteries which are as impressive on a small scale as the Roman water supplies of ancient times were on a large scale. In a Carthusian monastery of London, for example, water was pumped into a central cistern and then flowed by gravity through pipes to a laundry, a sacristan's washing basin, the monks' cells, the brewhouse, the kitchen, and finally out via a large conduit.[16, 17]

Medicine was practiced by the monks in a rudimentary sense, and they attended nearly all the hospitals as well as their own infirmaries where the sick monks and the disabled, crippled, and diseased in the community might find rest, a good meal, and, if needed, medical care. Many monasteries also had their own herbal gardens and pharmacies. The monks were eventually prohibited by Church edict from the practice of medicine outside their monasteries, but they were not prohibited from maintaining their infirmaries.

The Church itself sponsored a number of hospitals as a result of the Crusades, and many medieval communities also built and maintained their own hospitals, refuges, and nursing homes. From the twelfth to the fifteenth centuries more than 700 hospitals were founded in Great Britain alone, of which 217 were for lepers.

Hygienic Treatises

During the Middle Ages, a number of treatises appeared which discussed the principles of personal hygiene and how best to ensure that the reader live his life in health and happiness. The most famous of these is the didactic poem *Flos medicinae,* or *Regimen sanitatis Salernitanum,* which went through over 300 editions and has been translated from Latin into German, French, Italian, and English. By memorizing the 362 stanzas of the poem, the medieval physician learned how to treat his patient simply but efficiently. All aspects of personal hygiene were discussed in the treatise: how to wash and bathe, what foods to eat, and even when and how to purge and bleed a patient.[18] By modern scientific standards the *Regimen of the School of Salerno* does not constitute a text of medical treatment, but it did have the virtue of spreading useful, practical, and safe hygienic maxims throughout the civilized world.

THE SIXTEENTH AND SEVENTEENTH CENTURIES

The Renaissance

A great revival of learning occurred in Europe during the Middle Ages. Learning was the province of the monks, but a center for secular studies and medicine existed at Salerno. In Northern Europe, the encouragement bestowed on scholars by Charlemagne and Alfred also had given impetus to teaching. The faculties of law, medicine, theology, and philosophy existed at Bologna in the eleventh and twelfth centuries, and similar disciplines were taught at the Universities of Paris, Oxford, and Cambridge. Scholars such as John Scot, Peter Abelard, Isidore of Seville, Robert Grosseteste, Albertus Magnus, Thomas Aquinas, Roger Bacon, and Nicholas of Cusa, by their studies of theology, philosophy, the natural sciences, and scientific methodology, helped to open the door to the Renaissance.

The spirit of the Renaissance was particularly apparent in Italy and incorporated a number of dominant ideas and attitudes among which were optimism, naturalism, and especially humanism. Humanism, in its broadest sense, has been defined as the glorification of the natural as opposed to the divine or otherworldly. Art, literature, and philosophy were all eagerly studied in an endeavor to return to the classical way of life. The humanists examined manuscripts from North Africa, Egypt, Syria, and Spain and translated the works of Euclid, Aristotle, Plato, Ptolemy, and others into Latin in order to absorb the wisdom of the ancient world.

Mercantilism

Humanism was one stream that helped develop the spirit of the Renaissance; the rise of commerce and industry was another. With the rise of a new social class, the *bourgeoisie,* the notion developed of wealth consisting no longer of land but of commodities of trade. Concomitant to an increased economic activity was the rise of the nation state and the theory of mercantilism. Mercantilism is basically an economic theory, but as is so often the case, it developed also as a conception of society. The more money a state accumulated, the more powerful it became. To ensure a steady economic growth the state had to protect and care for its citizens. What was needed to increase the national wealth was a large population, provided for materially and basically obedient to the dictates of the state.[19]

Labor, for example, became a precious commodity and an essential element in the production of national wealth. Obviously, any loss of labor productivity owing to illness and death resulted in a significant economic problem. It became of paramount importance for the state to know how many citizens it had, their occupations, the number of laborers, and the number of soldiers under arms. The "statistics of the state" were the subject of many treatises published in the sixteenth and seventeenth centuries.

England: Political Arithmetic and the Nation's Health

In England the statistical analysis of production and population began in the seventeenth century with the works of John Graunt and William Petty. The Bills of Mortality, published weekly in London, date to the sixteenth century, when plague once again became epidemic. Eventually, the Bills became a measure of morbidity and mortality but were not used in a statistical sense until John Graunt's treatise on vital statistics appeared in 1662. Statistics is the science of numbers applied to the life-history of communities and nations, and the life-history of a community describes the numerical record of marriage, birth, death, and morbidity by which the health and growth of a community may be studied. It was Graunt who studied the Bills in this sense and observed a regularity of social phenomena when he determined the excess of male over female births, the high rate of mortality during the earlier years of life, the approximate numerical equality of the sexes, and the excess of the urban over the rural death rate.

Although Graunt appears to have grasped the importance of statistical analysis related to vital statistics, William Petty's "political arithmetic" was statistics by the classical definition. Petty repeatedly urged the collection of numerical data on population, education, diseases, revenues, and economic production in all his treatises relating to the statistics of the state. He was keenly aware of the importance of a healthy population as a factor in national wealth and power. In 1676, Petty presented a paper in Dublin which stressed the duty of the state to foster medical progress and, in 1687, advocated a Health Council for London. Isolation hospitals for plague patients, maternity hospitals, and a 1000-bed general hospital were also high on the list of Petty's recommendations. He discussed problems relating especially to medical care and medical manpower and recommended a statistical analysis of health needs which would have then made it possible to calculate the number of physicians, surgeons, and ancillary medical personnel necessary to satisfy these needs.

Samuel Hartlib, Daniel Defoe, Nehemiah Grew, and John Bellers were also among those who attempted to deal with public health problems on a national scale. In *An Essay Toward the Improvement of Physick,* which appeared in 1714, Bellers stated that illness and death, especially in children, resulted in a waste of human resources. Bellers considered that the health of the people was the responsibility of the state, whose task it was to establish and maintain hopitals and laboratories, erect a national health institute, and provide medical care for the sick.[1]

For the most part the sick poor remained the responsibility of the town or parish, and medical care was provided by physicians in hospitals at the expense of the community. When the monasteries were dissolved in England by Henry VIII in the sixteenth century, medical care, as dispensed in the monastery infirmary, was no longer possible. Local municipalities assumed the responsibility for a number of these infirmaries and, from that time until the rise of the voluntary hospital in the eighteenth century, the hospitals developed as a combination old-age home, almshouse, and clinic.

Various measures were presented to the English Parliament designed to deal with poverty. In 1601, these measures were consolidated in the Elizabethan Poor Law, which became the basis for the administration of the Poor Law until the Poor Law Amendment Act of 1834. The Elizabethan Law does not treat health matters specifically, but it was designed to relieve the "lame, impotent, old, blind, and such other among them being poor and not able to work." This statement, however, was interpreted rather leniently and, in time, was expanded to include the provision of medical and nursing care.

America: Diseases and Their Control in Early Colonial Times

The conditions which greeted the arriving colonist to the New World were stark at the very best. Epidemic diseases, hostile savages, and severe winters completely obliterated many of the early settlements. The settlers at Jamestown and Roanoke Island, for example, were ravaged by a severe smallpox epidemic. Many Indian tribes in the northeastern section of the country experienced severe epidemics of measles, and settlers and aborigines alike succumbed to yellow fever in the area of the Carolinas. Influenza, scarlet fever, diphtheria, and other highly contagious diseases were all rampant in the Colonies.[20]

To meet the threat of the epidemics the governor of a settlement would appoint a commission to control the spread of disease. Some physicians were appointed to the commission, but its chief function was care of the sick, provision for orphans, and burial of the dead. The only preventive measure which was effected at this time was to quarantine the sick individual and his family and, if necessary, to quarantine the community itself. The colonists passed a number of acts designed to control the noxious atmospheric influences which were thought to produce epidemic disease. Between 1692 and 1708, the cities of Boston, Salem, and Charlestown passed acts dealing with the nuisances and trades offensive to public health, and Massachusetts passed laws providing for the isolation of smallpox cases and for ship quarantine in 1701. Such administrative measures helped in part to control epidemics, but without a knowledge of the etiology of disease the colonists were impotent to prevent them.

Epidemic Diseases: Contagion and Miasma

The demonic and theologic theories of epidemic disease remained popular until the germ theory of disease was formulated in the nineteenth century. In the seventeenth century, however, the naturalistic conception of disease, which emphasized the atmospheric and telluric (i.e., miasmatic) factors as those responsible for epidemics, was a successful working hypothesis by which to understand the epidemic disease.

Plague continued as an endemic disease in Europe, and sporadic outbreaks of varying intensity occurred in all Near Eastern and Western countries. In 1603, an epidemic of plague claimed the lives of 33,300 residents of London, and in 1665, London experienced a plague epidemic of even greater severity which claimed the lives of 68,000 residents (see Fig. 1-4). Written records and illustrations are extant which describe and depict the great mortality, the suffering of the poor, the paralysis of business, and the mass burials.

The 1665 London epidemic was described by two eyewitnesses: Nathaniel Hodges [*] and William Boghurst.[†] Both discussed the plague in naturalistic terms, but differed in their approach to the disease. Hodges wrote in his *Loimologia* that the plague was contagious and transmissible by infected cotton and silk goods which had been imported from the Levant to London. Boghurst took a contrary view, believing that the disease was latent in London and had occurred three or four years before the 1665 outbreak.

The controversy of whether epidemic disease was contagious or miasmatic, that is, spreading from person to person or occurring locally owing to a number of peculiar atmospheric and telluric conditions, continued to confuse and confound physicians, epidemiologists, and sanitarians until the late nineteenth century. The miasmatic theory, as will be shown in a later section, profoundly affected the public health movement in the nineteenth century.

---

[*] Hodges, Nathaniel. *Loimologia, or an Historical Account of the Plague in London in 1665*, translated from Latin by John Quincy, 2nd ed. London, 1720.

[†] Boghurst, William. "Loimographia, or an Experimental Relation of the Last Plague of London." Edited by J. F. Payne. *Supplement, Transactions of the Epidemiological Society of London*, 13:1–99, 1894.

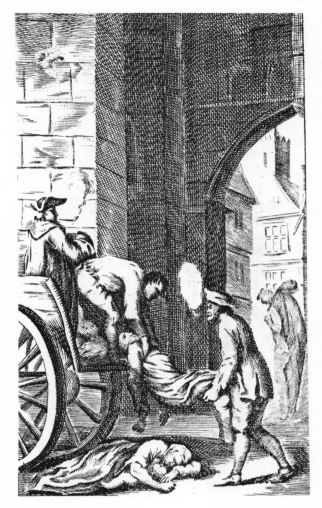

FIGURE 1-4. Plague in London, 1665. (Courtesy of the Wellcome Trustees, London, England.)

THE EIGHTEENTH AND NINETEENTH CENTURIES

Public health from the mid-eighteenth century to the present time has been greatly influenced by general scientific progress and an increasing social awareness. Intellectual enlightenment, the industrial revolution, evangelicalism, humanitarianism, utilitarianism, and the cholera pandemics of the nineteenth century—all served as catalysts in bringing about the first comprehensive and significant solutions to the social and health problems of the people.

Social Injustice and Humanitarianism

The eighteenth- and nineteenth-century attitudes toward sickness, suffering, and social injustice stand in marked contrast to those of the present time. High mortality rates, slum living conditions, and squalor were commonplace. The rapid industrialization and urbanization resulted in an increased callousness and insensitivity toward one's fellow man.

The Prevailing Economic Philosophy. The predominant economic theory was bound to the Industrial Revolution. Almost as soon as industrialism began in earnest, the new commercial classes began to defend their privileges. The entrepreneurs expressed a brazen confidence in their own rights and believed, as did the nobles before them, that property was sacred, that every man had a right to do with his own as he willed, and that poverty invariably was the result of laziness and incompetence. Some of the *nouveau riche* argued that poverty was beneficial because it taught the poor to respect their superiors and to be grateful to Providence for such blessings as they did receive.

This economic theory became known as *laissez faire,* which expressed the doctrines of economic individualism, obedience to natural law, freedom of contract, and competition and free trade. Controls or regulations imposed by government on business were considered anathema and self-defeating of the national purpose. The blatant fact that the wealth of the state was being built upon the backs of children, women, and men in ill health was of no concern to the parliamentarians or the industrialists.

This rigid economic philosophy was attacked on economic grounds by the Utilitarians, the Utopian Socialists, and the Marxian Socialists and also by men imbued with the motives of basic humanitarianism. It is not surprising that most of the men who called for social justice had been influenced by Evangelical Christianity. John Wesley's movement exerted enormous influence in bringing about a reaction to the inhuman doctrine of *laissez faire, laissez passer.* John Howard, for example, who wrote a classic study of prison,* was influenced by the Wesleyan movement, as were William Wilberforce and his associates, who were instrumental in the abolition of the slave trade.

Social Reforms. The children received the especial attention of the social reformers. Illegitimacy was common, and the infant mortality rate was high, even among those for whom care was provided. Many children were abandoned or sent to the parish authorities only to be farmed out to fill the laborers' rank in the factories and mines.

Thomas Coram, a wealthy merchant, established the Foundling Hospital of London in 1741 for the care of abandoned children (see Fig. 1-5). Jonas Hanway, perhaps better known for his advocacy of the umbrella and tea drinking, waged an important campaign against infant mortality and succeeded in 1769 in securing an act of parliament which made it compulsory for London parishes to send infants into the country to be nursed. Hanway also waged an active campaign to rehabilitate prostitutes.† In France and

---

* Howard, John. *The State of Prisons in England and Wales.* London, 1777–1780.

† Hanway, Jonas. *Letter V. to Robert Dingley, Esq. Being a Proposal for the Relief and Employment of Friendless Girls and Repenting Prostitutes.* R. and J. Dodsley, London, 1758.

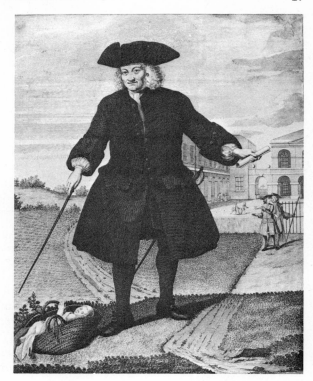

FIGURE 1-5. Thomas Coram and the Foundling Hospital. (Courtesy of the Wellcome Trustees, London, England.)

Germany, similar expressions of humanity and revulsion at the unnecessarily high mortality rate of children were voiced by Nicholas Andry and Jean Charles des Essartz, and also by Jean Jacques Rousseau, whose novel *Émile*, published in 1762, provided an extremely effective vehicle for social protest.

Elizabeth Barrett Browning's poem *The Cry of the Children* was suggested by an official report on the employment of children in mines and factories. The report appalled Mrs. Browning, and all England was stirred by the question which was expressed in her last stanza: "How long . . . how long, O cruel nation, will you stand, to move the world, on a child's heart. . . ?" Mrs. Browning's poem was published in 1843. By that time the English Parliament had passed in 1802 a "Health and Morals of Apprentices Act" limiting to 12 the laboring hours of children in factories and an 1833 Act forbidding the employment of children under 12 years of age for more than eight hours a day. As the result of a report appearing in the early 1840's, women, and children under ten years of age, were forbidden to work underground. The ten-hour working day for women and children was introduced in 1847, but despite the efforts of many social reformers, children under ten years of age were permitted to work in English factories until 1874 (see Fig. 1-6).

Reform in other areas was also apparent in the eighteenth and nineteenth centuries. As a reaction against the licentiousness of the urban masses, Gin

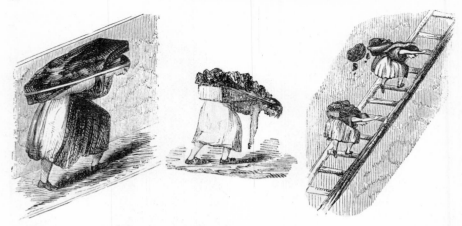

FIGURE 1-6. The physical and moral conditions of the children and young persons employed in mines and manufactures. (Courtesy of the Wellcome Trustees, London, England.)

Acts were passed by the English Parliament. Justices, physicians, and ordinary citizens who abhorred the great waste of human resources owing to the traffic in gin petitioned Parliament in an unprecedented attempt to sway the legislators. Hogarth's painting *Gin Lane* appeared at this time and was added to the propaganda attack. By 1751, the battle had been won and a final act was passed by Parliament which gave the control of licensing to the magistrates and limited the amount of spirits which could be consumed.

The social reformers also turned their attention to lunatic asylums and initiated reforms for the mentally ill. G. F. Jaegerschmid, Vincenzo Chiaurgi, Philipe Pinel, and William Tuke hypothesized that proper food, medical care, fresh air, and exercise were more effective than brutality and chains and proceeded to prove their beliefs by treating the mentally ill as patients rather than as prisoners.[1]

Continental Health Policies

In the German states, public health policy was formulated by political scientists whose desire was to fit the health needs of a nation within the framework of legislative policies and by physicians imbued with the principles of the humanitarian and the social reformer. The concept of "medical police," a policy conceived by Wolfgang Thomas Rau and expanded upon by Johann Peter Frank, both of whom were physicians, became the paradigm for the administration of health services on the Continent. The term was derived from the theory and practice of public administration, which was known as the "science of police"; the branch of the field dealing with public health administration was designated "medical police."[1]

The health of the people as a responsibility of the state had been an accepted principle since the rise of mercantilism and the nation state.

Frank believed firmly in this function of the state and, accordingly, directed his work to the governmental officials who were in a position to take his ideas and formulate them into a coherent policy. Frank's six-volume work, published between 1779 and 1819,* stands as the most comprehensive presentation of public health policy ever published by a physician before the present time. Frank dealt with all aspects relating to the health of a population, including procreation, marriage, midwifery, education, vital statistics, environmental sanitation, personal hygiene, control of communicable diseases, and nutrition. He explored systematically all aspects of community life and offered solutions to the health and social problems manifest in society.[21]

The one major fault of Frank's work was that it was built upon absolutism and an outmoded mercantilism. Although Frank's health and social policies were enlightened, they never became the basis for a national policy because they were associated with authoritarianism and reaction. Nevertheless, the principles he discussed formed the basis for determining the scope of health services offered in other countries.

Public Health in England

Some treatises on the subject of medical police were published in Great Britain,† but humanitarian ideals proved to be the most effective means of achieving health and social reform. In England, social reform was also aided by the cholera epidemics, which effectively exposed the health and social problems of the people.

The Cholera Epidemics. Cholera spread from India beginning in 1817. It reached Africa by 1820 and by 1823 was at the gateway to Russia and the West. The disease subsided for a time, and it was not until 1827 that it again began its inexorable movement westward. In 1831, it erupted with fearful intensity in the western provinces of Russia and from there moved into Germany and Austria. In July and August of 1831, the first cases of cholera were reported on board some vessels stationed in the Medway in England. By October 1831, the disease had spread to Northern England, Scotland, and Ireland, and it erupted in London in February 1832.

In 1831 the British government sent a commission to Russia to study the epidemic and to make recommendations as to its control and prevention. The commission was comprised of physicians, a member of the Board of Customs, and the superintendent-general of quarantine. Their report stated that the highest mortality was reported in slum districts and that the only

* Frank, Johann Peter. *System Einer Vollständigen Medicinischen Polizey.* 6 vols. 1779–1819. (Vols. 1–4 published in Mannheim by C. F. Schwan; Vol. 5 published in Tübingen by J. F. Cotta'schen; Vol. 6 (part 1–3) published in Vienna by Carl Schaumburg.)

† Roberton, John. *A Treatise on Medical Police.* Edinburgh, 1809.

means of preventing the disease was to enforce a strict quarantine. The quarantine proved effective in London for a period of about six months, but when the metropolis began to feel the effects of the dread disease in spite of the control measures, a loud protest against the restrictions of quarantine was heard from merchants and physicians. The merchants complained that they were suffering economic losses because their goods rotted on the docks. The physicians argued that quarantine was ineffective because the disease was miasmatic and associated with the filth and decay of the slum dwellings of the poor. If the living conditions of the poor were improved, went their argument, the disease could not be generated.[22]

When the epidemic occurred, local boards of health were created and ordered to attend to the slum conditions. Temporary acts were passed to regulate against foul odors, refuse, and the general unsanitary conditions of the poor, but mostly these were of no avail and the cholera took a heavy toll of life.

The epidemic, however, was not without significance for public health. The intelligentsia were forced to become more critically cognizant than ever before of the sanitary conditions under which the mass of the people had been living. It is true that after the 1832 cholera epidemic, no exact knowledge had been gained relating to the cause of the disease, but the physicians and the social reformers at least had become aware of the needy and of the squalor in which they lived.

Reform of the Poor Law and Passage of the Public Health Acts. The social reformer also became aware of the condition of the slum dweller by means of the reports of the Poor Law Commission. In 1832, Parliament appointed a royal commission to investigate the administration of the Poor Laws. Edwin Chadwick, an ardent Radical and close associate of Jeremy Bentham, was appointed to the commission, and with the assistance of Nassau Senior, an economist, he produced a report which became the basis for the Poor Law Amendment Act of 1834. The Act was designed primarily to reduce the poor-law rates and, more importantly, to force the laborer into the open market.

Chadwick became acutely aware of the living conditions of the laboring poor when he had gathered material for his report to the Poor Law Commission. The laborers' ill health appalled him, and the cholera epidemic of 1831–1832 convinced him that their poor standard of health had made them more susceptible to disease than the rest of the community.

Chadwick's classic survey of the health of the laboring class was begun in the mid-1830's. In his researches, Chadwick was assisted by three physicians, James Kay, Neil Arnott, and Thomas Southwood Smith. All three were extremely able: Kay had written a treatise on the health of laborers in Manchester, and Arnott and Smith were experienced in treating epidemic diseases. Smith, moreover, had written the medical section of Bentham's *Constitutional Code.*[23]

Reports of the living conditions of laborers were solicited from all over England, which were then analyzed, collated, and published in 1842 as the *Report on the Sanitary Condition of the Labouring Population and on the Means of its Improvement*.[24] The report proved to Chadwick's satisfaction that disease was related to the unsanitary environment in which the laborers lived. Lack of drainage, water supply, and means of removing refuse from homes and streets was the cause of the higher mortality rates in such areas.

It should be emphasized that the then-current theory of disease was miasmatic. Disease was thought to be generated in filth, decaying organic material, swamps, and cesspools. The miasmatists argued convincingly that if refuse was removed, cesspools drained, and houses properly ventilated, epidemic disease would no longer trouble the population. The fact that a heap of manure was considered as dangerous as a cesspool that was contaminating a well of drinking water was relatively unimportant for the reformers, who were convinced that the health of the people was an engineering rather than a medical problem. It was not until bacteriology became an exact science in the late nineteenth century that filth was assigned its rightful position as a vector rather than a nidus of epidemics.[25]

The immediate result of Chadwick's report was the appointment of a Royal Commission for the Inquiry into the State of the Large Towns. Chadwick drafted the major part of the first report, which helped to highlight the overcrowding, poverty, crime, ill health, and high mortality then rampant in the towns. This report, and two more subsequently, were submitted to Parliament recommending that the government supervise the general measures for regulating the sanitary condition of the larger towns. The Commission reports further proposed that in each locality drainage, paving and cleaning of streets, and the provision of potable supplies of water be placed under a single administrative body.

The recommendations expressed in the reports were included in a bill introduced to Parliament in 1846. The bill was hotly debated and did not pass into law until 1848, and then only in an emasculated form. The Public Health Act of 1848 created a General Board of Health empowered to establish local boards of health either when petitioned by one tenth of the taxpayers or by mandate when the average mortality rate in an area over a period of seven years exceeded 23 per 1000. Local boards were given the responsibility for water supply, drainage, offensive trades, and cemeteries. The Public Health Act was to last only five years and, for the most part, proved too permissive a piece of legislation owing to the opposition of the vested interests who owned the water and sewerage companies and who were not used to being told how to run their business. The provisions of the Public Health Act did not even apply to London, which remained autonomous. By 1854, the General Board of Health had become one of the most despised of governmental agencies, and it is not surprising that Parliament refused to renew the Public Health Act of 1848. However, the

General Board of Health was permitted to continue on an annual basis until 1858, when it was abolished by a new Public Health Act. The new act also transferred the supervision of public health to the Privy Council, where it remained until 1871.

During this time, John Simon came into prominence when he was appointed in 1848 as the first medical officer of health of London. Subsequently, he was appointed to the General Board of Health while it remained in existence until 1858, when he became the medical officer of the Privy Council. Simon proved to be a remarkably able administrator. In his yearly presentations to the Privy Council, he reported on the problem of communicable diseases, congested housing, occupational health, employment of mothers, and poor nutrition. From a social point of view, Simon grasped totally the community responsibility for public health.[26]

In 1869, Simon increased his efforts to effect a change in the administrative mechanism of public health. At his instigation, a royal commission was appointed to study the matter. A report was submitted to Parliament in 1871 recommending the creation of a government department which would combine the administration of the Poor Law and public health. The result was the creation of the Local Government Board, under whose aegis was placed the Poor Law Board and the Medical Department of the Privy Council.

The recommendations of the commission were accepted by Parliament and appeared as the Public Health Act of 1875.[27] This act divided England into urban and rural sanitary districts subject to the supervision of the Local Government Board. With the passage of this act, England possessed the administrative mechanism and cohesion necessary to deal with the problems of community health.

Public Health in the United States

The history of public health in the United States from the early colonial period to the end of the nineteenth century followed the same developmental pattern as occurred in England. The catalysts for sanitary reform in America were the yellow fever and cholera epidemics, which were believed to be caused by miasma and the unsanitary living conditions of large towns. As in England, municipal authorities learned that mortality rates could be lowered by establishing health boards, paving streets, draining marshes, and building waterworks.

Public Health Legislation. The threat of disease continued to be the major force which led to the initiation of health policy. Legislation for the establishment of state boards of health was passed in 1797 by New York and Massachusetts and in 1805 by Connecticut. The first of the larger cities to establish a board of health was New York in 1796. Baltimore established a board in 1798, Boston and Salem in 1799, Alexandria in 1804, Charleston in 1815, Philadelphia and New Orleans in 1818, and Providence in 1832.[28] New York City formed a public health committee which was concerned with provision of potable water, construction of sewers, drainage, and burial of the dead. At the same time, to provide for the care of sick and disabled merchant seamen, Congress created a Marine Hospital Service in 1798, which eventually became the United States Public Health Service.

Epidemics and Medical Provisions. In the nineteenth century, epidemic diseases continued to threaten the public health and welfare. The cholera epidemics which ravaged Great Britain in the mid-1800's also erupted in the United States. Smallpox, yellow fever, diphtheria, typhus, and typhoid all were highly prevalent, as were malaria and tuberculosis. In Massachusetts, the mortality rate for tuberculosis in 1850 was over 3 per cent, and the infant mortality was about 20 per cent.

The high mortality rates were a reflection not only of epidemic disease but also of the flagrant lack of proper medical care. Professional teaching facilities for physicians were few and inadequate, and a large number of those physicians practicing in America were trained as mere apprentices. The therapeutic agents available to physicians were usually ineffective for the treating of disease, and hospital gangrene and septicemia were prevalent among those patients who were hospitalized. The urban problems attendant upon the Industrial Revolution in England were also apparent in the United States.

The Shattuck Report. Reform was slow in coming but there were also Chadwicks, Smiths, Franks, and Simons to be found in America.[29] The most notable of the men to whom American public health is indebted is Lemuel Shattuck, whose *Report of the Sanitary Commission of Massachusetts*[30] bears a striking resemblance to Chadwick's famous report of 1842. Shattuck was a teacher, book dealer, statistician, and legislator who had a keen interest in sanitary reform. His interests in public health began when he collected and collated the vital statistics of the city of Boston. As a result of this activity he was appointed to a committee of the state legislature for the study of the health and sanitary problems of the Commonwealth.

Shattuck's report was at one and the same time historical, descriptive, and analytic. He described the sanitary movement in England, on the Continent, and in the United States, with special reference to the activities of Chadwick and Southwood Smith. The report also dealt with a plan for a sanitary survey of Massachusetts, and provided some 50 recommendations including the creation of state and local boards of health; the need for a registrar-general to collect and collate vital statistics; the supervision of housing, factories, sanitation, and foods; the provision of periodic vaccination; child health measures; and the teaching of public health and preventive medicine to students. Finally, the report discussed the practical, economic, charitable, and moral reasons why the recommendations should be accepted. The influence of Shattuck's recommendations cannot be over-estimated. Of the 50 recommendations which Shattuck listed, 36 have become accepted principles of public health practice.

National Quarantine and Sanitary Conventions. An attempt to establish a nationwide maritime quarantine code began in 1857 with the meeting of the first Quarantine Convention in Philadelphia. The Convention, attended by 73 delegates from nine states, discussed the nature of communicable disease and the means of best preventing epidemics. A tentative quarantine code was drawn up by Dr. Wilson Jewell—a member of the Philadelphia Board of Health and the first chairman of the Convention—which related to the quarantine of smallpox, cholera, and yellow fever. As a result of the Convention it was recommended that a full-time medical officer be appointed by local boards of health of port cities, who was to be given power to inspect all vessels, quarantine those found infected, remove and care for the sick, and cleanse and purify cargo removed from ships.

The second and third quarantine and sanitary conventions of 1858 and 1859 were extremely well attended by physicians, mayors, and legislators. Proposals for a uniform system of quarantine laws and the organization of a "Committee on Internal Hygiene" or the "Sanitary Arrangement of Cities" were put forward by the delegates. The delegates also debated the confusing issue of whether cholera and yellow fever were contagious or miasmatic. Eventually a resolution was passed which settled the problem, at least in the case of yellow fever. The resolution stated ". . . that in the absence of evidence establishing the conclusion that Yellow Fever has ever been conveyed by one person to another, it is the opinion of this Convention that personal quarantine in cases of Yellow Fever may be safely abolished." [31]

The American Public Health Association. The quarantine conventions, although resolving none of the major public health and medical issues, did plant the seed which grew into a national health association. In 1872, ten men, including Dr. Elisha Harris and Dr. Stephen Smith, met at the City Health Department in New York City for purposes of planning a public health conference on a national scale. A second meeting was held in New Jersey at which time a national organization, the American Public Health Association, was created. A constitution was drafted, and Dr. Stephen Smith was elected the first president. The Association since that time has continued to meet annually and to provide a forum for its members to discuss sanitation, communicable diseases, hospital hygiene, longevity, quarantine, and other health-related subjects.

National Board of Health. Discussions regarding the organization of a governmental health agency were often heard in the meetings of the quarantine conventions and the American Public Health Association. Dr. C. C. Cox, health officer of Washington, D.C., gave an excellent discourse on the necessity for a national health agency at the very first meeting of the American Public Health Association in 1872. In 1875, meetings were held in Washington, D.C., for the purpose of founding such a health organization, but the meetings proved fruitless, resulting mainly in jurisdictional disputes between the Army, the Navy, and the Marine Hospital Service. In 1878, a devastating yellow-fever epidemic erupted, and again an epidemic provided the necessary impetus for social action. The disease was reported to have entered the United States through the port of New Orleans, and local Louisiana authorities were blamed for their laxity. Public sentiment was aroused, and as a result the Army, the Marine Hospital Service, and the American Public Health Association sponsored bills to Congress for the establishment of a National Board of Health. The bill sponsored by the American Public Health Association passed Congress in 1879. By the articles of the act, the duties and powers of the Marine Hospital Service, including maritime quarantine, were transferred to the National Board. Seven physicians and representatives from the Armed Forces, the Marine Hospital Service, and the Department of Justice were appointed to the Board. A second act appropriated $500,000 for the Board to carry out its duties, but it also included an unfortunate clause which limited the Board to a period of four years.

The Board met the same resistance as its English counterpart which had been created in 1848. Opponents decried the Board's work as coercive and restrictive of trade, and one opponent objected to the presence of Board officers, calling them "federal agents and spies." Every opportunity was seized to belittle and misrepresent the Board's activities. The objections influenced Dr. John Hamilton, Surgeon General of the Marine Hospital Service, who realized that if the act which limited the duration of the Board was not re-enacted, its powers and functions would revert to his Service. Charging misuse of funds, extravagance, and incompetence, Hamilton succeeded in preventing re-enactment, and the National Board of Health came to an untimely end.

Wilson Smillie has written that the problem with the 1879 National Board of Health, from an administrative view, related to the controversy of state versus federal authority. The Board made the fatal mistake of encroaching upon the prerogatives of the individual states, and Congress at that time did not entertain the idea of centralization of power. The problem also related to the lack of cohesion of the Board itself. The members were experts who lived in different communities and merely attended meetings. There was no central authority and no real unity of opinion. Dr. Stephen Smith recognized this problem and suggested in 1883 that the Board be continued, but that the officers, the staff, and the activities of the Marine Hospital Service be incorporated into its structure. Smith foresaw that Congress would lose interest in a National Board of Health, but would continue to support a service agency which had full-time career officers and was incorporated as an integral part of the national government machinery.[29]

SCIENTIFIC ADVANCES AND THE
NEW PUBLIC HEALTH IN THE TWENTIETH CENTURY

Preceding sections of this chapter have shown that, over the centuries, there were conflicting theories regarding epidemic diseases: whether they were miasmatic or contagious and, thus, whether the most appropriate control measure consisted of sanitation or quarantine. The dilemma arose, of course, because scientific knowledge was lacking regarding the causes and modes of transmission of the prevalent diseases. Frequently in controversies, the "miasmatic-sanitation" theory won out, and although they were based on an incorrect hypothesis, the efforts to improve sanitary conditions in the nineteenth century were responsible at least in part for reducing mortality from diseases such as cholera, typhoid, malaria, and typhus. However, significant advances were not made until the late nineteenth century when sufficient scientific knowledge had been amassed to resolve the age-old conflict of theories; to put an end to the devastating epidemics, at least in the Western world; and to usher in a new and modern epoch in public health at the beginning of the twentieth century.

Development of Scientific Knowledge Concerning
the Cause and Control of Disease

The most significant scientific advances that occurred just before the beginning of the twentieth century consisted of the development of bacteriology, which established living particles, or microorganisms, as the cause of epidemic diseases; the development of immunology, which enabled prevention of disease through inoculation; the identification of sources and modes of transmission of disease; and the discovery of various techniques for the diagnosis and treatment of illness. These developments had roots going back many decades—even centuries—and the scientific advances of the late nineteenth century were the fruition of this long history.

Bacteriology. The problem of epidemic diseases related to whether or not a particular disease was caused by a living particle and whether or not this living particle was contagious, i.e., could be transferred from one person to another. If contagious diseases were caused by living particles, it was necessary to determine the characteristics of the particles and to find a way to destroy them.

In the sixteenth century, Gerolamo Fracastoro reasoned that a living contagious particle, which he called *semanaria*, was the cause of infection and that the *semanaria* spread by direct contact, by contaminated articles, and by atmospheric transfer.[32] However, the first man actually to have seen living particulate matter was Anton van Leeuwenhoek, of Delft. In the seventeenth century, Leeuwenhoek peered through a microscope of his own design and saw "little animacules of divers sorts." Leeuwenhoek, however, did not take the next conceptual step, which would have permitted him to determine the relationship between bacteria and disease. This was left for others who were seeking to prove or disprove the theory of spontaneous generation.

In Italy, Spallanzani proved that microbes were present in the air. He observed animacules in rotting hay, and in order to prove that they were not generated by this medium, he heated a flask containing an infusion of hay. If the flask was then sealed from the air, no animacules were observed in it; but animacules readily appeared in a similarly treated flask which was left unsealed.

In the 1830's, three significant developments occurred that profoundly affected bacteriology. First, the power and precision of the microscope was greatly improved. Second, French and German scientists were able to show that yeast was a living one-celled organism and that the fermentation of sugar into carbon dioxide and alcohol resulted from the activity of this organism; thus, fermentation was a living process, not a dead one. The third discovery was that a disease of silkworms was caused by a specific microbe. It remained for Louis Pasteur subsequently to demonstrate that silkworm disease and anthrax, a disease of cattle, sheep, and other animals, were definitely caused by living contagion. Microorganisms of other diseases were discovered soon after. Once a disease was found to be caused by microbes, scientists could then develop methods to combat them and thereby prevent and control disease.

Immunology. In the late seventeenth and early eighteenth century, reports reached England from the Near East, China, and Africa concerning a therapeutic procedure which would prevent smallpox before an epidemic occurred and attenuate the virulence of the disease if it had erupted. All the reports related the same technique, which came to be called inoculation. The process was relatively simple and easy to master. Smallpox matter was taken from a pustule of a natural case of smallpox, dried for a number of days, and then "inoculated" into the arm of a person who desired protection from the disease. Through the efforts of Lady Mary Wortley Montagu, a close friend of the English Royal family; Sir Hans Sloane, the Royal Physician; and Dr. James Jurin, Secretary of the Royal Society of London, the practice of inoculation was established in England and quickly spread to America and France.[33]

Certain problems were attendant upon inoculation, however, and it was practiced only intermittently in the eighteenth century. One problem was the definite threat that a person might die from the smallpox inoculation. Another problem arose from the belief that the inoculated person might serve as a source of infection for those who were not similarly protected. The third problem was religious in nature: "If God is the cause of life and death, is it not presumptuous of man to protect himself from the instrument of His Divine Will?" In France especially, the religious argument was used effectively against the practice. Voltaire, who himself had survived a case of smallpox, led the fight against such dogmatic and reactionary thinking, and inoculation became a *cause célèbre* of the Enlightenment.

At the end of the eighteenth century, the problem of deaths due to inoculation was solved by substituting cowpox matter for the smallpox virus. Benjamin Jetsy, empirically, and Edward Jenner,[34] more scientifically, proved that vaccination with cowpox was a safe and effective preventive against smallpox.

In the latter half of the nineteenth century, another advance in immunology was made, this time in connection with diphtheria. In 1888, Roux and Yersin discovered that the diphtheria bacillus produced a toxin, and in 1890, Behring and Kitasato prepared an antidote to this toxin, which they termed antitoxin. Large amounts of diphtheria antitoxin were prepared from horse serum and administered by Roux to some 300 children at the Hôpital des Enfant Malades in Paris. As a result of the antitoxin, the case mortality in children suffering from diphtheria in that hospital was reduced from 52 to 25 per cent.[35]

By the close of the nineteenth century, the principles of producing artificial immunity through inoculation were extended to diseases other than smallpox and diphtheria, including plague, tetanus, and bacillary dysentery.

Transmission of Disease. At the same time that bacteriology was demonstrating specific microorganisms as the cause of certain contagious diseases, advances were also being made in identifying the means by which disease was transmitted. Before the discoveries regarding transmission, there were still several puzzling questions concerning the disease process, such as why persons contracted a particular disease in the absence of contact with anyone who had it, and why some persons who were exposed to a particular disease did not contract it. These and other questions were answered when it was found that intermediaries transmitted some diseases. Depending on the disease, it was established that the intermediaries could be insects, animals, and even human beings who were apparently healthy. These discoveries provided further understanding of the infectious, or communicable, disease process and permitted new and more effective control measures.

Investigations of malaria and yellow fever provided the first significant discoveries about the mode of transmission of disease. A possible connection between malaria and mosquitoes was suggested as early as 1717 by Lancisi, in Italy, and the idea recurred from time to time during the nineteenth century. In 1880, the malarial microorganism was discovered by Laveran, and in 1885, Italian observers had shown that man became infected with malaria from the bites of mosquitoes. In the last decade of the nineteenth century, Manson and Ross proved that one species of mosquito was infested by parasites which proved to be the infecting microorganism in an early stage of development. With this knowledge, malaria could be prevented by interrupting the life cycle of the mosquito and destroying its larvae.

By the mid-1800's, the mosquito was also thought to be implicated in yellow fever, and its role in the transmission of that disease was proved about 1900 by Walter Reed and his associates. The investigation was carried out in Cuba, where Reed headed a commission to study an outbreak of yellow fever among the American troops that were occupying the island following the Spanish-American War. Another significant discovery made by the commission was that, although yellow fever was transmissible by way of the mosquito, it was not contagious; i.e., transmission did not occur through the contact of a well person with a sick one.

The possibility that human beings who were apparently in good health could be the carriers of disease organisms was suggested—but not demonstrated—in 1855 in connection with cholera.[1] In 1893, Park and Beebe, working in New York, definitely established the role of the "healthy" carrier, this time in diphtheria. Subsequently, it was found that other diseases, such as typhoid, cholera, malaria, meningitis, and poliomyelitis, may be harbored by healthy persons who would then transmit the infection to other people. This new concept of disease transmission eventually revolutionized control measures, but did not become fully established until the early twentieth century.[36]

Treatment of Disease. In the late nineteenth and early twentieth centuries, advances in the treatment of disease were made through the discovery of new drugs and the use of improved surgical procedures. In 1912, for example, Ehrlich, the founder of modern chemotherapy, announced his discovery of an arsenic compound which he named salvarsan. Salvarsan was said to destroy the *Spirochaeta pallida,* the cause of syphilis in man. In later years, a series of synthetic drugs based on sulfanilamide and sulfonamides were found effective in controlling streptococcus and pneumococcus infection. Penicillin, first prepared by Sir Alexander Fleming from the mold penicillium in 1929, and studied by Florey and others at Oxford, has been shown to be even more powerful than the sulfonamides.

Progress was also made in the treatment of the noninfectious diseases. After 1900, many deficiency conditions associated with malnutrition (beriberi and pellagra, for example) and endocrinal disorders (diabetes and hyperthyroidism, for example) were treated by regulating the diet and by artificially prepared endocrinal supplements.

Until the middle of the nineteenth century, the use of surgery as a method of treating disease was seriously restricted owing to the high probability of death from infection following surgery and to the lack of anesthetics. By 1867, Joseph Lister, an English surgeon, had developed the antiseptic method of treating wounds by using carbolic acid, and he also introduced the principle of asepsis to surgery. Effective, general anesthesia had been discovered as early as the 1840's, but it was not until the last decades of the nineteenth century that it was used together with the principles of antisepsis and asepsis, thereby making certain operations safe which hitherto had been thought to be quite impossible. Surgical progress in the nineteenth and twentieth centuries also was aided by the clinical pathologist, who furnished the clinician and surgeon with information about biopsy material, bacteriology, and the physics and chemistry of the body fluids and excretions, thus ensuring that a patient would be managed in the best possible way. In a similar fashion, certain technical discoveries aided the clinician and surgeon. The ophthalmoscope, laryngoscope, and other apparatus of various sorts, for example, permitted the examination of internal organs, thereby providing direct information concerning morbid processes. The detection of pathologic conditions also was aided enormously by the discovery of the roentgen rays in the year 1895.

Public Health in the Scientific Era in the United States

By the beginning of the twentieth century, the new knowledge of bacteriology and immunology was being applied to public health in the United States (as in England and on the Continent) with striking results: it became possible to control infectious diseases to an extent and with an effectiveness that theretofore were unknown. However, it soon became apparent that these measures provided only part of the solution to the problems of health and well-being. Various developing social phenomena had aspects which were proving to be deleterious to health, and new and increased public health efforts began to be directed toward their alleviation. Thus, new scientific knowledge, a growing social awareness, and the pressure of social circumstances all combined to lead to the vast expansion of activities which has come to characterize public health in the United States in the twentieth century. Accompanying this expansion was a developing basic ideology which embodied the various goals and the fundamental intent of public health, and these, too, broadened as time went by.

Expansion of Areas of Public Health Activity. By the 1900's, much of the new scientific knowledge about infectious disease was still to be applied in the United States, and although the hazards of epidemics were reduced, disease in general was by no means eradicated. In addition, the vast industrial and urban growth which the United States began experiencing early in the twentieth century became associated with a host of social problems, including poverty, malnutrition, high rates of maternal mortality, and the proliferation of congested slums. The health aspects of these and other similar problems soon became apparent, and public health began to expand its activities in order to provide for the rapidly increasing and pressing health needs of the population.

In the area of *infectious disease control*, immunization programs began to be undertaken in the United States early in the twentieth century. In connection with certain diseases such as smallpox, vaccination became a legal requirement by 1915 in most states, being either compulsory for school attendance or required under certain other conditions. However, a few states had regulations that stated circumstances under which vaccination was actually prohibited.[37] Subsequently, some states passed laws requiring immunization against other diseases such as diphtheria and typhoid. The age-old provision of quarantine as a method of infectious-disease control gradually was modified as the characteristics of various diseases became known, but as late as the 1920's, some communities still had stringent quarantine requirements for many diseases.[37] The prevention and control of disease were also advanced through other methods such as efficient sewerage systems; improved practices in connection with the purification of water and food supplies; and comprehensive programs to control insect, animal, and healthy-human carriers of disease.

Maternal and infant health * received intensive public health attention very early, with an emphasis on disease prevention, nutritional improvement, and prenatal care. When it was discovered that many young babies died as the result of contaminated milk, stations were established to dispense clean milk. Following some European models, a system of milk stations was established in New York in 1893 by the philanthropist Nathan Strauss; the stations continued to operate until 1919. Government action was also undertaken along these lines under the auspices of local health departments. In 1908, the New York City Health Department established a Division of Child Hygiene with a broad program aimed at teaching mothers the principles of child care, and four years later a child hygiene unit was established in the Louisiana state health department. In 1912, after six years of national agitation and discussion, the federal government created a Children's Bureau which was responsible for the welfare of children on a nation-wide basis. The Bureau also soon became concerned with maternal health, including maternal mortality and the health education of mothers. Subsequent federal legislation directed toward maternal and child health and welfare included the Maternity and Infancy Act (Sheppard-Towner) of 1921 and certain provisions of the Social Security Act of 1935.

Attention was also directed toward the *health of the school-age child* early in the twentieth century. Among the earliest provisions (as in Massachusetts) were physical examinations for schoolchildren, primarily aimed at controlling communicable diseases. In 1912, New York City provided free clinics for schoolchildren under the auspice of the health department,

---

* A number of the historical facts which are briefly summarized in the subsequent discussion of the development of specific public health program-areas appear, and are discussed considerably more extensively, in *A History of Public Health* by George Rosen (MD Publications, New York, 1957).

offering general medical services and attention to various special conditions. School lunch programs were also established during the first decade of the twentieth century in an effort to cope with malnutrition, and during the 1930's the federal government undertook a significant role in this area.

Occupational health was another area of expansion of public health activity during the early twentieth century, from roots going back to post-Civil War days. At that time, owing largely to pressure from labor unions, numerous states and the federal government established labor bureaus to investigate working conditions, including health matters. The U.S. Department of Labor was created in 1913, having evolved over a period of about twenty-five years. During the first decade of the twentieth century, a number of studies were made and reports prepared on health conditions in various industries highlighting a wide variety of health hazards. In the second decade of the century, several organizations were formed to promote occupational health, and physicians began to be employed by industries throughout the country to provide care for injured employees and sometimes to give medical examinations. Workmen's compensation laws began to be enacted about 1910. These laws at first covered only industrial accidents but later were extended to occupational diseases as well; by the late 1950's, a vast majority of the states had laws containing both provisions. Stimulated by the Social Security Act of 1935 and by the needs created during World War II, most state health departments had an occupational health program by the 1950's, and cities and counties began to follow suit.

Needs for the provision of *medical care* were recognized in the United States as early as the colonial period, when physicians and midwives were paid by town governments to offer care to the sick poor. In the twentieth century, provision for the poor remained a concern in medical care, but owing to a combination of social factors and the advances of medical science, the problem began to extend to increasingly larger segments of the population. If illness occurred, there were new and improved diagnostic and treatment procedures available, including better-equipped and -operated hospitals, but these advances increased the cost of medical care. As industrialization proceeded, more people worked for wages which, for many, did not keep pace with increasing medical costs, and the matter was particularly aggravated when wages were subject to interruption by periods of unemployment. Thus, how to make medical care accessible when it was needed and not just when the individual could afford it was a problem that emerged early in the twentieth century. As a solution, the provision of health insurance developed and followed two divergent paths: compulsory provisions and voluntary provisions. The first movement to enact government-sponsored, compulsory health insurance occurred in 1912, and efforts persisted sporadically thereafter, increasing in intensity as a result of the severe economic depression of the 1930's. However, it was not until 1965 that the first compulsory health insurance was finally enacted when the

United States Congress amended the Social Security Act and created Medicare, which provided benefits to persons age 65 or older. Voluntary, or private, prepaid health insurance plans existed on a limited and not very effective scale during the first decade of the twentieth century under the auspice of groups such as fraternal orders, trade unions, and lodges. However, voluntary plans were given strong impetus by the depression of the 1930's when the relationship between economics and medical care became strikingly apparent, and the growth of such plans was particularly rapid after 1937.

The preceding discussion illustrates the range of expansion of public health activities since the turn of the century, the different courses of development that the various areas of concern have undergone, and the gradually increasing responsibility that government has assumed for health matters. In addition to the examples just reviewed, public health has also undertaken numerous other activities during the twentieth century, including programs in mental health, chronic disease, nutrition, health education, rehabilitation, and several new facets of environmental health. Attention also has been directed toward improving the mechanisms for delivering services to the population, such as through the consolidation of health and welfare services and the provision of community health centers where a number of different services may be grouped under one roof.

Along with the growth of activities in the present century, the field of public health has also acquired a large number of professional specialties which contribute to its mission, including public health nursing, dentistry, veterinary medicine, medical technology, pharmacology, and occupational and physical therapy. These and many other specialists now perform vital tasks in several different organizational settings, including official agencies, voluntary agencies, and international health organizations. In addition, although public health has developed its own body of knowledge and language, a large number of different disciplines contribute to its scientific nature. Thus, various branches of medical science such as bacteriology, virology, and genetics are of fundamental importance. Related to these are other disciplines such as epidemiology and biostatistics which have developed to serve the particular needs of public health. As the social nature of public health became recognized, attention was directed toward the analysis of the social dimensions of health problems, and the utility of various social science disciplines became apparent, including sociology, psychology, anthropology, political science, economics, education, and law.

Public Health Ideology. Paralleling the expanding public health activities of the twentieth century and influencing their direction was a developing basic ideology pertaining to various goals and to fundamental intent. This ideology, or philosophy, embodied the principles, values, ideas, attitudes, and institutions of public health that were emerging in the course of the historical development which has been described in this chapter.

Society's attitudes toward health and disease have been shown to change in time depending on the prevalent theologic, economic, or social ideas. By the late nineteenth century, attitudes toward disease were beginning to be influenced by scientific knowledge, so that new concepts regarding disease causation, prevention, and cure began to mitigate ancient fears and superstitions. It has also been shown that, over time, public health advances and reforms have been based on different motives: sometimes they were idealistic, as was the case with the humanitarians and social reformers; and sometimes they were pragmatic, arising from threats to the security of man and society. Public health in the twentieth century has also been subject to a variety of external influences which have caused it to change over time, and several facets of ideology have emerged as a consequence.

Public health has developed a basic concern for the conservation of life and health, and thus its activities have become essentially humane and protective. In the past, this concept was sometimes misinterpreted to mean that it was concerned primarily with saving the weak and unfit of society. The evolution of public health, however, has clearly shown that its activities are directed toward promoting the health and well-being of the total of society and all of its segments—rich and poor, strong and weak, healthy and infirm. C.-E. A. Winslow, in defining the mission and scope of public health in 1920, stated that it "is the Science and Art of (1) preventing disease, (2) prolonging life, and (3) promoting health and efficiency through organized community effort," and that it encompasses numerous specific areas of activity ranging from environmental sanitation and communicable disease control to the organization of medical services and the development of means to ensure a standard of living adequate for maintaining health.[38] In general terms, public health has come to be regarded as that body of knowledge and those practices which contribute to maintaining the health of the individual or of the population in the aggregate. Maintenance of health is viewed as being accomplished through the application of preventive measures or of curative measures, or both, and thus has come to include detection or diagnosis of disease, treatment, and rehabilitation.

An awareness has grown in public health of the significance of applying medical knowledge to the benefit of man in his social state, a concept which is known as social medicine. This branch of knowledge has been the subject of many treatises, written mainly by Europeans in the eighteenth, nineteenth, and twentieth centuries,[39] but also by members of the health professions in the United States, including Lemuel Shattuck, Stephen Smith, Edgar Sydenstricker, Joseph Mountin, Henry E. Sigerist, and C.-E. A. Winslow.[37] There are two principles of social medicine: (1) to regard human subjects as persons who are integral parts of families and communities, and (2) to use medical knowledge for the benefit of these persons within the context of their society.[40] Studies in the field of social medicine, therefore, would include the influence of housing, poverty, occupation, nutrition, and other factors as they affect the health of a person or community. Since man interacts with his environment and with society, his physical and mental illnesses may be more easily defined, prevented, and cured by an analysis of this interaction.

The view regarding society's role in and responsibility for health promotion and maintenance has become broadened as public health concepts have developed. In the past, health matters were considered the responsibility of the individual except for certain aspects that were clearly outside his purview. The latter were the responsibility of the local community and were fairly narrowly defined to include such matters as sanitation and the prevention and control of epidemics. This definition of society's role and responsibility in health reflected the social philosophy of individualism that prevailed in the United States for many generations. It gradually became modified by the recognition that there were many dimensions to health; that many health-promoting activities were beyond the scope of the individual; and that many social problems had health aspects and thereby required a broad and concerted attack. Thus, the concept of society's responsibility for health became expanded and was accompanied by an increased recognition of the role of the national government in health matters. As a central, unified authority representing the people, the national government was viewed as the appropriate agent for fulfilling an increasing number of society's responsibilities for health and well-being.

The concept of health as a global concern gradually emerged as a further extension of the view regarding society's responsibilities for health. Distances between nations have continually shrunk, and the health problems of individual nations are now considered as reflecting upon the health of all nations. Problems of inadequate medical care, epidemic disease, overpopulation, nutritional diseases, and tropical diseases, for example, are still found in several parts of the world. Such problems are no longer viewed as the sole concern of the particular nations which suffer from them. Rather, present objectives are to utilize the scientific and technologic resources of all nations in the solution of health problems wherever they occur in the world.

SUMMARY

The evolution of public health has been characterized by the interaction of several phenomena: the nature and severity of disease; the status of knowledge regarding the cause, control, and treatment of disease; and the prevailing social ideology and situational factors. These phenomena have interacted in a particular time and place throughout history, and also, they have changed historically.

The earliest known health-related concepts were restricted to matters of personal hygiene and were based largely on religious precepts. By Greco-Roman times, public health began to acquire institutional aspects; thus, although personal hygiene was still emphasized, programs in environmental sanitation, medical care, and administration of health services were undertaken as civil activities.

In the Middle Ages, bubonic plague and leprosy took a staggering toll of lives. During this period, concepts as to the cause of disease included divine or demonic wrath, climate, conjunction of the stars and planets, corruption of dead bodies, and exhalations by the sick. Medieval cities contributed markedly to the prevalence of disease, but they also had significant military, political, economic, and social functions. Infirmaries, hospitals, and other facilities to care for the sick were provided by monasteries, the Church, and many medieval communities.

From the sixteenth to the nineteenth centuries, epidemic diseases continued to besiege the inhabited parts of the world, cholera being one of the most devastating in the nineteenth century. During much of this time, controversy raged over the cause and control of these diseases: whether they were contagious (i.e., spread from person to person) and thus controllable by quarantine; or whether they were miasmatic (i.e., due to various atmospheric or telluric conditions) and controllable by sanitation measures. Both kinds of control measures were instituted from time to time.

During the same four centuries, the evolution of society also influenced the course of public health. In England in the seventeenth century, the rise of mercantilism and the nation state made the health of the people of economic and political import, and in the eighteenth century views were expressed in both England and Germany that health was the responsibility of the state. However, disease, poverty, and unsanitary living conditions became the by-products of the industrial revolution and of urban growth in the eighteenth and nineteenth centuries; these conditions were mitigated only by prolonged efforts of ardent humanitarians and social reformers. In the nineteenth century, reports by Edwin Chadwick in England and Lemuel Shattuck in the United States highlighted the interaction of physical ills and social ills in the population. A General Board of Health and a National Board of Health were established in England and in the United States, respectively, and although both were eventually abolished, they reflected the beginning of organized efforts on the part of national government to promote public health. Meantime, in the United States the enactment of legislation to establish boards of health in the states and the larger cities had been under way since the late eighteenth century.

In the middle and late nineteenth century, concepts regarding the cause, prevention, treatment, and control of disease were revolutionized by the advent of scientific knowledge, from roots going back many decades. Bacteriology established microorganisms as the cause of epidemic diseases; immunology provided means of preventing disease by vaccination; and identification of various carriers of disease made control measures possible. These and other significant scientific discoveries ushered in a new epoch in public health in the Western world. In the United States, public health activities expanded markedly, in both breadth and depth, after the beginning of the twentieth century, and government began to assume an important role in the promotion of health and the control of disease. The basic ideology of public health also underwent maturation and now includes several facets: a basic concern with the conservation of life and health; an awareness of the need to apply medical knowledge to man in his social state; a broadened view of society's role in and responsibility for health matters; and a recognition of health as a global concern.

REFERENCES

1. ROSEN, GEORGE. *A History of Public Health.* MD Publications, New York, 1957.

2. ————. Purposes and value of medical history. In: Galdston, I., ed. *On the Utility of Medical History.* Monograph I, Institute on Social and Historical Medicine. International Universities Press, New York, 1957.

3. TREVELYAN, G. M. *An Autobiography.* Longmans, Green and Company, London, 1949.

4. SIGERIST, HENRY E. *A History of Medicine,* 2nd ed. 1. Oxford University Press, New York, 1955.

5. ————. The philosophy of hygiene. *Bull Inst Hist Med,* 1:323–31, 1933.

6. SEXTUS JULIUS FRONTINUS. *The Two Books on the Water Supply of the City of Rome . . . A Photographic Reproduction of the Sole Original Latin Manuscript.* Translated by C. Herschel, 2nd ed. Longmans, Green and Company, London, 1913.

7. GARRISON, FIELDING H. The history of drainage, irrigation, sewerage-disposal and water-supply. *Bull NY Acad Med,* 5:887–938, 1929.

8. RICHMOND, I. A., ed. *The Aqueducts of Ancient Rome by Thomas Ashby.* Clarendon Press, Oxford, 1935.

9. WOODHEAD, A. G. The state health service in ancient Greece. *Cambridge Hist J,* 10:234–53, 1952.

10. MUNDY, JOHN H., and RIESENBURG, PETER. *The Medieval Town.* N. J. Van Nostrand, Princeton, 1958.

11. SIGERIST, HENRY E. *Civilization and Disease.* Cornell University Press, Ithaca, 1945.

12. CAMPBELL, ANNA. *The Black Death and Men of Learning.* Columbia University Press, New York, 1931.

13. NOHL, JACQUES. *The Black Death.* Unwin Books, London, 1961.

14. MAJOR, RALPH H. *Classic Descriptions of Disease,* 3rd ed. Charles C Thomas, Springfield, Ill., 1959.

15. WINSLOW, CHARLES-EDWARD AMORY. *The Conquest of Epidemic Disease.* Princeton University Press, Princeton, 1944.

16. HALE, THE VENERABLE ARCHDEACON. The Carthusian Monastery of London. *Trans London and Middlesex Archeolog Soc,* 3:309–31, 1870.

17. AMULREE, RT. HON. LORD. Monastic infirmaries. In: Poynter, F. N. L., ed. *The Evolution of Hospitals in Britain.* Pitman Medical Publishing Co., London, 1964.

18. PACKARD, FRANCIS R., ed. *Regimen Sanitatis Salernitanum. The School of Salernum,* the English Version by Sir John Harington. Oxford University Press, London, 1922.

19. ROSEN, GEORGE. Cameralism and the concept of medical police. *Bull Hist Med,* 27:21–42, 1953.

20. DUFFY, JOHN. *Epidemics in Colonial America.* Louisiana State University Press, Baton Rouge, 1953.

21. BAUMGARTNER, LEONA, and RAMSEY, ELIZABETH, M. Johann Peter Frank and his "System Einer Vollständigen Medicinischen Polizey." *Ann Med Hist,* **5**:525–32 and **6**:66–90, 1953.

22. SIMON, SIR JOHN. *English Sanitary Institutions.* Cassell, London, 1890.

23. POYNTER, F. N. L. Thomas Southwood Smith—the man (1788–1861). *Proc Roy Soc Med* (Section of the History of Medicine), **55**:381–92, 1962.

24. FLINN, M. W., ed. *Report on the Sanitary Conditions of the Labouring Population of Great Britain by Edwin Chadwick, 1842.* Edinburgh University Press, Edinburgh, 1965.

25. HIRST, L. FABIAN. *The Conquest of Plague.* Clarendon Press, Oxford, 1953.

26. LAMBERT, ROYSTON. *Sir John Simon.* Macgibbon and Kee, London, 1963.

27. SIMES, E., and SCHOLEFIELD, C. E., eds. *The Public Health Acts by W. G. Lumley and Edmund Lumley,* 12th ed. Butterworth and Co., London, 1950.

28. KRAMER, HOWARD D. Early municipal and state boards of health. *Bull Hist Med,* **24**:504, 1950.

29. SMILLIE, WILSON. *Public Health, Its Promise for the Future; A Chronicle of the Development of Public Health in the United States, 1607–1914.* Macmillan Company, New York, 1955.

30. SHATTUCK, LEMUEL. *Report of a General Plan for the Promotion of Public and Personal Health, Devised, Prepared and Recommended by the Commissioners Appointed Under a Resolve of the Legislature of Massachusetts, Relating to a Sanitary Survey of the State.* Dutton and Wentworth, Boston, 1850.

31. *Proceedings and Debates of the Third National Quarantine and Sanitary Convention.* Edward Jones and Co., New York, 1859.

32. FRACASTORO, GEROLAMO. *De Contagione et Contagiosis Morbis et Eorum Curatione, Libri III.* Translation and notes by Wilma Cave Wright. B. P. Putnam's Sons, New York, 1930.

33. MILLER, GENEVIEVE. *The Adoption of Inoculation for Smallpox in England and France.* University of Pennsylvania Press, Philadelphia, 1957.

34. JENNER, EDWARD. *An Inquiry into the Causes and Effects of the Variolae Vaccine.* Low, London, 1798.

35. PARISH, H. J. *A History of Immunization.* E. & S. Livingstone, Ltd., Edinburgh, 1965.

36. CHAPIN, CHARLES V. *The Sources and Modes of Infection.* John Wiley & Sons, New York, 1910.

37. HANLON, JOHN J. *Principles of Public Health Administration,* 4th ed. The C. V. Mosby Company, St. Louis, 1964.

38. WINSLOW, CHARLES-EDWARD AMORY. The untilled field of public health. *Mod Med,* **2**:183, 1920.

39. ROSEN, GEORGE. The evolution of social medicine. In: Freeman, H. E., Levine, S., and Reeder, L., eds. *Handbook of Medical Sociology.* Prentice-Hall, Inc., Englewood Cliffs, N.J., 1963.

40. ANDERSON, J. A. D. *A New Look at Social Medicine.* Pitman Medical Publishing Company, London, 1965.

CHAPTER 2

ORGANIZATION FOR HEALTH

Contemporary modes of organization for health are described in this chapter, and the development, goals, functions, and trends with respect to various organized health efforts are discussed.

The first two sections of the chapter comment on the general goals and status of health organization and the various forces which influence the organizational process. In subsequent sections of the chapter a distinction is made among three basic kinds of organized health agencies: official agencies in the United States, which are operated by the federal, state, or local governments and are supported through tax resources; voluntary agencies in the United States, which are supported by endowments, donations, campaign subscriptions, patient fees, membership dues, or contracts and are operated by a nongovernmental staff under an independent board; and international agencies, which are concerned with worldwide health problems and are operated cooperatively by combinations of several nations or instigated by one or more of the most advanced countries. Information on the level, sources, and objects of health expenditures in the United States is also presented.

GENERAL GOALS AND STATUS
OF HEALTH ORGANIZATION

In the course of development and adaptation, mankind has generated an intellectual ability to change rapidly and even to control much of the physical and some of the biologic environment. Although in this process marked gains have been made in the solution of many health problems, at the same time various "diseases of civilization" have emerged and proliferated, and some aspects of the environment have been manipulated to the detriment of health largely because of failure to meet efficiently and realistically the emerging problems associated with advancing technology. The fundamental goals of health organization are to find solutions for these problems and to develop successful or acceptable plans to meet health needs in an epoch of constant change. The challenge today is not so much survival, per se, but the quality of being. Present concern is with the mode of organization which can best enhance the pursuit of, and the opportunity for, optimal health and increased longevity.

Contemporary health efforts are organized on the basis of common interests and objectives related to improving the physical and mental well-being of a defined population group. Organizations for health services differ from one nation to another, and in the United States from one state to another; some state organizations may be comparable to those of emerging nations as far as basic concepts, the actual provision of environmental health protection, and the delivery of medical care services are concerned. For long periods in history, progress in organization for health—whether on the community, national, or international level—has been the result of repeated emergencies and crises rather than long-range representative planning. The American people have been slow to express their concern for systematic group health protection and services through representative government at the several levels. Similarly, international health efforts which depend on cooperative action among nations have evolved slowly and haltingly. However, in recent decades the pattern began to be altered by the emergence of several influential factors, including higher levels of education, increased communication and travel, rising standards of living, and heightened expectations of health and social benefits. The result is a trend toward action by increasingly larger representative units of government and of population groups for the purpose of creating broader and more effective organization for health.

INFLUENCES ON THE
ORGANIZATIONAL PROCESS

Several factors have a bearing on the kinds of health organizations which predominate within a geographic area or period of time. The organizational process to meet needs involves human expectations as to levels of health, longevity, and equality and the means of their attainment. The relative weight or priority of expectation of individuals and populations is influenced by many elements, including socioeconomic levels (e.g., education and income), ideology (e.g., concepts and attitudes), and degree of acceptance of individual responsibility through the exercise of citizenship, leadership, and political endeavors.

There are many philosophies which are expressed in the history of national, religious, and ethnic groups, but one most prominent in recent centuries is the organization of the multicultural group in order to meet the problems of physical health, mental health, and environmental control. In the United States, as well as in many other countries, responsibility for health is shifting to an ever broader base. Furthermore, there is an increasing appreciation of the interrelationship and interdependence of world population groups and recognition that no subgroup can survive in isolation. A realization is growing that efforts for the advancement of health and longevity are best achieved through unified action and sharing of resources.

Health organization and administration are, therefore, influenced by the philosophy, aspirations, and objectives of population groups and reflect the acceptable implementation which emerges and ultimately survives in pursuit of various goals. The mid-twentieth century is a dynamic period of program development, organization, and administration, and the approach to organization of health services must be based on the pressures of changing need. Current and continuous study founded on clues from the past will help to evaluate the present and to predict and plan for the future.

THE LEGAL AND GOVERNMENTAL FRAMEWORK OF PUBLIC HEALTH IN THE UNITED STATES

Constitutional Powers and Organization of the Federal Government *

The role of the federal government in health activities is determined by the framework of the United States Constitution within which both the national and the state governments operate. The authors of the Constitution used certain broad and general phrases which have permitted considerable latitude in interpretation with respect to matters of public health. An example of such phrasing is the basic mandate to the federal government to "promote the general welfare," which occurs in the Preamble to the Constitution.[1] In addition, the body of the Constitution grants several powers to the federal government which have been interpreted to include

* This section, pp. 45–46, is based on a paper by William H. Stewart entitled "Health Services in the Structure of the United States Government" and presented at the Public Health Colloquium, UCLA School of Public Health, January 8, 1963.

health activities. Thus, the power to regulate commerce with foreign nations and among the several states (Art. I, sec. 8, par. 1) has been construed as including such matters as international and interstate quarantine, sanitary supervision, and vital statistics.[1] The power to levy taxes "to provide for the common defense and general welfare" (Art. I, sec. 8, par. 3) permits, for example, federal government activity in maternal and child health and the subsidization of state and local health programs.[1] The power to raise and support armies, to provide and maintain a navy, and to make rules for the government and regulation of the land and naval forces (Art. III, sec. 8, pars. 12–14) has given to federal agencies the responsibility for maintaining the health of the Armed Forces.[1] Still other opportunities for health activities are provided by the power to exercise exclusive legislation in federal territory (i.e., the District of Columbia, military bases, national parks, Indian reservations, etc.; Art. I, sec. 8, par. 17) and by the power to make treaties (Art. II, sec. 2, par. 2). Finally, an omnibus provision grants the federal government the authority "to make all Laws which shall be necessary and proper for carrying into Execution the foregoing Powers, and all other Powers vested by this Constitution in the Government of the United States, or in any Department or Officer thereof" (Art. III, sec. 8, par. 18).

The roles and responsibilities of the United States government are established by the Constitution through the organization of three branches with separate powers: *the Congress,* a bicameral legislature to make national laws and to appropriate tax monies for support of the government (this function underlies all federal activities, including, of course, those of a health and welfare nature); *the executive branch,* headed by the President and aided by a cabinet of secretaries who are administratively responsible for carrying out the intent of the Constitution, its amendments, national legislation, and court and executive interpretations; and *the judicial branch,* composed of the Supreme Court and lower federal courts which interpret the Constitution, amendments, and national laws as they may affect the health and welfare of individuals and groups. This distribution of functions among three branches of government—executive, legislative, and judicial—is found typically, also, at state and local levels.

The powers vested in the federal government by the Constitution are considerable and permit opportunity for the exercise of leadership in developing and implementing policy based on changing concepts, philosophy, and community needs. Over the years, the original Constitution and Bill of Rights have remained the same, but intent, interpretation, and application have changed. These changes have come about through Constitutional amendments, Supreme Court decision, unchallenged state laws and administrative law, and socially accepted practices. As a consequence, there has been an accelerated rate of increase in the role and influence of federal law and administration on state and local governments in meeting health and social problems.

The Nature and Intent of Federal Health Legislation

The twentieth century has been marked by an expansion not only in the quantity but also in the variety of federal health legislation generated by the United States government. The Congress has enacted several general kinds of measures, including the creation of new services and programs; the training of personnel for the health professions; the support of basic and applied research on a vast array of health related topics; and, periodically when required, the organization and reorganization of administrative structures in an effort to optimize the delivery of health services.

A basic aim of federal health and health-related legislation enacted in recent years has been to establish integrated, federal-state-local programs which will strengthen the roles of the lower-echelon governments as effective instruments of public policy. The intention is to stimulate the development of better community health programs by supporting local governments in health activities and by encouraging the growth of regional jurisdictions to solve the health and social problems of modern America. The following brief review of several laws passed by the Eighty-ninth United States Congress during the 1965–1966 session illustrates the nature and intent of contemporary health legislation.

Emphasis on regional development is embodied in Public Law 89–239, which provides for the establishment of regional centers to attack the problems of heart disease, cancer, and stroke; the regions involved do not necessarily bear any relationship to existing political jurisdictions. The development of comprehensive metropolitan, areawide, and regional approaches to water pollution problems and the disposal of wastes is provided in the Water Quality Act (Public Law 89–234). Public Law 89–105 augments an enactment by the Eighty-eighth Congress (Public Law 88–164) which authorized the creation of community mental health centers in order to provide a continuum of mental health services locally and to serve as a major alternative to existing, massive mental hospitals. Basic health services in state and local public health organizations are extended through Public Law 89–109, which includes the authorization of mass immunization programs, special aid for the chronically ill, and formula grants for general services by local public health departments. The Appalachian Regional Development Act (Public Law 89–4) involves 360 counties in 11 states in the Appalachian area and includes programs in transportation; health facilities construction, equipment, and operation; land stabilization; conservation and erosion control; vocational education facilities; sewage treatment construction facilities; comprehensive housing programs; and supplements to existing federal grant-in-aid programs. The Older Americans Act (Public Law 89–73) declares joint federal, state, and local governmental responsibility for older persons; creates an Administration on Aging as a coordinating center for state and local government services; and sets goals for the health and welfare of older people including adequate income, optimal physical and mental health, suitable housing, and the provision of restorative services.

The intent of the Comprehensive Health Planning and Public Health Services Amendments of 1966 (Public Law 89–749) as stated in the Act, is to promote and assure "the highest level of health attainable for every person" through "effective partnership involving close intergovernmental collaboration, official and voluntary efforts, and participation of individuals and organizations." The Act recognizes that "comprehensive planning for health services, health manpower, and health facilities is essential at every level of government; that desirable administration requires strengthening the leadership and capacities of State health agencies; and that support of health services provided people in their communities should be broadened and made more flexible." To accomplish these purposes, the law provides for federal grants to the states for comprehensive health planning at the state level through a designated state agency. In addition to the state health planning agency, there must also be a state health planning council to include representatives of state and local agencies, nongovernmental organizations, and other groups concerned with health, but with representatives of consumers of health services as the majority of the membership. Grants are also available for areawide comprehensive health planning (regional, metropolitan, or other local areas), and for training health planners. In addition, the law provides for federal grants to the states for a flexible program of public health services based on the state's comprehensive plans, and there is also provision for support for studies, demonstrations, or training to develop or improve methods of providing services.

The enactment of federal laws such as those summarized above may be viewed as a significant form of "creative federalism" which extends and expands the partnership of federal, state, and local agencies. Federal programs of this nature rely on local initiative and the strengths of local government and local officials to solve the more pressing social and other domestic problems that confront America in the last third of the twentieth century. In the process, the federal income tax dollar is returned to the states, regional bodies, and local governments in order that these governments can, by a concerted and well-organized effort, attack their own problems and, in doing so, improve the health and welfare of the entire nation.

Federal-State Relationships and Powers of the States °

In the United States, federal-state relationships are based on (1) the principle that the states are inseparable units of one nation rather than independent governments and (2) provisions of the Constitution whereby

° This section, pp. 48–49, is based on a paper by William H. Stewart entitled "Health Services in the Structure of the United States Government" and presented at the Public Health Colloquium, UCLA School of Public Health, January 8, 1963.

certain powers are delegated to the federal government, certain powers are prohibited to the states, and all powers not so delegated or prohibited are reserved for the people and their states. Around these constitutional provisions the so-called "states' rights" issue has arisen frequently from the earliest years of the nation to the present time. The "reserved" powers of the states are not clearly defined, and from time to time controversy arises as to whether a power asserted by the federal government or by a state is valid under the Constitution. No state may determine such issues for itself. The United States Supreme Court determines the line between federal and state powers, and its decisions have the force of national law.

The states have broad powers to organize their own government, to generate programs to meet social needs, and to raise revenues to support these programs. They also have the power to organize *local* governments and to authorize the levy of local taxes. The federal government intervenes in state activities when foods, drugs, and biologic products are sold in interstate commerce or when certain problems arise that are beyond the control of an individual state. A good example is the interstate pollution of common waterways by cities and industries. When cities and states pollute water or use an inequitable amount of any natural resources to the detriment or disadvantage of surrounding states, the federal government has the power to intervene for mutual protection of all population groups. Thus, when one level of government fails to meet the needs of the people, the next higher level undertakes action through policy legislation and financing of programs.

State and Local Health Legislation

Each state, as a sovereign power, has responsibility for and authority to protect the health of the people within its geographic boundaries. State constitutions provide for general responsibility and authority, but new issues are met by adoption of specific health laws or statutes by the state legislature. There has been a trend for general policy, philosophy, and intent to be established by the state legislature followed by implementation through the adoption of regulations by the governing body of the state health department (i.e., the board of health); these regulations then are enforced or monitored by state or local health agencies. In the event that a city or county fails, refuses, or is otherwise unable to cope with its health problems, the state may lend assistance, or it may even assume control, although it seldom does.

No two states have the same system of resolution of problems of health and social need, and few states are consistent in the application of their sovereign powers to specific issues. In fact, the exercise of these powers has resulted in 50 different state sanitary codes, 50 different requirements for marriage and divorce, legal adoption, education and employment of children, licensure of practitioners of the healing arts, safety of buildings, eligibility for public assistance and medical care, procedures for handling the mentally ill and retarded, etc.

Local government has only the authority which the state delegates, but on this basis it adopts ordinances as well as supplementary rules and regulations. Through federal, state, and local governmental mechanisms, there is now some sort of legal provision for the principal aspects of health in almost every community, including the reporting of births and deaths, the reporting of certain communicable diseases, food and milk control, and environmental sanitation. Such provisions are considered to be the minimum, basic public health laws needed to monitor and protect the health of the community. Many communities now have or are striving to develop laws either directly or indirectly related to health which go well beyond these minimum requirements. Financial support by the federal government to the states and by the states to local governments influences the quality and kinds of health programs and the administration of services by local health agencies.

With the launching of programs characterized by "creative federalism," units of state, regional, and local government undoubtedly will develop new relationships with the federal government as the result of attempts to team the federal effort with that governmental unit which is most appropriate to resolve each domestic problem. Stronger, better organized, and more effectively administered state, local, and regional official health departments will be required in order to fulfill the responsibilities they will be given for carrying out the new health programs.

HEALTH ROLES AND ORGANIZATION OF THE UNITED STATES GOVERNMENT

Health Programs of the Federal Government

The health activities of the United States government are authorized by laws designed to achieve particular purposes. The programs are financed by appropriations passed by the Congress each year, and they are administered by various federal departments and other executive bodies. The specific functions may be classified broadly as dealing with the health of the general population, with the health of special population groups, and with international health.*

Functions Dealing with the General Population. Health functions which the federal government undertakes for the general population include: (1) protection against hazards affecting the entire population which can-

---

* Portions of this section, pp. 50–52, are based on a paper by William H. Stewart entitled "Health Services in the Structure of the United States Government" and presented at the Public Health Colloquium, UCLA School of Public Health, January 8, 1963.

not be provided by the states; (2) collection and dissemination of national vital and health statistics and related data; (3) advancement of the biological, medical, and environmental sciences; (4) augmentation of health facilities and certain categories of health personnel; (5) support of state and local governments in the maintenance of public health services; and (6) organization and support of disaster relief and civil defense.

Functions Dealing with Special Population Groups. The special population groups and the kinds of health measures provided for them by the federal government are: (1) protection of certain classes of workers against hazardous occupations and adverse conditions of work; (2) provision of categorical and special services by state and local governments for children, the aged, the mentally ill and retarded, the economically deprived, vocationally handicapped adults, and blind persons; (3) purchase of medical care by state and local governments for certain financially dependent population groups; (4) provision of special services for farm families; (5) provision of hospital and medical care to veterans, merchant seamen, American Indians and Alaska natives, federal prisoners, narcotic addicts, persons with leprosy, members of the "uniformed services" (e.g., the Army, Navy, Coast Guard, and commissioned officers of the Public Health Service) and their dependents, and civil service employees of the government injured as a result of their employment; and (6) hospital and medical insurance for civil service employees of the federal government.

This rather extensive array of health functions which the federal government undertakes for the general population and for special groups in the United States is based on the recognition that, although American public health resources need rarely be mobilized in this half-century for anything as severe as the classical epidemics, the frequency of occurrence of certain other kinds of health conditions necessitates a high degree of specialized organization for health services by the national government as well as by the states and local communities. These contemporary needs may be illustrated by a few facts pertaining to the nation's health status. For example, in one year recently, noninstitutionalized civilians in the United States experienced an estimated 387 million *acute illnesses or injuries* requiring medical attention or causing restriction of activity for at least one day; about half (53 per cent) of these illnesses were of a respiratory nature. At least one *chronic condition* had been reported by 84 million persons or 45 per cent of the civilian population, and about 23 million of these persons were limited in their activities as a result. In a year, the average American experiences about 16 days of restricted activity from *chronic or acute conditions,* six days of which are spent in bed. More *deaths* are due to the major cardiovascular-renal diseases than to all other causes together, and their relative importance in causing death has not changed greatly in the past ten years.[2]

Functions Dealing with International Health. Participation of the United States government in international health activities is based on a sense of responsibility to make this country's public health knowledge available to other nations, particularly those developing countries where there are still high disease and death rates owing to malnutrition, poor environmental sanitation, and inadequate health care programs. Toward this end, the federal government maintains membership in the United Nations and cooperates with all of its specialized agencies, as well as participating in the health activities of such international organizations as the Pan-American Union, the Organization of American States, the North Atlantic Treaty Organization, and the Southeast Asia Treaty Organization. In addition, the government participates in the conduct of health programs through bilateral treaties with the governments of Canada and Mexico and certain countries in Central and South America, Africa, the Eastern Mediterranean, Southeast Asia, and the Southwest Pacific. The federal government also makes financial grants for the conduct of research in the health sciences *in* foreign countries and of fellowships for the training of health personnel *from* foreign countries.

Organization and Distribution of Federal Health Functions

The health functions described above are widely dispersed in the structure of the United States government, as are counterpart activities in state and local governments. The federal government has usually applied the principle of grouping health and medical activities for the population with its programs in the fields of social insurance, public assistance, and education. The U.S. Department of Health, Education, and Welfare is the principal organizational unit for this large functional grouping.

The U.S. Department of Health, Education, and Welfare. Created in 1953, the U.S. Department of Health, Education, and Welfare took over the functions and components of the Federal Security Agency, which was then abolished. The purpose of the new department was to improve the administration of those agencies of the federal government which have major responsibility in promoting the general welfare in the fields of health, education, and social security.[3]

The programs of the Department of Health, Education, and Welfare are currently administered by *eight operating agencies;* the Department is also responsible for *three federally aided corporations* (American Printing House for the Blind, Gallaudet College, and Howard University). The operating agencies, as shown in Figure 2-1, are: Public Health Service, Office of Education, Vocational Rehabilitation Administration, Food and Drug Administration, Social Security Administration, Welfare Administration, Saint Elizabeths Hospital, and Administration on Aging, the latter having

been newly authorized in the 1966 fiscal year.[4] Three of these agencies—
Public Health Service, Food and Drug Administration, and Social Security
Administration—maintain field organizations throughout the country. Department regional offices (Fig. 2-1) are maintained in each of nine regional
areas in the United States, as shown in Figure 2-2. Each office is headed by
a Regional Director who is responsible for carrying out department policies
of providing leadership, coordination, evaluation, and general administrative supervision of all program representatives located in the regional
offices.[4]

In the years since it was created, the U.S. Department of Health, Education, and Welfare has been given vastly increased responsibilities. This
is indicated by the fact that congressional appropriations to the Department
rose from $3.5 billion in the fiscal year ending June 30, 1960, to $7.1 billion
for the 1965 fiscal year. The total available for fiscal year 1966 was approximately $9.2 billion.[4]

The Public Health Service. Although all of the various operating agencies of the U.S. Department of Health, Education, and Welfare have health-
related elements in their programs, the Public Health Service is the one
specifically charged with responsibilities for protecting and improving the
health of the nation. It is also responsible for collaborating with governments of other countries and with international organizations in world
health activities.[3]

The major responsibilities of the Public Health Service are: (1) to conduct and support research and training in the medical and related sciences
and in public health methods and administration; (2) to provide medical
and hospital services to persons authorized to receive care from the Service,
to aid in the development of the nation's hospital and related facilities, and
to prevent the introduction of communicable diseases into the United States
and its possessions; and (3) to assist the states and other governments in
the application of new knowledge for the prevention and control of disease,
the maintenance of a healthful environment, and the development of community health services.[3]

These general functions have expanded rapidly in recent years and countless new specific programs have been added. Annual congressional appropriations to the Public Health Service have increased in order to keep

° Effective August 15, 1967, the Department of Health, Education, and Welfare
merged three of these agencies—Welfare Administration, Vocational Rehabilitation Administration, and Administration on Aging—into a new agency called the Social and
Rehabilitation Service. Further reorganization placed two of the original eight operating
agencies in the Public Health Service: the Food and Drug Administration and Saint
Elizabeth's Hospital (which was transferred to the National Institute of Mental Health).
Thus, as shown by the organizational chart in the Appendix, the operating agencies of
the Department of Health, Education and Welfare were reduced to four: Public Health
Service, Social and Rehabilitation Service, Social Security Administration, and Office of
Education.

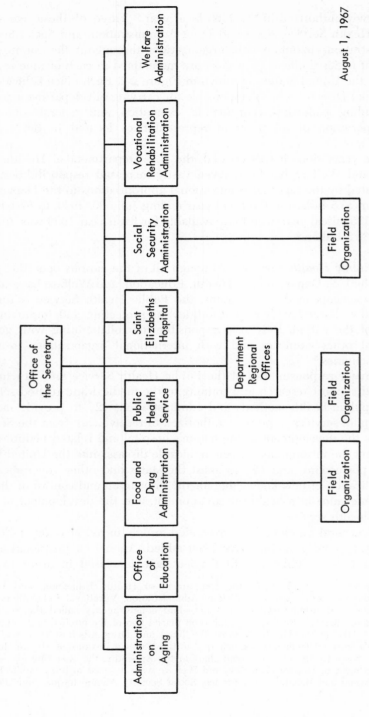

U.S. Department of Health, Education, and Welfare

August 1, 1967

FIGURE 2-1.

U. S. Department of Health, Education, and Welfare

Regional Boundaries and Offices

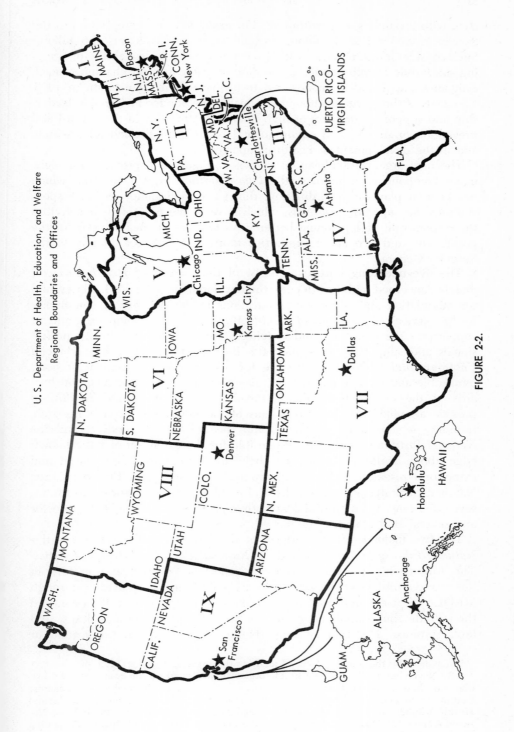

FIGURE 2-2.

55

pace with expanding responsibilities. For example, the appropriation to the Service in 1953 was $222 million; ten years later, in 1963, it was $1.6 billion.[5] Such considerations, together with a recognition of the desirability of bringing the Public Health Service up to date in order to meet changing social, economic, and health demands, led to an over-all reorganization in 1966. The goals of the reorganization are to enable the Service to "provide leadership and support in delivery of high quality health care, in the control and prevention of disease and environmental hazards, in biomedical research, and in the development of health manpower." [*]

The new organization plan, as shown in Figure 2-3, provides for eight major components as follows: the *Office of the Surgeon General,* which has general planning, coordinating, directorial, and policy-setting responsibilities; *five operating bureaus,* which have at the core of their activities the responsibility for planning better ways to meet the health needs of the population; and *two major supportive units,* which report directly to the Surgeon General.

The five operating bureaus[†] consist of the *Bureau of Health Services,* mainly concerned with health care, the development of health facilities, and the stimulation and support of innovations in the delivery of community health services; the *Bureau of Health Manpower,* to develop programs of support for the education and training of urgently needed health professionals and supporting personnel; the *Bureau of Disease Prevention and Environmental Control,* responsible for activities in the control of communicable and chronic diseases, injuries resulting from accidents, and hazards of the environment; the *National Institute of Mental Health,* to provide a unified attack on problems of mental illness through research, training, demonstration programs, and the delivery of services; and the *National Institutes of Health,* responsible for the extension of basic knowledge about health problems and their solutions through intramural and extramural research and training programs. As shown in Figure 2-3, the National Institutes of Health consist of eight separate categorical institutes, seven divisions, and a clinical center; there are also the office of the director and several staff offices.

The two major supportive units[†] of the Public Health Service are the *National Library of Medicine* and the *National Center for Health Statistics.* The Library has the most extensive collection of medical literature in the world. Bibliographic access to its collections is provided through MEDLARS, a computerized information storage and retrieval system, and through the publication of guides in the form of catalogs, indexes, and bibliographies. The Library supports the translation and publication of

---

[*] Statement by the Surgeon General made to the press on October 11, 1966.

[†] By November 1968, as shown by the organizational chart on the endpapers, the five operating bureaus of the Public Health Service had been reduced to three components: Consumer Protection and Environmental Health Service, Health Services and Mental Health Administration (including the National Institute of Mental Health and the National Center for Health Statistics), and the National Institutes of Health (including the Bureau of Health Manpower and the National Library of Medicine).

biomedical literature and administers a program for the support of medical library development.[3] The National Center for Health Statistics serves as the principal statistical arm of the Public Health Service. It conducts continuing surveys and special studies of the nation's population to determine the extent of illness and disability and to gather information related to these conditions. The Center is also the primary instrument of federal government cooperation with the states in the collection of vital statistics (births, deaths, marriages, and divorces) and is the only source of national tabulation and analysis of such data.[3]

Other Federal Agencies with Health Functions. Many other federal agencies have health functions which are secondary or supplementary to their main mission. Thus, the Departments of the Army, Navy, and Air Force administer medical services for military personnel and their dependents; the Veterans Administration has a corresponding function for war veterans; the Department of Justice provides medical care for federal prisoners; and the Department of State operates a medical program for Foreign Service personnel on duty outside the United States.

The Department of Labor administers federal laws related to conditions of work, including industrial health, safety standards, and the employment of children. In the administration of these laws, the Department works with the labor departments of the various states in order to coordinate the enforcement of federal and state regulations.

The federal government also exercises regulatory powers over certain specific industries which directly affect the public health and safety.[3] Thus, the Bureau of Mines (Department of the Interior) has responsibility for safety and healthful working conditions in the mineral industries. The Atomic Energy Commission has responsibility to protect the health and safety of the public in matters concerning the development, use, and control of atomic energy. The Federal Aviation Agency promulgates a variety of safety regulations with respect to air commerce; the U.S. Coast Guard (Department of the Treasury) is responsible for maritime safety; and the Interstate Commerce Commission enforces safety regulations pertaining to common carriers by railroad and highway, including the transportation of explosives and other dangerous items. The Department of Agriculture regulates livestock in an attempt to eradicate animal diseases and inspects domestic and imported meat and meat products.

STATE AND LOCAL HEALTH SERVICES AND ORGANIZATION

Basic Tasks and Range of Services

Official health agencies customarily perform several basic tasks, including planning of programs, organization and administration in connection with agency operation and the delivery of services, and evaluation of the

OFFICE OF THE SURGEON GENERAL

Surgeon General
Deputy Surgeon General
Associate Surgeon General
Executive Officer

Office of Program Planning and
  Evaluation
Office of Legislation
Office of Extramural Programs
Office of International Health
Office of Administrative Management
Office of Personnel
Office of Equal Health Opportunity
Office of Information
Office of Comprehensive Health
  Planning and Development

ASG for Special Projects
Chief Dental Officer
Chief Nurse Officer
Chief Sanitary Engineering Officer
Deputy Equal Employment Opportunity
  Officer
Special Assistants to Surgeon General

NATIONAL LIBRARY OF MEDICINE

BUREAU OF HEALTH SERVICES

Office of Program Planning and Evaluation
Office of Health Economics
Office of Research and Development
Office of Administrative Management
Office of Information

Div. of Community Health Services
Div. of Direct Health Services
Div. of Federal Employee Health
Div. of Health Mobilization
Div. of Hospital and Medical Facilities
Div. of Indian Health
Div. of Medical Care Administration
Div. of Mental Retardation

Medical Programs: Bureau of Prisons, Peace Corps,
  Bureau of Employees' Compensation, U. S. Coast
  Guard
Appalachian Health Program

BUREAU OF HEALTH MANPOWER

Office of Program Planning and Evaluation
Office of International Health Manpower
Office of Administrative Management
Office of Educational and Training
  Communications
Office of Information

Div. of Allied Health Manpower
Div. of Dental Health
Div. of Health Manpower Educational Services
Div. of Nursing
Div. of Physician Manpower

**BUREAU OF DISEASE PREVENTION AND
ENVIRONMENTAL CONTROL**

Office of Compliance and Control
Office of Administrative Management
Office of Program Planning and Evaluation
Office of Research and Development
Office of Standards and Intelligence
Office of Information

National Center for Air Pollution Control
National Center for Chronic Disease Control
National Communicable Disease Center
National Center for Radiological Health
National Center for Urban and Industrial Health

PHS REGIONAL ORGANIZATION

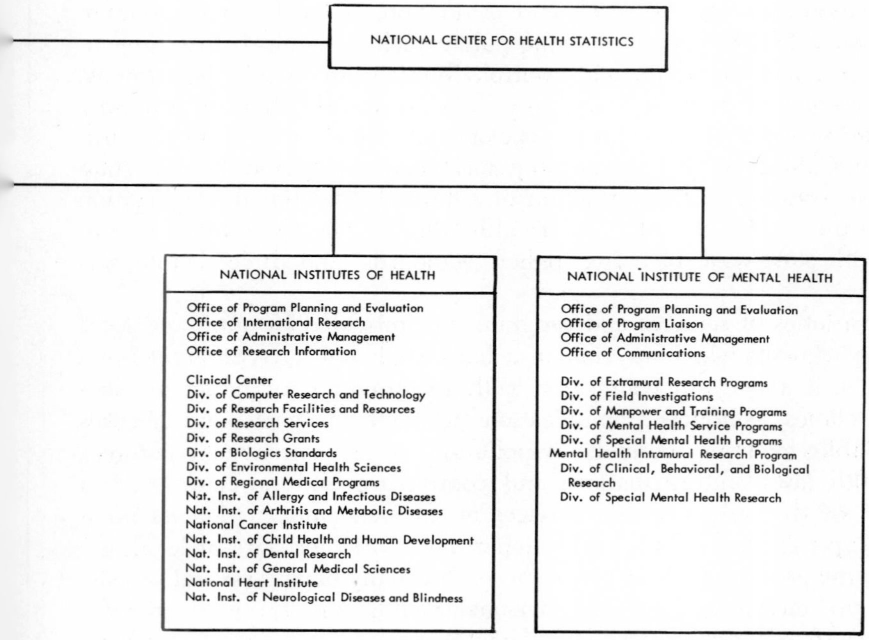

NATIONAL CENTER FOR HEALTH STATISTICS

NATIONAL INSTITUTES OF HEALTH

Office of Program Planning and Evaluation
Office of International Research
Office of Administrative Management
Office of Research Information

Clinical Center
Div. of Computer Research and Technology
Div. of Research Facilities and Resources
Div. of Research Services
Div. of Research Grants
Div. of Biologics Standards
Div. of Environmental Health Sciences
Div. of Regional Medical Programs
Nat. Inst. of Allergy and Infectious Diseases
Nat. Inst. of Arthritis and Metabolic Diseases
National Cancer Institute
Nat. Inst. of Child Health and Human Development
Nat. Inst. of Dental Research
Nat. Inst. of General Medical Sciences
National Heart Institute
Nat. Inst. of Neurological Diseases and Blindness

NATIONAL INSTITUTE OF MENTAL HEALTH

Office of Program Planning and Evaluation
Office of Program Liaison
Office of Administrative Management
Office of Communications

Div. of Extramural Research Programs
Div. of Field Investigations
Div. of Manpower and Training Programs
Div. of Mental Health Service Programs
Div. of Special Mental Health Programs
Mental Health Intramural Research Program
  Div. of Clinical, Behavioral, and Biological
    Research
  Div. of Special Mental Health Research

FIGURE 2-3. U.S. Department of Health, Education, and Welfare, Public Health Service (January 1, 1967).

programs which are in operation. *Planning* generally involves the assessment of health needs and already existing resources, the definition of purposes and objectives of a proposed new program, and the determination of which of several possible needs is most pressing. *Organizational and administrative* tasks consist of policy making, implementation of program plans, internal management of the agency (e.g., personnel and finances), and coordination of activities both internally and with outside agencies. Through *evaluation,* the agency assesses the quality and effectiveness of its programs, and the results of such activity in turn influence planning and organization; evaluation is generally accomplished through the assembly and assessment of various kinds of information which may either be accumulated on an ongoing basis or through special studies.

These basic tasks are performed to some extent by health agencies at both the state and local (county and metropolitan) levels. However, a state agency is more likely to be concerned with policy, planning, legislation, consultation to local agencies, indirect services, financial support, organizational relationships, and research and evaluation. A local agency is more likely to provide direct services to the public such as medical care, preventive services, and environmental control. Many state health departments have provision within their organization for the coordination of planning, policy, and services with the lower-echelon units which implement the programs. In California, this relationship has been recognized by the state legislature resulting in the formation of a formal operational organization known as the Conference of Local Health Officers. The Conference is concerned with state-wide planning, policy, standards, and direct health services.

Wide varieties of services and programs are provided by state and local health departments which are similar at both levels but have different functions. A local agency in connection with its provision of direct services operates clinics, conducts immunization programs, inspects and licenses certain public facilities, monitors air pollution, etc. A state agency enforces state health laws and regulations and coordinates and provides over-all direction for the programs and services of all local units within its jurisdiction. Typically found in a health department, whether state or local, are the following general kinds of programs, each usually having several specific aspects: preventive medical and personal health care services; environmental health services; patient care facilities and services; and supportive services, including certain professional specialties, research, and laboratory and administrative services.

Preventive Medical and Personal Health Care Services. Several programs of state and local health departments emphasize prevention (although they may have other functions as well) and are directed essentially toward personal health care. *Communicable disease services* and *chronic disease services* deal with disease entities and are concerned with etiology, prevention, detection, treatment, and rehabilitation. *Maternal and child health services,* in addition to providing programs for maintaining the health and preventing illness of mother and child, are also concerned with maternal and infant mortality, prematurity, school health problems, and the mentally or physically handicapped child (services for crippled children are sometimes in a separate organizational unit). *Occupational health services* exercise surveillance of the work environment in order to prevent illness, injury, and disability and to improve the physical and mental health of various categories of workers. *Nutritional services* are concerned with educational programs to improve nutrition and with the provision of consultation on nutritional matters to other programs such as maternal and child health, chronic disease, and occupational health. *Dental health services* are involved with public education regarding the need for fluoridation of public water supplies, promotion of individual dental health, local dental health programs, clinics, and increased availability of private and public dental services. *Alcoholism services,* sometimes including narcotic addiction, are concerned both with prevention and rehabilitation.

Environmental Health Services. Programs and services in this category are responsible for achieving and maintaining a physical and biologic environment for the entire population which will enhance survival, prevent disease and disability, and improve health, safety, and comfort. The environmental health activities of state and local health departments are often subdivided into several programs. *Sanitary engineering services* deal with purity of domestic water supplies, disposal of various kinds of wastes, and prevention of contamination of recreational resources (swimming pools, lakes, streams, and coastal areas). *Food and drug control programs* are concerned with standards of safety and purity in the production and processing of foods and the manufacture and sale of drugs and cosmetics. *Air pollution control services* involve the assessment of the hazards to human, animal, and plant life that come from the increasing discharges into the air of chemical gases and dusts from sources such as industry and motor vehicles; the goal of such activity is to develop legislation which will minimize air pollutants. *Vector control services* deal with the control of insects and rodents when they are sources of the transmission of disease, and more recently, these services have also become concerned with the hazards arising from the overuse or improper use of pesticides. *Radiologic health services* are responsible for monitoring air, water, food, and soil for possible contamination that may result from various practices associated with the use of ionizing radiation. *General sanitation services* include the inspection and sometimes licensing of various establishments such as restaurants, recreational areas, and jails; programs related to the sanitation of milk supplies may also be included. *Housing quality and urban planning services* are concerned with broad programs aimed at improvement of the physical environment through better housing and urban facilities (e.g., medical care, transportation, and recreation) and the elimination of blighted areas.

Patient Care Facilities and Services. Inspection and licensing of general hospitals, chronic disease facilities, and convalescent and nursing homes are traditional responsibilities of state and local health departments. As the result of federal legislation during the past few years, programs for hospital planning and the allocation of federal-state financial support have been added to the responsibilities of the state agency. These responsibilities will be expanded still further as the result of federal legislation providing medical care for the aged, and programs will need to take into account the relationship between institutional care facilities, outpatient clinics, home care services, and even the availability of physician services.

Supportive Services. State and local health departments customarily have supportive programs involving one or more basic *professional specialties*, the most usual being public health nursing, health education, and social services. *Research* is another type of supportive program and may include vital and health statistics, data processing, research planning, statistical consultation, and research training. *Laboratory services* may include specialized units for serology, bacteriology, virology, and parasitology; in general, these services support the other health department programs, engage in research, sometimes provide direct services to physicians and private laboratories, and at the state level are responsible for licensing and certification. *Administrative services* include basic business and administrative "housekeeping," including fiscal and personnel management, personnel training, management analysis and auditing, and the provision of health information to the public.

Among the 50 state and the many local health departments in the United States, there is great variety in the actual organization of the specific services just described, i.e., in the way they are grouped administratively. In general, however, most program areas are represented as divisions or bureaus of state and local health departments, although a few may still be missing in some health agencies. Figure 2-4 shows how one state health department has organized its programs and services; Figure 2-5 shows the organization of a county health department.

It should also be kept in mind that many of the health department's programs and services are shared by other agencies of government; by medical, dental, and allied professions; by citizens' groups; and by private enterprise. With respect to governmental agencies, efforts are being made in some states to consolidate related programs in a single organization. In California, for example, the state health department is part of the Health and Welfare Agency, as shown in Figure 2-4. Similar efforts to consolidate are being made on the local level in some areas.

Health Department Organization

Both state and local health departments generally have an executive officer or health officer, a board of health, and a number of divisions or bureaus to conduct programs and services; they may also have various advisory committees and consultants.

In state health departments, the health officer is usually appointed by the governor on recommendation of the board of health, but in most cases he remains in office indefinitely. As chief administrator, the state health officer has far-reaching responsibilities within the department, and he also has a key role in maintaining relationships with the governor's office, the legislature, other department heads, and nongovernmental organizations that have an interest in health affairs. The state board of health has from five to ten members, appointed by the governor in most states, and may consist of members of the medical profession only, although the trend is to broaden representation to include other professions and the lay public. The board generally serves in an advisory capacity, helps to establish policy, holds hearings, acts as liaison between the health department and the public, and sometimes works with the state legislature and professional organizations. In order better to carry out its various programs and services particularly in a large and populous state, the health department may subdivide the state into regions, placing a departmental representative in each subdivision.

In local health departments, the health officer is appointed by the mayor, the county governing body (commissioners, supervisors, etc.), or the board of health; or he may be selected from a civil service list. The health officer in turn may appoint subordinate personnel or they, too, may be selected through civil service procedures. A large metropolitan or county health department may subdivide its area into health districts in order to facilitate the delivery of services to the public. Each subdivision has a district health officer and appropriate personnel and facilities and is directly responsible to the health officer of the local department.

VOLUNTARY HEALTH AGENCIES

Voluntary health agencies have, traditionally, come into existence in the United States when a citizen or group of citizens has felt that there is an unmet need for a health service or a need for new knowledge in a particular health field. The resulting organization may be on a local, state, or national basis; a national agency may have state and local units, chapters, or affiliates. Voluntary health agencies are not tax supported, and are responsible only to their members and to public opinion, although they are chartered and licensed by appropriate state and local governmental agencies.

In addition to voluntary health agencies, there are also, of course, voluntary organizations which deal with welfare matters, such as the provision of family, youth, and recreation services. In 1958, it was estimated that there were more than 100,000 health and welfare organizations altogether,[6] a large number of these being concerned with health matters, either exclusively or partly. In the same year, voluntary health and welfare agencies raised an estimated total of $1.5 billion, of which $570 million went to organizations that had a *primary* interest in health.[6]

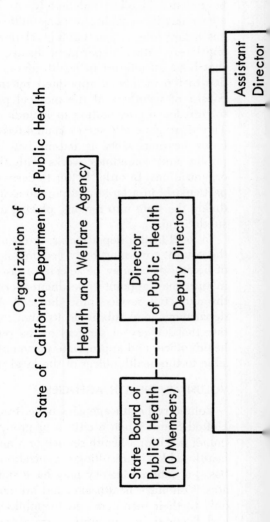

Organization of
State of California Department of Public Health

Health and Welfare Agency

State Board of
Public Health
(10 Members)

Director
of Public Health
Deputy Director

Assistant
Director

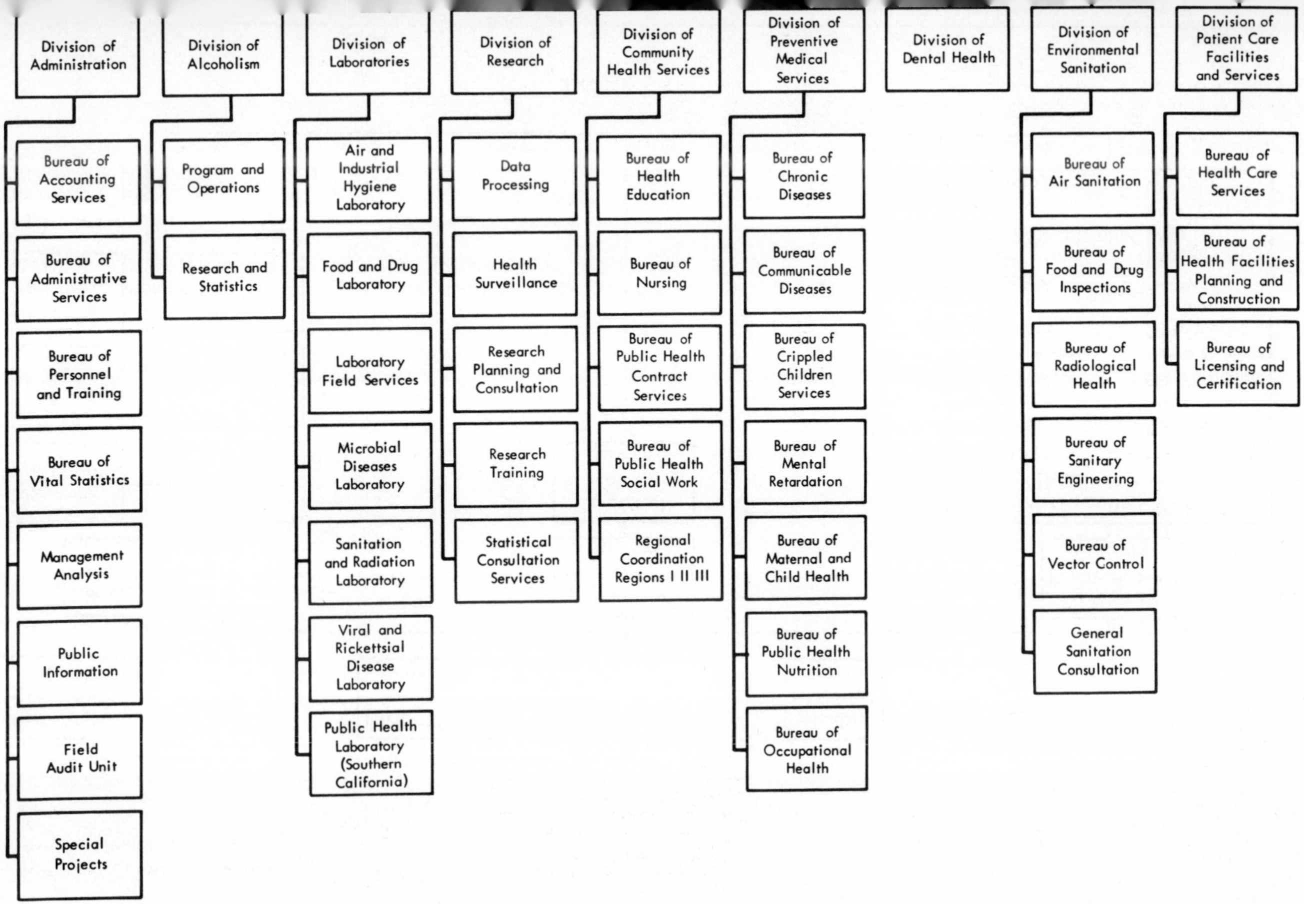

Division of Administration
- Bureau of Accounting Services
- Bureau of Administrative Services
- Bureau of Personnel and Training
- Bureau of Vital Statistics
- Management Analysis
- Public Information
- Field Audit Unit
- Special Projects

Division of Alcoholism
- Program and Operations
- Research and Statistics

Division of Laboratories
- Air and Industrial Hygiene Laboratory
- Food and Drug Laboratory
- Laboratory Field Services
- Microbial Diseases Laboratory
- Sanitation and Radiation Laboratory
- Viral and Rickettsial Disease Laboratory
- Public Health Laboratory (Southern California)

Division of Research
- Data Processing
- Health Surveillance
- Research Planning and Consultation
- Research Training
- Statistical Consultation Services

Division of Community Health Services
- Bureau of Health Education
- Bureau of Nursing
- Bureau of Public Health Contract Services
- Bureau of Public Health Social Work
- Regional Coordination Regions I II III

Division of Preventive Medical Services
- Bureau of Chronic Diseases
- Bureau of Communicable Diseases
- Bureau of Crippled Children Services
- Bureau of Mental Retardation
- Bureau of Maternal and Child Health
- Bureau of Public Health Nutrition
- Bureau of Occupational Health

Division of Dental Health

Division of Environmental Sanitation
- Bureau of Air Sanitation
- Bureau of Food and Drug Inspections
- Bureau of Radiological Health
- Bureau of Sanitary Engineering
- Bureau of Vector Control
- General Sanitation Consultation

Division of Patient Care Facilities and Services
- Bureau of Health Care Services
- Bureau of Health Facilities Planning and Construction
- Bureau of Licensing and Certification

FIGURE 2-4.

65

Organization of
Los Angeles County Health Department

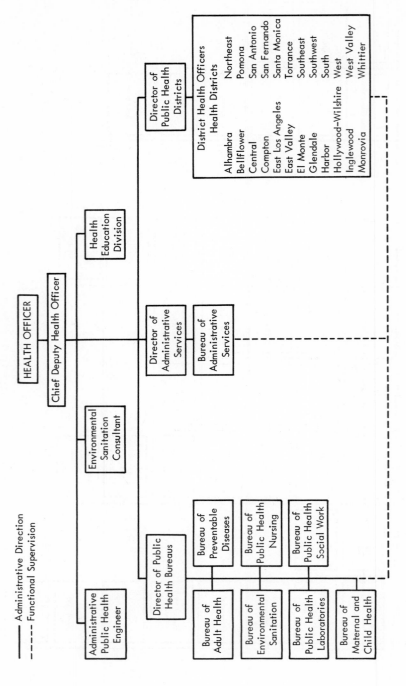

FIGURE 2-5.

History of Voluntary Health Agencies

There was scarcely a local voluntary health agency at the turn of the century with the exception of the American Red Cross and a few tuberculosis societies. Late in the nineteenth and early in the twentieth centuries, a combination of several factors initiated a marked and persistent growth of voluntary health agencies.[7] First, new knowledge about, and attitudes toward, physical health emerged as a result of scientific advances of the nineteenth century; second, rapid economic expansion through industrialization provided more financial resources and free time for activities other than mere daily subsistence; and third, government-sponsored health programs were still sporadic, rudimentary, and struggling to emerge as organized public efforts. These scientific, economic, and political realities found a favorable climate in emerging humanitarian impulses to alleviate suffering and privation and in the prevailing American tradition of freedom of enterprise and aggressive individual (rather than governmental) action to solve problems. The result was a gradual acceleration in the number and kinds of organized voluntary health agencies, culminating in particularly rapid growth since 1940.[6]

The voluntary health movement began in the United States with the founding of the Anti-tuberculosis Society of Philadelphia in 1892, followed by the formation of the National Association for the Study and Prevention of Tuberculosis in 1904. This organization is now known as the National Tuberculosis Association and has 50 state associations and some 3000 local affiliates. Other problem areas were recognized, stimulating local, and later national, organizations. In New York City, the concern with venereal diseases and prostitution led to the development in 1914 of the American Social Hygiene Association. There was developing interest in mental hygiene, and by 1910 concern arose over excessive illness and deaths of infants and mothers. During the next decade, national movements were initiated for cancer control, for prevention of blindness, for maternal hygiene, for the hard of hearing, and for public health nursing. Subsequently, national organizations were formed which were concerned with child health, crippled children, infantile paralysis, diabetes, and heart disease.

Among the vast number of voluntary health agencies in the United States, the American Red Cross has a particularly unique history and position, especially since it is the only one which has quasiofficial status. It originated during the Civil War through the efforts of Clara Barton, who aroused national and international attention to the need for organized medical care for soldiers on the battlefields. Her activities led to the recognition of the International Red Cross in 1882 and to the granting of a charter to the American Red Cross by the United States Congress in 1900. The President of the United States serves as the president of the organization, and it has diverse peace and wartime functions, including service as the official disaster relief agency of the nation.

Principal Categories and Activities of Voluntary Health Agencies

Some understanding of the range of the programs and activities of voluntary health organizations may be gleaned by classifying them according to major types, although it should be kept in mind that such classification is unavoidably somewhat arbitrary.

The first and most important group which may be singled out consists of the voluntary health agencies which are essentially categorical and are supported by financial contributions and donations. Gunn and Platt [7] have subdivided this group into three classes: (1) those concerned with *specific diseases* such as tuberculosis, venereal diseases, cancer, poliomyelitis, and diabetes (e.g., the National Tuberculosis Association, the American Social Health Association, the American Cancer Society, the American Diabetes Association); (2) those concerned with *special organs and structures of the body* such as diseases of the heart, loss of vision or hearing, and dental, locomotor, or skeletal defects (e.g., the American Heart Association, the National Society for the Prevention of Blindness, the National Society for Crippled Children and Adults); and (3) those concerned with *the health and welfare of special groups or of society as a whole,* including maternal and child hygiene, planned parenthood, mental hygiene, and environmental hazards (e.g., the Maternity Center Association, the Planned Parenthood Federation of America, the National Association for Mental Health, the National Safety Council). Direct service to the public is provided by a few of the categorical voluntary health agencies but is not the major objective of most. Rather, the principal activity is usually the conduct of public and professional educational programs to improve the utilization of health services and to raise the quality of personnel and facilities. Other activities may include assessment of community health needs; support of demonstration and experimental projects as pioneering ventures into new health fields; encouragement of research; cooperation with other agencies, both voluntary and official, in the planning and coordination of health activities; provision of advisory services to official health agencies; and support of beneficial health legislation.

Besides the major group of categorical voluntary health organizations just described, several other kinds have been categorized by Hanlon,[1] including foundations, professional associations, integrating or coordinating agencies, and certain kinds of private, proprietary and nonprofit institutions and organizations.

Foundations undertake a variety of activities including the promotion and subsidy of local health programs (particularly in rural areas), basic research, and public and professional education. Among the more prominent organizations are the Rockefeller Foundation, the Ford Foundation, the W. K. Kellogg Foundation, the Commonwealth Fund, the Milbank Memorial Fund, the Markle Foundation, and many others.

Professional associations, usually organized on a national basis with state and local affiliates, provide an arena for the exchange of information and ideas among members of the various health professions, promote improved standards and programs, and encourage basic and applied research. The American Public Health Association, the American Medical Association, the American Dental Association, and the American Hospital Association are a few of the countless organizations in this category.

Integrating or coordinating agencies, organized on national, state, and local levels, are concerned with community and areawide planning to reduce overlapping interests and objectives of the many specialized voluntary agencies. Examples of such organizations are health councils, community chests, and community councils. The most prominent organization in this category is the National Health Council, which has the mission of coordinating the activities of all the separate and specialized nongovernmental groups which are in the health field nationally.

Private proprietary and nonprofit institutions and organizations of certain kinds constitute a final category of voluntary health agencies and include voluntary health insurance organizations (e.g., Blue Cross and Blue Shield), private hospitals, nursing homes, privately sponsored clinics, and others whose objectives are primarily to contribute to improved health services.

Organization and Financing of Voluntary Health Agencies

The typical national voluntary health agency has a board of directors frequently composed of prominent persons from industry, business, the arts, professions, and politics. The size of some boards prevents frequent meetings, and much of the day-to-day work is performed by a paid professional staff subject to review by an executive committee. Many of the state and larger metropolitan organizations operate in the same manner.

Principal responsibilities at the national level include development of general policies; creation of a public image; exercise of leadership, coordination, and guidance; and promotion of research and public interest in the specific area of concern. The state level provides broad leadership, stimulation, and guidance to the local affiliates, exerting some influence on program planning and administration, budgets, and fund raising. The local health associations raise money, develop program plans, and determine priorities for activities. Generally, the local organizations are more attuned to immediate community needs, and the state and national levels are more concerned with long-range planning.

The large group of voluntary health agencies which depends on financial contributions and donations obtains such support mainly from individual citizens and to a lesser extent from corporations.[6] Some agencies have other sources of income as well, including payments by clients for services, membership dues, and investment earnings.[6] Contributions and donations are obtained through fund-raising campaigns conducted by local committees as part of a national drive at some designated time of the year. Portions of the funds thus collected on the local level are channeled to the next higher echelons; the actual proportional distribution between local, state, and national levels varies with the organization concerned. The proliferation in recent years of the number of voluntary agencies and hence of the number of individual fund-raising campaigns has led to the formation of community chests and united funds. These are federations of agencies that undertake a single drive or appeal for funds and subsequently distribute the proceeds among the participating organizations. The result in numerous communities has been a considerable lessening of the number of different requests for contributions that are made upon the public in a given year.

Problems and Trends in the Voluntary Agency Movement

Voluntary agencies—health and welfare alike, and particularly the large group of categorical health organizations—have been experiencing an increasing number of problems during the past decade or so. Some problems are internal and not unlike those experienced by official health and welfare agencies; for example, issues involving the nature and goals of programs, efficiency of administrative organization and management, shortages of trained personnel, etc. A second group of problems is essentially intra-agency and includes the existence of overlap and duplications in programs which still persist in spite of efforts to coordinate activities. A third category of problems pertains to financial matters, and although these might appear to be largely internal concerns, they assume an added dimension because the public, as the source of funds, is involved. In addition to being the object of criticism for generating a multiplicity of fund-raising campaigns, voluntary agencies have been under scrutiny in connection with the expenditure of funds obtained through public contributions. An analysis [6] of 56 national voluntary agencies with a primary interest in health revealed that 52.3 per cent of agency expenditures went for organizational expenses and fund raising, public and professional information, and other expenditures such as cost of goods sold, capital expenditures, and special projects; the remaining 47.7 per cent went for services to patients, professionals, and the public and for professional training and research.

Added to this considerable array of problems is the trend toward increasing governmental participation in health and welfare programs, as described earlier in this chapter. Increased taxes to finance this participation may make inroads on public resources which in the past have supported voluntary agencies. In fact, the rate of increase of support for many agencies is already at or below the rate of population increase. At present, there is pressure for regional and areawide coordinated planning for the advancement of health and welfare services through the most efficient use of total available funds from all sources, whether local, state, or national taxes, or the financial resources of voluntary agencies.

The pressures and forces being exerted on voluntary agencies are leading to re-evaluation of programs and are resulting in shifts in emphasis and broadening of activities. Changes may be expected to continue to take place for many years to come, particularly if voluntary agencies are to maintain a role in the organized health-and-welfare effort.

EXPENDITURES FOR HEALTH IN THE UNITED STATES

Preceding sections of this chapter have described organized health efforts in the United States—through official agencies on the federal, state, and local levels and through voluntary agencies. In addition, reference has been made to the fact that both kinds of agencies are supported by revenues (from taxes, contributions, etc.) which amount to considerable sums of money. Does the *expenditure* of these funds constitute a major element in the nation's *total* expenditures for health purposes, or are there other sources which are of greater magnitude? For what specific health purposes are expenditures made? How much, in fact, have total expenditures amounted to over the years? Information which illuminates these questions is provided in Tables 2-1, 2-2, and 2-3.

In 1964, a total of $36.8 billion was expended for health purposes, the funds coming from several sources in varying magnitudes, as shown in Table 2-1. Almost three fourths of the total, or $27.2 billion, came from *pri-*

TABLE 2-1 National Health Expenditures by Source of Funds, 1964

Source of Funds	Amount (in Millions)
Private: Total	$27,232
Consumers	24,842
Philanthropy	1,421
Other	969
Public: Total	9,531
Federal	4,756
State and local	4,775
Total	$36,763

Source: Adapted from Social Security Administration, U.S. Department of Health, Education, and Welfare. National Health Expenditures, 1950–64. *Social Security Bulletin,* **29:**3–19, January 1966, Table 1.

vate funds, most of this amount being spent by consumers, i.e., the American public. The remaining $9.5 billion expended were *public funds,* which came from federal and state-local sources in almost equal proportions. Thus, in contrast to governmental, philanthropic, and other sources, *consumers* directly were, and still are, by far the major spenders of funds for health purposes.

Regarding the specific purposes for which funds are spent, 91 per cent ($33.4 billion) of all national health expenditures in 1964 was for currently consumed *health services and supplies* such as hospital care and physicians' and dentists' services (Table 2-2). The remaining $3.3 billion was spent

TABLE 2-2   National Health Expenditures by Object of Expenditure, 1964

Object of Expenditure	Amount (in Millions)
Health services and supplies: Total	$33,431
Hospital care	12,713
Physicians' services	7,293
Dentists' services	2,368
Other professional services	903
Drugs and drug sundries	4,463
Eyeglasses and appliances	1,082
Nursing-home care	1,214
Net cost of insurance	1,151
Medical activities in federal units other than hospitals	707
Government public health activities	804
Private voluntary health agencies	275
School health services	133
Industrial in-plant health services	325
Research and medical-facilities construction: Total	3,332
Research	1,329
Medical-facilities construction	2,003
Total	$36,763

Source: Adapted from Social Security Administration, U.S. Department of Health, Education, and Welfare. National Health Expenditures, 1950–64. *Social Security Bulletin,* 29:3–19, January 1966, Table 1.

for *medical research* and the *construction of hospitals and related facilities.* Of the expenditures for health services and supplies, 77 per cent came from private funds, again mostly consumers; but of expenditures for medical research, 88 per cent derived from public funds, primarily federal sources.

Trends in national expenditures for health purposes are shown in Table 2-3. The estimates presented reveal substantial increases since 1950, from $12.9 billion in that year to $36.8 billion spent in 1964, as mentioned previously. In the same period of time, per capita expenditures for all health purposes increased from $84.49 to $191.32, or by 126 per cent. Even when these estimates are adjusted to take into account the increase in living costs, the per capita expenditures have increased 75 per cent in the period from 1950 to 1964. This would indicate a true increment in the utilization of health facilities and services, and it also reflects advances in technology and changes in the content of services.[8]

TABLE 2-3   Total and per Capita National Health Expenditures, Selected Years, 1950–1964

	Total (in Millions)	Per Capita *	
		Actual	Adjusted †
1950	$12,867	$ 84.49	$109.02
1955	18,036	108.67	125.93
1960	26,892	148.81	155.99
1961	28,811	156.76	162.62
1962	31,263	167.46	171.76
1963	33,703	177.90	180.24
1964	36,763	191.32	191.32

Source: Adapted from Social Security Administration, U.S. Department of Health, Education, and Welfare. National Health Expenditures, 1950–64. *Social Security Bulletin*, 29:3–19, January 1966, Table 5 and Table 6.
* Based on total population, including Armed Forces and federal civilian employees abroad, as of July 1.
† Adjusted to 1964 price levels in order to take into account changes in purchasing power of the dollar as shown by the Bureau of Labor Statistics consumer price index for all items.

INTERNATIONAL HEALTH AGENCIES

The Need for International Health Work

By now, every country in the world has some kind of health program even if minimal or rudimentary. However, local-national health activities frequently are not sufficient to bring twentieth-century scientific technology to bear on health problems, and as a consequence a good deal of impetus has been given to the protection of health everywhere by international health work, which in a sense transcends local boundaries. A considerable number of international health activities are sponsored by the technically more advanced and economically more advantaged nations, either on a direct country-to-country basis or through participation in organizations that have developed an administrative apparatus for conducting health programs on a broad scale.

Organized international health work is of particular importance in the developing countries of the world where the greatest lag occurs in the application of medical and health technology. Higher death rates and shortened life expectancy are among the consequences of this lag, as illustrated in Table 2-4. Thus, it will be observed that in contrast to more developed countries, the African nations in particular have a higher rate of deaths per 1000 population and a lower average number of years of life expectancy at birth. Table 2-4 also illustrates the variations in death rates and life expectancy that can occur even within a continent (e.g., North America, South America, and Asia).

TABLE 2-4   Death Rate and Life Expectancy, Selected Countries

	Crude Death Rate *		Life Expectancy †		
	Year	Rate	Date	Male	Female
North America					
United States	1965	9.4	1964	66.9	73.7
Canada	1965	7.5	1960–62	68.3	74.1
Mexico	1965	9.5	1956	55.1	57.9
South America					
Argentina	1964	8.3	1959–61	63.1	68.8
Peru	1959–61	‾ .–15 ‡	1961	. . . 50	. . .
Europe					
Sweden	1965	10.1	1962	71.3	75.3
England an .,ales	1965	11.5	1961–63	67.9	73.9
Asia					
China (Taiwan)	1965	5.5	1959–60	61.3	65.6
Japan	1965	7.1	1964	67.6	72.8
India	1963–64	12.9 ‡	1951–60	41.8	40.5
Cambodia	1959	19.7 ‡	1958–59	44.2	43.3
Africa					
Southern Rhodesia	1961	14.0 ‡	1961	. . . 50	. . .
Morocco	1962	18.7 ‡	1960	. . . 49.6	. . . ‡
Kenya	1962	20 ‡	1962	. . . 40–45	. . . ‡
Central African Republic	1959–60	30 ‡	1959–60	33	36

Source: Adapted from United Nations. *Demographic Yearbook, 1965,* Table 3.
* Number of deaths per 1000 population.
† Average number of years of expectation of life at birth, for years given.
‡ Data are estimates or are from civil registers which are incomplete or of unknown reliability.

In spite of inequities in longevity and general health status, the world as a whole is experiencing a phenomenal increase in population, and this fact has become a major concern in international health work. In many countries, including some developing nations, the control of infectious diseases has reduced the death rate, but the birth rate has not declined proportionally or has even remained stationary. The resulting large net gain in population has produced serious problems in meeting the needs for food, clothing, shelter, and many other necessities of life, and the economic strain is particularly great on nations which already have limited resources. A major effort in international health work is directed toward the application of scientific knowledge to control population increase and to find means for sharing world resources.

History of International Health Organization

The devastating and recurring epidemics which began many centuries ago, as described in Chapter 1, may be considered as marking the advent of international health problems, since the diseases frequently spread from one country to another. However, prior to the mid-nineteenth century, protection and control activities were primarily on a national rather than an international scale. The beginning of serious efforts at organized international health activity occurred between 1851 and 1909 when a series of meetings known as International Sanitary Conferences [9] took place in various parts of the world. The principal topics for these meetings were the control of epidemics through quarantine and the exploration of the origin of infections.[10] The first conference, held in Paris with representation of 12 nations, developed a treaty to limit the spread of epidemic disease through the regulation of international commerce, but it was never ratified by the participating nations. The subsequent conferences had similar limited practical results except for one significant accomplishment, which was the creation of the first permanent, worldwide organization dealing with international health.[9, 10] This body was known as the International Office of Public Health (l'Office International d'Hygiène Publique) and came into being in Paris in 1909.

The *International Office of Public Health*, popularly known as the "Paris Office," had a small full-time staff and responsibilities which were concerned mainly with quarantinable diseases: to gather information, revise international regulations, and arbitrate differences.[10] Over a period of time, the Paris Office broadened the range of international regulations, including, for example, obtaining agreement by 14 countries on measures to control the spread of venereal diseases along the shipping routes.[10] It also began the standardization of serums and the control of drug traffic and created several committees to study a wide range of public health problems.[10]

Aside from establishment of the Paris Office, the creation of two other international health organizations constituted notable accomplishments of the early twentieth century. These were the Pan-American Sanitary Bureau, created in Washington, D.C., in 1902, and the Health Section of the League of Nations, established in Geneva in 1923.

The *Pan-American Sanitary Bureau*, in contrast to the Paris Office, was more limited in scope geographically since its activities were confined to the Western hemisphere, but the history and development of the two organizations were similar. The Bureau was organized by a Pan-American Sanitary Conference as an agency of the 21 American republics, and its original purpose was merely to serve as an information center for keeping the participating nations informed about outbreaks of epidemic diseases.[9] Subsequently, the Bureau's activities expanded considerably and included the stimulation of all American countries to make greater efforts for the prevention, control, and eradication of disease;[9] the development of a vigorous program in epidemiology; the training of professional personnel; and the encouragement and support of research.

The *Health Section of the League of Nations*, known popularly as the "Geneva Office," functioned alongside the Paris Office until World War

II.[10] Its mandate under the Covenant of the League of Nations was to undertake international activity in the prevention and control of disease. The Geneva Office established a system of epidemic intelligence with a center in Singapore; carried on the work of international standardization and control of drug traffic begun by the Paris Office; established "expert committees" which considered a wide range of subjects including malaria, cancer, housing, and the teaching of medicine; sponsored international conferences which produced well-documented statements about health needs in developing countries; and provided medical services in the field, although these were limited because of meager financial resources.[10]

Principal Contemporary International Health Agencies

Prior to the establishment of the Health Section of the League of Nations, efforts to develop international cooperation in health matters were directed mainly toward finding an international sanitary code strict enough to prevent transmission of disease from one nation to another, but not so strict that it interfered with commerce. It was not until the mid-twentieth century that significant change occurred in prevailing ideas about the true concerns of international health, the translation of these ideas into programs, and the provision of means to make the programs effective and far-reaching. The turning point was reached in 1948 when the World Health Organization was created as a specialized agency of the United Nations.

The World Health Organization. The stage was set for the establishment of the World Health Organization as an agent for more effective international health work, first, by the scientific and technical developments which had occurred between the end of World War I and the end of World War II; and, second, by the determination of governments and peoples following World War II to rebuild world peace, the means for which, it was felt, would be provided by scientific knowledge.[11]

During the United Nations Conference on International Organization held in San Francisco in 1945, the presentation of a memorandum by the Brazilian delegation led to the inclusion of health as a problem to be considered by the United Nations. As plans for the establishment of a formal international health organization proceeded through a series of conferences and committees, the conception of health became broadened, and the health of all peoples was seen as fundamental to the attainment of peace and security.[11] This philosophy was amplified in the constitution of the World Health Organization, which states that "health is a state of complete physical, mental and social well being, and not merely the absence of disease or infirmity"; that "enjoyment of the highest attainable standard of health is one of the fundamental rights of every human being without distinction of race, religion, political belief, economic or social condition"; and that "achievement of any state in the promotion and protection of health is of value to all."

The WHO has over 120 member countries which contribute to its budget; a nation may be a member of WHO without being a member of the United Nations. It provides epidemic and statistical service; develops international quarantine measures; promotes the international standardization of drugs, vaccines, and other biologics; stimulates health research; and prepares and distributes many publications. Technical and program-planning assistance is available for participating nations and includes: (1) strengthening individual national health services; (2) training health workers and developing training programs; (3) aiding the attack on major diseases such as malaria, tuberculosis, venereal diseases, and parasitic and virus diseases, especially those which can be controlled environmentally; (4) protecting maternal and child health; (5) improving sanitation and water supplies; (6) promoting mental health; (7) improving nutrition in cooperation with other international agencies; and (8) providing general administrative and technical program assistance. The WHO also is concerned with health education of public and professional groups, exchange of information on dental health, and collaboration with the International Labor Organization to improve occupational health.

The International Office of Public Health (Paris Office) became part of the WHO shortly after the latter was established. The Pan-American Sanitary Bureau (now renamed the Pan-American Health Organization) became a regional office of the WHO in 1949, although it still maintains its own organizational identity. The WHO has an executive board composed of 24 health experts who are designated by, but do not represent, their governments. Proposals and issues are presented to the annual World Health Assembly composed of delegations from all member countries. An administrative and technical staff of approximately 2600 people from more than 70 countries is stationed at the Geneva headquarters, in the regional offices, and with operational field projects in every continent. There are six WHO regional offices, as follows:

African Region: headquarters at Brazzaville—25 member nations and three associate members representing a population of over 153 million;

Region of the Americas: headquarters at Washington, D.C., at the Pan-American Health Organization—24 member nations with a population of 405 million;

Southeast Asia Region: headquarters at New Delhi—eight member nations representing a population of 617 million;

European Region: headquarters at Copenhagen—32 member nations representing 678 million people;

Eastern Mediterranean Region: headquarters at Alexandria—17 member nations and a population of 207 million;

Western Pacific Region: headquarters at Manila—11 member nations representing a population of 198 million.

Other Sponsors of International Health Programs. The United Nations Children's Fund, known as UNICEF at the time it was established, was organized originally as a temporary, emergency agency to assist children in war-torn countries. It later expanded its program to provide food and supplies for child and maternal welfare throughout the world and particularly in developing countries. It has also been concerned with programs of vaccination and the control of yaws, syphilis, and malaria. In 1953, the Fund was granted permanent status by the United Nations.

The Agency for International Development emerged in 1961—after a series of reorganizations and name changes since the end of World War II—as the international assistance program of the United States. Organizationally, it is within the State Department, but it is semi-independent inasmuch as its funds are appropriated separately. The Agency provides military, economic, and technical assistance to other nations. A significant part of the technical assistance provided involves public health matters through direct services, consultation, and fellowships for training in the United States and in other countries.

There are many nongovernmental agencies which have also made major contributions to international health work. These include foundations such as the Rockefeller Foundation, the Kellogg Foundation, and the Ford Foundation; and numerous religious organizations. These international voluntary organizations have provided direct service to population groups throughout the world, contributed to the control of infectious diseases, and supported the training of health workers.

SUMMARY

Organization for health is concerned with the search for, and implementation of, plans which will enhance optimal health and increase longevity. The nature of the organization is influenced by the philosophy, expectations, and objectives of the population groups involved in the planning.

The role of *official health agencies* in the United States is determined by the United States Constitution and by the constitutions of the various states which have certain sovereign powers. On these bases, the federal government and the individual state governments enact specific health legislation; local governments (i.e., county, municipal, etc.) adopt ordinances on the basis of authority delegated by the state. Guided by socially and politically conscious motives, the federal government increasingly has assumed leadership for health programs of benefit to the individual as well as to the national and local populations through legislative enactments designed to stimulate and support regional and local planning, services, and research.

The United States government carries forward a wide variety of health programs directed toward the general population, special population groups, and international cooperative efforts. The principal health agency of the federal government is the Public Health Service, which is one of eight operating agencies within the U.S. Department of Health, Education, and Welfare.

State and local activities are conducted through their respective health departments. Generally, the state level is concerned with policy, planning, legislation, consultation, indirect services, financial support, organizational relationships, and research; the local level is concerned with direct health services such as medical care, preventive services, and environmental control. Although the functions differ according to the level of the agency, a state or local health department typically has several general kinds of programs, including preventive medical and personal health care services, environmental health services, patient care facilities and services, and various supportive services.

Voluntary health agencies, which were almost nonexistent in the United States at the turn of the century, have increased markedly in recent years. Several kinds of voluntary health agencies are distinguishable, the major group consisting of those which are essentially categorical and supported by financial contributions and donations. An agency may be organized on a local, state, or national basis; it usually has a board of directors and may have a paid professional staff. Currently, voluntary agencies are striving to solve several basic problems with which they are beset, including the nature and goals of programs, overlap and duplication of effort, and various financial dilemmas.

Even though official and voluntary health agencies both make large financial expenditures for health, the largest spender of all is the United States consumer. The vast bulk of all national health expenditures goes for currently consumed health services and supplies, and trends over the past several years reveal a true increment in the utilization of health facilities and services.

International health agencies conduct programs which transcend local boundaries and have a primary mission of bringing modern scientific technology to bear on health problems everywhere, but particularly in countries where the greatest lag occurs in health matters. International health agencies are confronted by complex and paradoxical problems such as, on the one hand, excessively high disease and mortality rates in some countries and, on the other, the threat of severe overpopulation in the world as a whole. Early international health efforts consisted largely of attempts by a particular nation to protect itself from the transmission of disease from other nations, and this approach did not undergo significant change until the World Health Organization was created in the mid-twentieth century. The WHO, as the principal agency engaged in international health work, has comprehensive and many-faceted programs and carries on its activities through a vast worldwide network of member countries and field installations.

REFERENCES

1. HANLON, JOHN J. *Principles of Public Health Administration,* 4th ed. The C. V. Mosby Company, St. Louis, 1964.

2. U.S. DEPARTMENT OF HEALTH, EDUCATION, AND WELFARE. *Annual Report, 1965.* U.S. Government Printing Office, Washington, D.C.

3. OFFICE OF THE FEDERAL REGISTER, National Archives and Records Service, General Services Administration. *United States Government Organization Manual, 1965–66.* U.S. Government Printing Office, Washington, D.C.

4. U.S. DEPARTMENT OF HEALTH, EDUCATION, AND WELFARE. *Handbook on Programs of the U.S. Department of Health, Education, and Welfare,* 1964–

65 ed.: Part I and Part II. U.S. Government Printing Office, Washington, D.C.

5. PUBLIC HEALTH SERVICE, U.S. Department of Health, Education, and Welfare. *The Public Health Service: Background Material Concerning the Mission and Organization of the Public Health Service.* Prepared for the Interstate and Foreign Commerce Committee, United States House of Representatives. U.S. Government Printing Office, Washington, D.C., 1963.

6. HAMLIN, ROBERT H. *Voluntary Health and Welfare Agencies in the United States.* The Schoolmasters' Press, New York, 1961.

7. GUNN, SELSKAR M., and PLATT, PHILIP S. *Voluntary Health Agencies.* The Ronald Press Company, New York, 1945.

8. SOCIAL SECURITY ADMINISTRATION, U.S. Department of Health, Education, and Welfare. National health expenditures, 1950–64. *Social Security Bull,* 29:3–19, January 1966.

9. GOODMAN, NEVILLE M. *International Health Organizations and Their Work.* J. & A. Churchill Ltd., London, 1952.

10. BROCKINGTON, FRASER. *World Health.* The Whitefriars Press, Ltd., London and Tonbridge, 1958.

11. WORLD HEALTH ORGANIZATION. *The First Ten Years of the World Health Organization.* The Organization, Geneva, 1958.

THE TOOLS
OF PUBLIC HEALTH

CHAPTER 3

DEMOGRAPHIC DATA AND VITAL STATISTICS

The components of demographic data and vital statistics
Census or enumeration information
Vital registration data

Morbidity statistics
Uses of demographic data and vital statistics in public health
Summary

This chapter describes what demographic data are, where they originate, and how they are combined to produce statistical measures such as distributions, averages, rates, and ratios. These measures are used in public health for a variety of purposes, including program planning, research, and general surveillance of the health status of the population.

The first section of the chapter defines demographic data and vital statistics. The next two sections provide more detailed discussion of the sources of, and the statistics derived from, the two main components of demographic data, namely, population size and characteristics, and vital events. The fourth section describes the common measures that are made of the amount of illness, or morbidity, in a population. The utilization of the various kinds of data and statistics in public health activities at the local, state, and national level is described in the final section of the chapter.

THE COMPONENTS OF DEMOGRAPHIC DATA AND VITAL STATISTICS

All human populations experience the fundamental or "vital" events of birth, death, marriage, divorce. Over time these events, together with migration, determine the size and composition of a population, whether its numbers grow, decline, or stay about the same; whether its peculiar combination of fertility and mortality results in a young or an old population.

Demographic data consist of the numbers which describe the size of a population and its vital events. Information on population size is derived from census enumeration of the number and characteristics of persons living in a specified area at a particular time. Information on vital events is obtained from official registration records of births, deaths, marriages, and divorces. *Vital statistics* relate the total numbers of various kinds of vital events which occur over a period of time (usually one calendar year) to the size of the affected population.

The number of occurrences of a vital event has little meaning unless it is related either to the total population within which the event occurs or to that segment of the population which is subject to the risk of the event. For example, only females age 15 to 49 rather than those of all ages are usually considered to be at risk for the occurrence of pregnancy. Because vital events, to be meaningful, must be related to population size, people within the relevant geographic area must be counted, and each individual's age, sex, and other characteristics enumerated. The resulting information describes the composition of the population, and the evaluation of vital statistics must be made in light of this composition; a population's death rates, for example, are influenced by age distribution, sex ratio, racial components, etc.

Although the main sources of demographic information * are the records of vital registration and enumeration of the census, many agencies, institutions, and individuals also conduct sample surveys in order to obtain demographic data. In addition, special health surveys of particular diseases such as coronary heart disease are sometimes used to supplement knowledge in specific areas. These surveys are needed when more detailed information is required from individuals and when that information is not collected in the desired detail from large aggregates of individuals. The public health worker is likely to use sampling techniques in a study to gain health information which he may then relate to census and vital registration data.

CENSUS OR ENUMERATION INFORMATION

The Decennial Census

The Constitution of the United States provides that a regular census be taken of the country's inhabitants. The first count was made in 1790. Though the U.S. Census is not the oldest, it has the longest continuous record of any census in history. Originally the count was made to determine the number of representatives each state was entitled to send to the House of Representatives. As time went by, the usefulness of census information to government, business, welfare workers, and numerous other individuals, groups, and agencies became obvious. The volume and variety of informa-

* There are other sources, which are demographically interesting, but are not directly relevant to public health problems; for example, information from the Immigration and Naturalization Service.

tion collected have grown tremendously, and the requests for additional data remain unabated.

Kinds of Information Obtained and Methods Used. Every ten years the Bureau of the Census (U.S. Department of Commerce) takes on the herculean task of counting every man, woman, and child in the United States. The age, sex, race, and marital status of each individual are recorded, and data are obtained about the number and make-up of households. Additional information, such as condition of housing, income, education, occupation, distance traveled to and from work, and length of stay in present residence, is acquired from representative samples of the population. In the 1960 Census, a 25 per cent sample of households was asked these additional questions. Data obtained by the sampling procedures employed by the Census may be used with confidence. Undoubtedly sampling will be used more and more in future Census counts. Among other advantages, it enables the Bureau to obtain more information per given cost than could be obtained with complete enumeration. To obtain useful information within small geographic areas, however, complete enumeration is necessary. This is one of the reasons for retaining a complete count of some items in the Census.

In the past, an enumerator visited every household to ask for information, which he recorded on the standard Census schedule (questionnaire form) of population and housing. In 1960, an "Advance Census Report," mailed to all homes, asked for information about the dwelling and the individuals who lived there. This was to be completed and made ready for the enumerator who transferred the information to the Census schedule. The 1970 Census may rely even more on a mailed questionnaire, sending enumerators only when a household head fails to return his questionnaire within a prescribed time period or returns it incomplete.

Much preliminary planning is essential if an individual from every household is to be interviewed within a period of a few weeks. This involves choosing the questions to be asked and checking the legal authority for asking them. Needs of government have top priority, but the needs of businessmen, labor leaders, and research workers in all fields using census data are considered. Attention is given to recommendations of the United Nations, which tries to encourage greater comparability among the population statistics of all nations. Furthermore, the questions to be asked must be pretested and geographic areas must be defined; instructions must be prepared for the enumerators, crew leaders, and district supervisors. For the 1960 Census, about 170,000 field workers were hired as temporary employees of the Bureau of the Census.

Geographic Units for Data Collection. For purposes of collecting information on population and housing, the United States is divided into enumeration districts. These districts are carefully mapped by the Census

Bureau, often after consultation with local authorities. Care is taken that these small, well-defined areas are delineated in such a way as to take account of the boundaries of various governmental units. Local governments rely heavily on census information for such needs as planning health, welfare, and education programs; planning construction and development projects (schools and hospitals, for example); and determining legislative representation. Some federal funds are allocated to states on a per-person basis; the estimated number of persons and thus the amount of money are based on census counts. When the information which has been collected by enumeration districts appears in published form, it is summarized in tables for various geographic and governmental units.

Geographic Units for Tabulating and Reporting. For purposes of tabulating and reporting Census information, the United States is divided into a series of progressively smaller units. The largest units consist of four *regions* and nine *divisions* within the regions, as follows:

A. Northeast
   1. New England
   2. Middle Atlantic
B. North Central
   3. West North Central
   4. East North Central
C. South
   5. East South Central
   6. South Atlantic
   7. West South Atlantic
D. West
   8. Mountain
   9. Pacific

Each *state* falls within one of the nine divisions. Information is published for regions, for divisions, and for each state. Within states, information is prepared for *counties* when appropriate. For some kinds of information, an *urban-nonurban* classification may be preferable. Information for the urban areas is available by *census tract* for all areas which have been tracted. Census tracts are small geographic units into which metropolitan areas are divided for purposes of reporting population characteristics, and these characteristics tend to be quite homogeneous within tracts. Requests have been made to the Census Bureau that future censuses obtain more detailed information for very small areas; this type of information has been very limited or completely lacking from past censuses. One of the problems in providing information for small areas, e.g., for a city block, is that of protecting individuals' rights to privacy. Areas must be kept large enough so that data can be made available in aggregates that will not betray information about particular individuals or households.

The Census must take account of changing patterns of population distribution and growth while preserving as much continuity and comparability as possible with earlier census data. One of the more obvious patterns of population change has been the movement of people in large numbers to the densely settled urban centers. An example of a parallel change made by the Census is its alteration of the definition of "urban." Before the 1950 Census, anyone living in an incorporated place of more than 2500 inhabitants was classified as living in an urban area. However, as movement to the cities progressed, many people lived in an "urban fringe" which was characteristically urban, but because it was not incorporated was classified by the Census as "rural." The 1950 Census changed this, and certain tables for 1950 and for 1960 Census data show one column labeled "previous urban definition" and another "current urban definition." The "previous urban definition" column is provided for purposes of comparability with earlier censuses; the "current urban definition" column takes into account the increment from including the population residing in urban-fringe areas and in unincorporated places of 2500 or more.[1] Figure 3-1 shows the differences that occur when the two definitions are applied to 1950 and 1960 population data; the figure also shows the general increases in the population of the United States and the shifts from rural to urban that have taken place since 1890.

The Nature of Census Data Reporting. Census information is readily available to everyone. Improvements in the speed of processing data have been made so that preliminary information obtained by a census is available within a few months after the enumeration is completed. Data that are compiled for each state are broken down by counties, by urban-rural areas, and by the large metropolitan areas. The census volume published for each state is divided into four sections:

1. Number of inhabitants,
2. General population characteristics,
3. General social and economic characteristics, and
4. Detailed characteristics.

More detailed information, which is not generally demanded by users, is available on computer tapes from the Census Bureau. These can be made available for research or other legitimate needs, always with the requirement that information about particular individuals must remain confidential.

Census data, like most demographic information, are collected and presented as aggregates of large numbers. To make them comprehensible and useful they must be expressed in statistical terms such as averages, frequency distributions (e.g., age distributions), percentages, or ratios. Some examples of the statistics which can be obtained from census enumeration are given in the remainder of this section. Only those which have some relevance to public health are included.

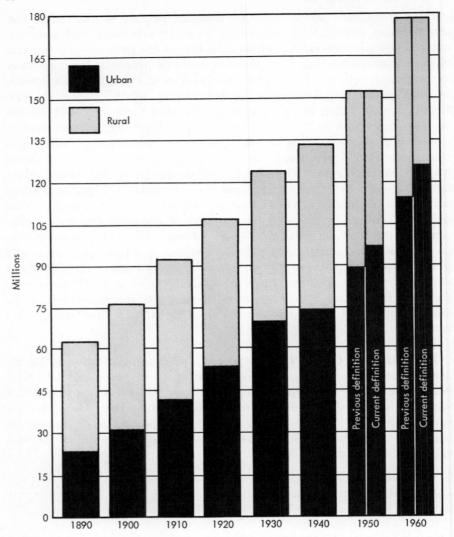

FIGURE 3-1. Population, urban and rural: 1890 to 1960. (Source: U.S. Bureau of the Census, *Statistical Abstract of the United States, 1965,* p. 4.)

Age Distribution

Within a large geographic area, the age distribution of a population will have its impact on almost everything, from television programs to voting patterns. For the United States as a whole, there are two significant aspects of the age distribution. First, the relative number of people in the older age groups has been increasing. This has been accompanied by greater emphasis on old-age social security, including, for example, the provision for medical needs under Medicare. Second, there are also increasingly large numbers of people under 20 years of age (about 69.0 million in 1960). This increase has followed the World War II "baby boom" and has been accompanied by the greatest demand on educational resources the country has ever known.

Table 3-1 provides an example of age distribution derived from census enumeration data; the table shows the relative proportions, or *percentages*, of persons in various age categories in the United States in 1960. Another way to assess age composition is by computing the *median*, which consists of the middle value of the age distribution; exactly half the cases lie on either side of the median. Median age of the total population increased steadily over the years through 1950, but by 1960 a very slight decrease had occurred for the first time since 1820, which is the earliest that appropriate data are available. Thus, for example, median age was 19.4 in 1860, 22.0 in 1890, 25.3 in 1920, and 30.2 in 1950—but 29.6 in 1960.[1] Such changes in age composition over periods of time are one of several indicators of changing needs of the population.

TABLE 3-1 Age Distribution of the Population of the United States, 1960

Age Interval	Percentage Distribution
Under 1 year	2.3
1–4	9.0
5–9	10.4
10–14	9.4
15–19	7.4
20–34	18.7
35–49	19.5
50–64	14.0
65–69	3.5
70–74	2.6
75 and over	3.1
All ages	100.0

Source: United Nations, *Demographic Yearbook,* 1961 (pp. 146–47).

The relative proportions of the young and the old within the population are of interest to public health because they influence the way health and welfare resources are employed and distributed for the country as a whole, for individual states, and for local areas. One would anticipate, for example, rather different public health needs in Alaska as compared to Massachusetts. For Alaska in 1960, the median age was 23 years and only 2.4 per cent of the population was 65 years of age and over.[2] In the same year the population of Massachusetts had a median age of 32.1 years and 11.2 per cent of its population was 65 years of age and over.[2] Similarly, a particular city may have some areas with a preponderance of elderly persons, other areas of housing developments with mostly young married couples and children, and still other areas made up largely of employed adults with few children. Planning for and meeting the needs of these various areas within the city will be influenced in part by the age distribution of people living there.

The age distribution of a population by sex and race is very useful from a health point of view, particularly when it is related to age distributions of disease incidence and causes of death. For example, the increasing control over causes of maternal death has altered the age distribution of females. Differences between the age distributions of males and females have changed with advances in all fields of medicine, permitting the apparent biologic superiority of the females to assert itself in a longer life expectancy at birth and lower death rates for females in all age groups, both white and nonwhite, in the United States.

Sex Ratio

The sex ratio is the number of males per 100 females. When the ratio is more than 100, there are more males than females; when it is less than 100, the reverse is true. At the time of the 1960 Census there were about 88,331,494 males in the United States and 90,991,681 females, giving a total average sex ratio of 97.1, thus:

$$\text{1960 sex ratio} = \frac{88,331,494}{90,991,681} \times 100 = 97.1 \text{ men per 100 women.}$$

The number of males per 100 females has declined steadily over the years. For example, in 1910 the sex ratio was 106.2, in 1930 it was 102.6, and in 1950 it was 98.7.[1] At present, the sex ratio is over 100 in the younger age groups because more male infants are born than female infants, but the ratio declines with age, giving further evidence of the higher death rates of males in all age categories.

Dependency Ratio

The dependency ratio is related to the age distribution. It indicates, as its name implies, the relative importance of the dependent age segments to the productively active age segments of a population. The dependency ratio takes account of three main age groups: dependent children, the active population, and the dependent aged. The size of the ratio will depend on the numbers in each group and how one chooses to define dependency. In the past, the dependency ratio has usually been defined as the number of persons under age 15, plus the number of persons 65 years and over, divided by the number of persons in the 15-through-64-year age group. The ratio, multiplied by the constant 100, estimates the number of dependent persons for every 100 in the active population, thus:

$$\text{Dep. ratio} = \frac{\text{No. of persons less than 15 years} + \text{no. of persons 65 and over}}{\text{No. of persons 15 through 64 years of age}} \times 100.$$

However, when children stay in school longer and many are dependent on parents until the completion of college, the age 15 years may be too low. Some suggest the dependent youth category should include all persons under 20 years. Such an increase in the size of the dependency category in the numerator of the ratio, with an equal decrease in its denominator, would produce an increase in the size of the dependency ratio.

The following example, using 1960 Census figures (in thousands), presents information about size of various age categories and the resulting dependency ratios:

The total number of persons under 15 years of age	55,786
The total number of persons under 20 years of age	69,005
The total number of persons 65 years and over	16,560
The total number of persons 15 through 64 years	106,977
The total number of persons 20 through 64 years	96,176

Dependency ratio (when dep. youth is 0–14 yrs.)
$$= \frac{55,786 + 16,560}{106,977} \times 100 = 68 \text{ "dependent" persons per 100 "active" persons.}$$

Dependency ratio (when dep. youth is 0–19 yrs.)
$$= \frac{69,005 + 16,560}{96,176} \times 100 = 89 \text{ "dependent" persons per 100 "active" persons.}$$

Child-Woman Ratio

The child-woman ratio is the ratio of children under five years of age to women in the childbearing ages 15 through 44 years (sometimes 15 through 49 years). This ratio gives some indication of the incidence of childbearing. Its greatest advantage is that it depends only on census data. For a country that does take a census but has a poor vital registration system or does not register vital events at all, the child-woman ratio gives a rough estimate of fertility. However, much better measures of childbearing incidence are obtained when the relevant vital registration data on births can be used with census estimates of population in the appropriate age categories.

At the time of the 1960 Census, the number of women 15 through 44 years of age was 36,079,000, and the number of children under five years of age was about 20,321,000. From these figures, the child-woman ratio is computed as follows:

Child-woman ratio (1960)
$$= \frac{20,321}{36,079} \times 100 = 56 \text{ children under 5 years of age per 100 women in the childbearing ages.}$$

Income, Education, and Employment

Income distribution, median income, educational attainment, and employment are population characteristics often referred to as socioeconomic variables. They may be classified by age, sex, race, location, or other characteristics, and are frequently considered in connection with indicators of health and well-being. There are relationships between health and socioeconomic status which have been observed for so long that some individuals tend to assign a "causal" relationship, even though the relationship may not persist indefinitely. For example, mortality differences based on income, education, and occupation are much smaller now than they once were and are declining with time.

From Census data, distributions of income by age, sex, race, educational attainment, and employment are available in numerous combinations. They are useful in planning health and other public programs, and have assumed great importance in the current attack on poverty.

VITAL REGISTRATION DATA

Historically, there were very early attempts (dating back to the pre-Christian era in Greece, Rome, and Egypt) to count the population, usually for military conscription or for taxing purposes. There are also examples, as far back as the Middle Ages, of records from which crude estimates of vital events can be made. These are the church registers, which recorded, not births, marriages, and deaths, but baptisms, weddings, and funerals and the gratuities which were received for performance of these sacraments. The problem of incompleteness in such records is obvious, as are the other disadvantages of recording ceremonies rather than vital events. The first civil registration in the Christian world occurred in the Massachusetts Bay and New Plymouth colonies in the first half of the seventeenth century.[3]

Registration of vital events means legally recording their occurrence in a permanent place. To meet today's requirements, registration of the vital events of birth, death, marriage, and divorce must be compulsory, and the individual responsible for registering each event must be clearly designated. Usually time limits are set within which the individual who is responsible must register the event. Unless these time limits are enforced, events may be forgotten and registration will be incomplete.

Past experience has demonstrated that vital registration is the most effective method of obtaining information about vital events. Attempts to get estimates of births and deaths from early United States censuses were grossly unsuccessful and were abandoned after 1900.

Registration Areas of the United States

Many years ago, the federal government undertook to establish a mechanism for collecting data from the states on the occurrence of births and deaths and to set standards for exactness, completeness, and promptness of reporting by the states. Toward this end, the national government passed model registration laws, and the states were urged to adopt them. Subsequently, as a state developed satisfactory birth and death registration laws and achieved 90 per cent completeness in reporting, it was admitted to membership in the "Registration Area for Births" and the "Registration Area for Deaths."

The death registration area was established in 1880, but the collection of mortality information did not begin until 1900 and then for only ten states, plus the District of Columbia and a number of cities located in nonregistration states. The birth registration area was established in 1915, and also included ten states and the District of Columbia; not all the states were the same as the ten contained in the death registration area. It was not until 1933 that all states in the Union had officially met the minimum requirements for membership in both the birth and the death registration areas.

Governmental Registration Functions

Registration of vital events in the United States has remained a function of the states and of local governmental units. Standard recommended certificates are provided by the National Center for Health Statistics, but the state legislatures must approve them for adoption. States usually modify the proposed standard certificates to conform to state needs and legal requirements.

Certificates of a vital event are filed with a local registrar, whose geographic area may be a city, county, town, or other civil unit. He checks them for completeness and sends them to the state registrar of vital statistics, where they are again checked for completeness. Transcripts or microfilm copies are prepared in the state offices for transmittal to the National Vital Statistics Division of the Public Health Service. At the National Office the certificates are put on microfilm and information from them is compiled for publication.

Care is taken in compilation for publication and in making records available to the public that the individual's right to privacy is preserved. There is a confidential section on the certificates of many states where additional medical information is recorded. More detailed information on immediate and underlying causes of death, complications of pregnancy and labor, congenital malformations and anomalies, and illegitimacy, for example, are valuable pieces of information. The great advantages of accurate reporting by physicians and the acceptance by legislatures of a confidential section can be continued only when privacy of the individual is strictly maintained. The confidential sections are among the most useful to the fields of medical research and public health.

Death Registration

That death was the first and most' adequately registered vital event probably was because of its unambiguous nature. For purposes of registration, death is an incontrovertible fact, and difficulties of agreeing on a definition were not so great as for definitions of other vital events. In 1953, the United Nations [3] proposed an international statistical definition as follows:

Death is the permanent disappearance of all evidence of life at any time after live birth has taken place. (Post natal cessation of vital functions without capability of resuscitation.) This definition therefore excludes fetal deaths.

The purpose of the definition was not so much to provide criteria of death, per se, but rather to distinguish postnatal deaths—for statistical and registration purposes—from fetal and prenatal deaths, which are separately defined and registered. The absence of conflict over the definition of death, and the fact that this event cannot occur more than once in the life of the same individual, have made treatment of mortality data easier and more successful than that of other vital events.

Not only the fact of death but also its cause is an important element of death registration. In order to standardize the nomenclature as to cause of death, the World Health Organization publishes a manual entitled *International Statistical Classification of Diseases, Injuries, and Causes of Death.* The purpose of the manual is to establish international usage of comparable terms. The manual is revised about every ten years and is used routinely by health departments.

The Death Certificate. In case of death, the funeral director fills out that part of the certificate (see Fig. 3-2) having to do with demographic facts about the deceased. He takes the certificate to the physician, or other appropriate professional, who completes the medical certification of death and affixes his signature. The funeral director then delivers the completed certificate to the local registrar from whom he obtains a burial permit.

Fetal Death Certification and Definition. In the certification of fetal death, the procedure and roles of funeral director and physician are essentially the same as those in the completion and filing of the death certificate. There are, however, some problems as to what constitutes a fetal death. In 1950, the Third World Health Assembly approved the following defi-

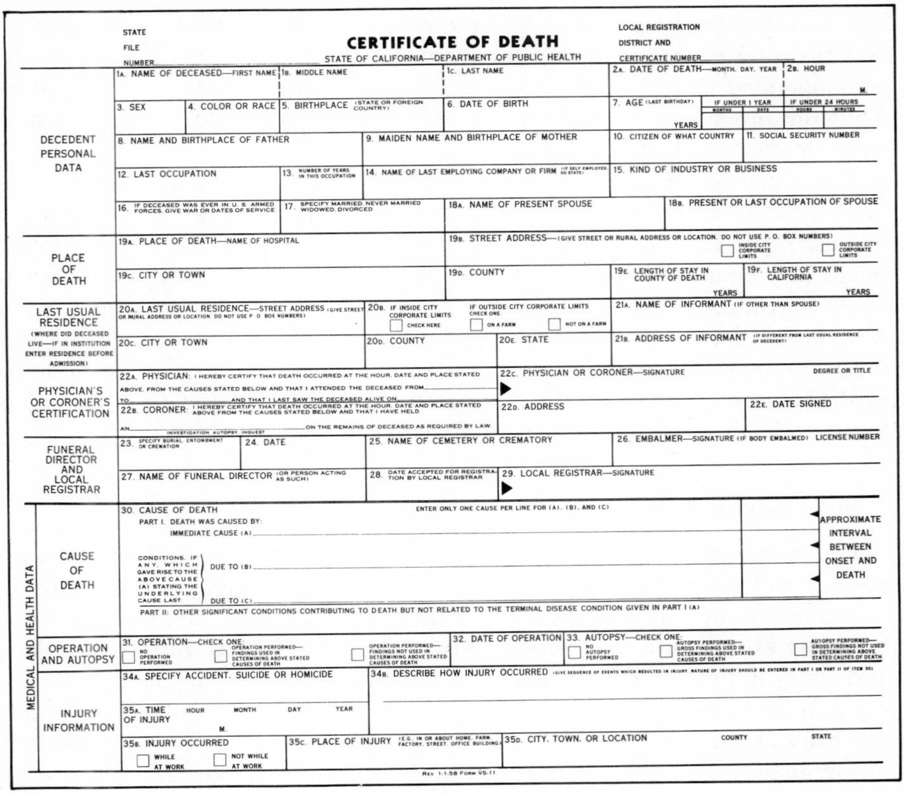

CERTIFICATE OF DEATH
STATE OF CALIFORNIA—DEPARTMENT OF PUBLIC HEALTH

STATE FILE NUMBER

LOCAL REGISTRATION DISTRICT AND CERTIFICATE NUMBER

DECEDENT PERSONAL DATA
- 1A. NAME OF DECEASED—FIRST NAME | 1B. MIDDLE NAME | 1C. LAST NAME | 2A. DATE OF DEATH—MONTH, DAY, YEAR | 2B. HOUR
- 3. SEX | 4. COLOR OR RACE | 5. BIRTHPLACE (STATE OR FOREIGN COUNTRY) | 6. DATE OF BIRTH | 7. AGE (LAST BIRTHDAY) | IF UNDER 1 YEAR | IF UNDER 24 HOURS
- 8. NAME AND BIRTHPLACE OF FATHER | 9. MAIDEN NAME AND BIRTHPLACE OF MOTHER | 10. CITIZEN OF WHAT COUNTRY | 11. SOCIAL SECURITY NUMBER
- 12. LAST OCCUPATION | 13. NUMBER OF YEARS IN THIS OCCUPATION | 14. NAME OF LAST EMPLOYING COMPANY OR FIRM (IF SELF EMPLOYED SO STATE) | 15. KIND OF INDUSTRY OR BUSINESS
- 16. IF DECEASED WAS EVER IN U. S. ARMED FORCES, GIVE WAR OR DATES OF SERVICE | 17. SPECIFY MARRIED, NEVER MARRIED WIDOWED, DIVORCED | 18A. NAME OF PRESENT SPOUSE | 18B. PRESENT OR LAST OCCUPATION OF SPOUSE

PLACE OF DEATH
- 19A. PLACE OF DEATH—NAME OF HOSPITAL | 19B. STREET ADDRESS—(GIVE STREET OR RURAL ADDRESS OR LOCATION. DO NOT USE P. O. BOX NUMBERS) | INSIDE CITY CORPORATE LIMITS | OUTSIDE CITY CORPORATE LIMITS
- 19C. CITY OR TOWN | 19D. COUNTY | 19E. LENGTH OF STAY IN COUNTY OF DEATH | 19F. LENGTH OF STAY IN CALIFORNIA

LAST USUAL RESIDENCE (WHERE DID DECEASED LIVE—IF IN INSTITUTION ENTER RESIDENCE BEFORE ADMISSION)
- 20A. LAST USUAL RESIDENCE—STREET ADDRESS (GIVE STREET OR RURAL ADDRESS OR LOCATION DO NOT USE P. O. BOX NUMBERS) | 20B. IF INSIDE CITY CORPORATE LIMITS CHECK HERE | IF OUTSIDE CITY CORPORATE LIMITS CHECK ONE | ON A FARM | NOT ON A FARM | 21A. NAME OF INFORMANT (IF OTHER THAN SPOUSE)
- 20C. CITY OR TOWN | 20D. COUNTY | 20E. STATE | 21B. ADDRESS OF INFORMANT (IF DIFFERENT FROM LAST USUAL RESIDENCE OF DECEDENT)

PHYSICIAN'S OR CORONER'S CERTIFICATION
- 22A. PHYSICIAN: I HEREBY CERTIFY THAT DEATH OCCURRED AT THE HOUR, DATE AND PLACE STATED ABOVE, FROM THE CAUSES STATED BELOW AND THAT I ATTENDED THE DECEASED FROM ___ AND THAT I LAST SAW THE DECEASED ALIVE ON ___ | 22C. PHYSICIAN OR CORONER—SIGNATURE | DEGREE OR TITLE
- 22B. CORONER: I HEREBY CERTIFY THAT DEATH OCCURRED AT THE HOUR, DATE AND PLACE STATED ABOVE FROM THE CAUSES STATED BELOW AND THAT I HAVE HELD ___ INVESTIGATION AUTOPSY INQUEST ___ ON THE REMAINS OF DECEASED AS REQUIRED BY LAW | 22D. ADDRESS | 22E. DATE SIGNED

FUNERAL DIRECTOR AND LOCAL REGISTRAR
- 23. SPECIFY BURIAL, ENTOMBMENT OR CREMATION | 24. DATE | 25. NAME OF CEMETERY OR CREMATORY | 26. EMBALMER—SIGNATURE (IF BODY EMBALMED) LICENSE NUMBER
- 27. NAME OF FUNERAL DIRECTOR (OR PERSON ACTING AS SUCH) | 28. DATE ACCEPTED FOR REGISTRATION BY LOCAL REGISTRAR | 29. LOCAL REGISTRAR—SIGNATURE

MEDICAL AND HEALTH DATA

CAUSE OF DEATH
- 30. CAUSE OF DEATH — ENTER ONLY ONE CAUSE PER LINE FOR (A), (B), AND (C) | APPROXIMATE INTERVAL BETWEEN ONSET AND DEATH
- PART I. DEATH WAS CAUSED BY: IMMEDIATE CAUSE (A) ___
- CONDITIONS, IF ANY, WHICH GAVE RISE TO THE ABOVE CAUSE (A) STATING THE UNDERLYING CAUSE LAST | DUE TO (B) ___ | DUE TO (C) ___
- PART II. OTHER SIGNIFICANT CONDITIONS CONTRIBUTING TO DEATH BUT NOT RELATED TO THE TERMINAL DISEASE CONDITION GIVEN IN PART I (A)

OPERATION AND AUTOPSY
- 31. OPERATION—CHECK ONE | NO OPERATION PERFORMED | OPERATION PERFORMED—FINDINGS USED IN DETERMINING ABOVE STATED | OPERATION PERFORMED—FINDINGS NOT USED IN DETERMINING ABOVE STATED CAUSES OF DEATH | 32. DATE OF OPERATION | 33. AUTOPSY—CHECK ONE | NO AUTOPSY PERFORMED | AUTOPSY PERFORMED—GROSS FINDINGS USED IN DETERMINING ABOVE | AUTOPSY PERFORMED—GROSS FINDINGS NOT USED IN DETERMINING ABOVE STATED CAUSES OF DEATH

INJURY INFORMATION
- 34A. SPECIFY ACCIDENT, SUICIDE OR HOMICIDE | 34B. DESCRIBE HOW INJURY OCCURRED (GIVE SEQUENCE OF EVENTS WHICH RESULTED IN INJURY. NATURE OF INJURY SHOULD BE ENTERED IN PART I OR PART II OF ITEM 30)
- 35A. TIME OF INJURY | HOUR | MONTH | DAY | YEAR
- 35B. INJURY OCCURRED | WHILE AT WORK | NOT WHILE AT WORK | 35C. PLACE OF INJURY (E.G. IN OR ABOUT HOME, FARM, FACTORY, STREET, OFFICE BUILDING) | 35D. CITY, TOWN, OR LOCATION | COUNTY | STATE

Rev. 1-1-58 Form VS-11

FIGURE 3-2.

nition of fetal death, which was subsequently adopted by the United Nations Statistical Commission in 1953: [4]

Fetal death is death prior to the complete expulsion from its mother of a product of conception, irrespective of the duration of pregnancy; the death is indicated by the fact that after such separation the fetus does not breathe or show any other evidence of life, such as beating of the heart, pulsation of the umbilical cord, or definite movement of voluntary muscles. . . . If a child breathes or shows any other evidence of life after complete birth, even though it be only momentary, the birth should be registered as a live birth and a death certificate also should be filed.

This definition was recommended for use in the United States, and in 1955 the Standard Certificate of Fetal Death was adopted, replacing a certificate which required only the reporting of stillbirths. However, in spite of the new definition's phrase, "irrespective of the duration of pregnancy," certain states in the United States still retain some minimum gestation period in their specification of fetal death. For example, fetal death may apply only to products of conception having a minimum gestation period of 20 weeks, and no other pregnancy wastage is registered in those states. Estimates of pregnancy wastage, at best, are very rough. Even states that use the recommended definition of fetal death undoubtedly obtain only gross estimates of pregnancy wastage, especially for the early abortions (i.e., prenatal deaths).

When comparing fetal death rates it is important that one check definitions used, or he may not be comparing the same things. Differences in definitions of fetal deaths may also influence the recorded number of live births and infant deaths. For example, a country which includes in its fetal death registrations all infants born alive, but dead before registration, could conceivably have a lower infant mortality rate than a country which used the recommended definition of fetal death. The latter would register some of the former country's fetal deaths as live births for which death registrations would be made shortly thereafter.

Birth Registration

The Certificate of Live Birth. The physician is responsible for completing and filing the Certificate of Live Birth (see Fig. 3-3). Consulting with the parents, he records demographic and personal information about them; he also records the name and sex of the child, birth order, and place and date of birth. The medical and health sections of the certificate are separate from the rest of the certificate and can be kept confidential. Facts recorded about prematurity, birth injuries, methods of delivery, conditions of pregnancy and labor, legitimacy, etc., provide important information which is used for medical and health purposes.

Definition of Live Birth. Every infant born alive must be registered as a live birth. If he is born alive, according to official definition, but subsequently dies, the death must also be registered. There is not universal agreement as to how a live birth should be defined, and before taking published birth and infant mortality rates at face value, one should compare the definitions of live birth and fetal death, particularly when comparing rates among different countries.

The following definition of live birth has been adopted by the World Health Assembly and is recommended for use in the United States: [4]

Live birth is the complete expulsion or extraction from its mother of a product of conception, irrespective of the duration of pregnancy, which, after such separation, breathes or shows any other evidence of life, such as beating of the heart, pulsation of the umbilical cord, or definite movement of voluntary muscles, whether or not the umbilical cord has been cut or the placenta is attached; each product of such a birth is considered liveborn.

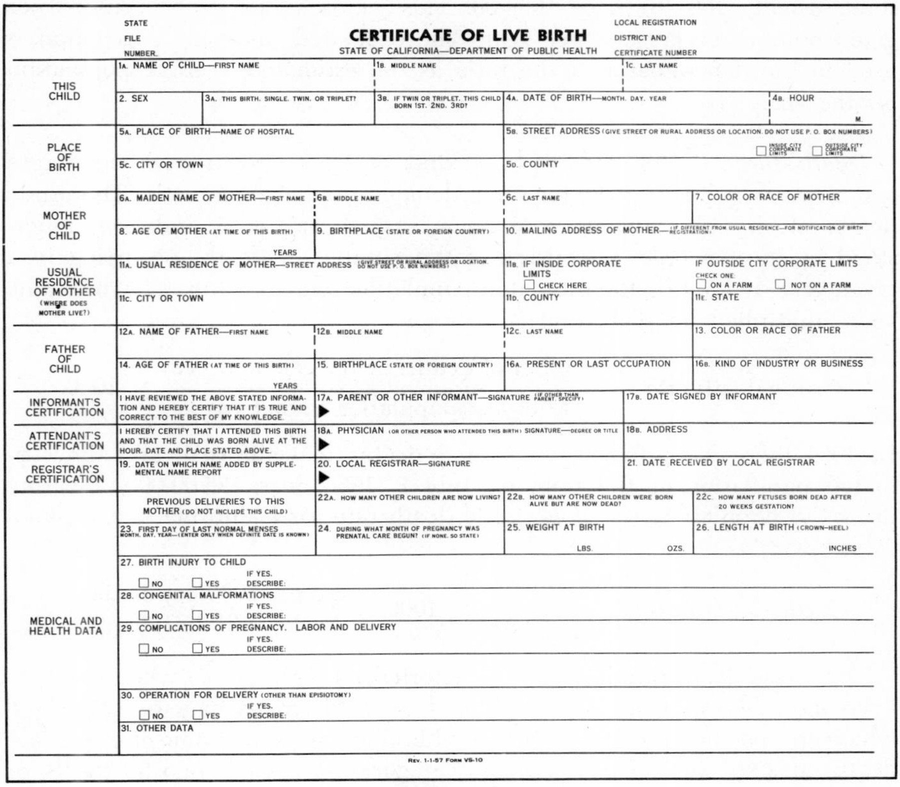

STATE

FILE

NUMBER

CERTIFICATE OF LIVE BIRTH

STATE OF CALIFORNIA—DEPARTMENT OF PUBLIC HEALTH

LOCAL REGISTRATION

DISTRICT AND

CERTIFICATE NUMBER

THIS CHILD

1A. NAME OF CHILD—FIRST NAME | 1B. MIDDLE NAME | 1C. LAST NAME

2. SEX | 3A. THIS BIRTH. SINGLE. TWIN. OR TRIPLET? | 3B. IF TWIN OR TRIPLET, THIS CHILD BORN 1ST. 2ND. 3RD? | 4A. DATE OF BIRTH—MONTH. DAY. YEAR | 4B. HOUR M.

PLACE OF BIRTH

5A. PLACE OF BIRTH—NAME OF HOSPITAL | 5B. STREET ADDRESS (GIVE STREET OR RURAL ADDRESS OR LOCATION. DO NOT USE P. O. BOX NUMBERS) INSIDE CITY CORPORATE LIMITS / OUTSIDE CITY CORPORATE LIMITS

5C. CITY OR TOWN | 5D. COUNTY

MOTHER OF CHILD

6A. MAIDEN NAME OF MOTHER—FIRST NAME | 6B. MIDDLE NAME | 6C. LAST NAME | 7. COLOR OR RACE OF MOTHER

8. AGE OF MOTHER (AT TIME OF THIS BIRTH) YEARS | 9. BIRTHPLACE (STATE OR FOREIGN COUNTRY) | 10. MAILING ADDRESS OF MOTHER—IF DIFFERENT FROM USUAL RESIDENCE—FOR NOTIFICATION OF BIRTH REGISTRATION

USUAL RESIDENCE OF MOTHER (WHERE DOES MOTHER LIVE?)

11A. USUAL RESIDENCE OF MOTHER—STREET ADDRESS (GIVE STREET OR RURAL ADDRESS OR LOCATION. DO NOT USE P. O. BOX NUMBERS) | 11B. IF INSIDE CORPORATE LIMITS — CHECK HERE | IF OUTSIDE CITY CORPORATE LIMITS CHECK ONE: ON A FARM / NOT ON A FARM

11C. CITY OR TOWN | 11D. COUNTY | 11E. STATE

FATHER OF CHILD

12A. NAME OF FATHER—FIRST NAME | 12B. MIDDLE NAME | 12C. LAST NAME | 13. COLOR OR RACE OF FATHER

14. AGE OF FATHER (AT TIME OF THIS BIRTH) YEARS | 15. BIRTHPLACE (STATE OR FOREIGN COUNTRY) | 16A. PRESENT OR LAST OCCUPATION | 16B. KIND OF INDUSTRY OR BUSINESS

INFORMANT'S CERTIFICATION

I HAVE REVIEWED THE ABOVE STATED INFORMATION AND HEREBY CERTIFY THAT IT IS TRUE AND CORRECT TO THE BEST OF MY KNOWLEDGE. | 17A. PARENT OR OTHER INFORMANT—SIGNATURE (IF OTHER THAN PARENT, EXPLAIN) | 17B. DATE SIGNED BY INFORMANT

ATTENDANT'S CERTIFICATION

I HEREBY CERTIFY THAT I ATTENDED THIS BIRTH AND THAT THE CHILD WAS BORN ALIVE AT THE HOUR. DATE AND PLACE STATED ABOVE. | 18A. PHYSICIAN (OR OTHER PERSON WHO ATTENDED THIS BIRTH) SIGNATURE—DEGREE OR TITLE | 18B. ADDRESS

REGISTRAR'S CERTIFICATION

19. DATE ON WHICH NAME ADDED BY SUPPLEMENTAL NAME REPORT | 20. LOCAL REGISTRAR—SIGNATURE | 21. DATE RECEIVED BY LOCAL REGISTRAR

MEDICAL AND HEALTH DATA

PREVIOUS DELIVERIES TO THIS MOTHER (DO NOT INCLUDE THIS CHILD) | 22A. HOW MANY OTHER CHILDREN ARE NOW LIVING? | 22B. HOW MANY OTHER CHILDREN WERE BORN ALIVE BUT ARE NOW DEAD? | 22C. HOW MANY FETUSES BORN DEAD AFTER 20 WEEKS GESTATION?

23. FIRST DAY OF LAST NORMAL MENSES (MONTH. DAY. YEAR—ENTER ONLY WHEN DEFINITE DATE IS KNOWN) | 24. DURING WHAT MONTH OF PREGNANCY WAS PRENATAL CARE BEGUN? (IF NONE, SO STATE) | 25. WEIGHT AT BIRTH LBS. OZS. | 26. LENGTH AT BIRTH (CROWN—HEEL) INCHES

27. BIRTH INJURY TO CHILD □ NO □ YES IF YES, DESCRIBE:

28. CONGENITAL MALFORMATIONS □ NO □ YES IF YES, DESCRIBE:

29. COMPLICATIONS OF PREGNANCY. LABOR AND DELIVERY □ NO □ YES IF YES, DESCRIBE:

30. OPERATION FOR DELIVERY (OTHER THAN EPISIOTOMY) □ NO □ YES IF YES, DESCRIBE:

31. OTHER DATA

REV. 1-1-57 FORM VS-10

FIGURE 3-3.

Vital Statistics Rates

Most demographic data are collected in the form of actual numerical counts by categories. There are times when it is desirable to know the actual numbers, but the very large aggregates that make up demographic data are not always useful in themselves. The earlier section of this chapter which discussed the Census used some examples of averages (the median age), distributions (the age distribution of a population), and ratios (the sex ratio, the child-woman ratio, etc.). These illustrated some ways in which enumeration data are systematically compiled and manipulated to make them understandable and useful.

The information about the vital events which occur during a year's time is expressed most meaningfully as vital rates. A vital rate may be defined as the number of occurrences of a vital event which takes place during a year's time divided by the average, or mid-year population "at risk" to the event. Vital registration data appear in the numerator, enumeration data are used in the denominator.* The resulting ratio is multiplied by a con-

---

* There are exceptions to this rule. For example, the infant mortality rate uses vital registration data in both numerator and denominator.[5]

stant, usually 100, 1000, or 100,000. This yields a rate of occurrence per given number of persons per year. The estimated mid-year population is used in the denominator of the ratio as the estimated average population for the year.

Death Rates. There are two basic kinds of death rates, a crude death rate and a rate which is specific for some demographic characteristic. The crude death rate has the advantage of being easy to calculate, and it is understood by most people. It consists of the number of deaths occurring in a given year divided by the estimated population living on July 1 of that same year, multiplied by 1000, thus:

$$\text{Crude death rate} = \frac{\text{Number of deaths in one calendar year}}{\text{Mid-year population in that year}} \times 1000.$$

In 1964 there were 150,793 registered deaths in California, and the estimated population of the state on July 1, 1964, was 18,209,000. Relating deaths to population, the 1964 crude death rate for California is calculated as follows:

$$\text{Crude death rate} = \frac{150,793}{18,209,000} \times 1000 = \frac{8.3 \text{ per 1000 population}}{\text{in Calif. in 1964.}}$$

The crude death rate may give a distorted picture, and so when more refined mortality statistics are considered desirable, rates may be calculated which are specific for various demographic characteristics. Some examples are death rates specific for different age categories, sex, race, marital status, or any other characteristic for which the appropriate information is available.

The age-specific death rate is frequently of interest, not only at a given time, but for changes that may occur over time. It is also enlightening when comparisons are made among countries having populations with different age structures. It is possible, for example, for country A to have a higher crude death rate than country B while enjoying lower age-specific death rates at all ages. Differences in age structure could very reasonably account for what at first appears paradoxical. The age-specific death rate is calculated as follows:

$$\text{Age-specific death rate} = \frac{\text{Number of deaths in a stated age group occurring in a calendar year}}{\text{Estimated mid-year population of that age group}} \times 1000.$$

Thus, for example, in the United States in 1960, there were 22,818,000 persons of age 25 to 34, and 33,414 deaths occurred among persons in this age group, so that:

$$\text{Age-specific death rate} = \frac{33,414}{22,818,000} \times 1000 = \frac{1.4 \text{ deaths per 1000}}{\text{population age}} \atop {25\text{--}34 \text{ years.}}$$

TABLE 3-2 Age-Specific Death Rates and Crude Death Rates, France and Japan, 1959

Age Group	France (Deaths per 1000)	Japan (Deaths per 1000)
Under 1 year	30.3	33.9
1–4	1.4	2.8
5–9	0.5	1.0
10–14	0.4	0.6
15–19	0.7	1.0
20–24	1.0	1.8
25–29	1.3	2.0
30–34	1.6	2.2
35–39	2.2	2.7
40–44	3.3	3.6
45–49	5.0	5.4
50–54	8.0	8.4
55–59	12.1	13.6
60–64	17.7	20.7
65–69	26.2	33.8
70–74	42.6	55.4
75–79	71.2	89.4
80–84	120.7	137.2
85 and over	213.5	212.8
Crude Death Rate	11.4	7.4

Source: United Nations, Demographic Yearbook, 1961 (pp. 374, 380).

Table 3-2 contrasts age-specific and crude death rates in two countries, France and Japan. Compared to Japan, age-specific death rates in France are lower for most age groups, but its crude death rate is higher. France's lower age-specific death rates are not sufficient to compensate for its larger number of older persons whose higher mortality rates so appreciably influence the country's crude rate. Japan's larger proportion of persons in the younger age categories, where death rates tend to be lower, explains its lower crude rate.

Death rates may be still further refined by specifying more than one category or characteristic. For example, death rates may be made specific for age, sex, and race simultaneously, as follows:

$$\text{Death rate for white males, age 20–24 years, U.S., 1960} = \frac{\text{8191 deaths in specified population}}{\text{Mid-year population of 5,272,340}} \times 1000 = \text{1.6 deaths per 1000 white males age 20–24 years.}$$

Birth Rates. Data on number of births are used in several vital statistics rates, including the crude birth rate, the general fertility rate, age-specific birth rates, and the infant mortality rate. The best known and most commonly used measure of the incidence of births and fertility is *the crude birth rate*. This consists of the number of registered live births occurring in a specified area during a calendar year, divided by the mid-year population, as follows:

$$\text{Crude birth rate} = \frac{\text{Number of births occurring during one calendar year}}{\text{Mid-year population}} \times 1000.$$

There were 4,257,850 registered live births in the United States in 1960, occurring among an estimated mid-year population of 179,323,000, so that:

$$\text{Crude birth rate} = \frac{4,257,850}{179,323,000} \times 1000 = \frac{23.7 \text{ live births per}}{1000 \text{ population.}}$$

Since the crude birth rate relates births to total population, its size will be influenced by such demographic characteristics as age distribution and sex ratio of the relevant population. Crude birth rates tend to be higher among young than among old populations.* Relative to total population size, the *total* number of women in the childbearing ages and the number of *married* women in the childbearing ages have an important influence on number of births and thereby on the crude birth rate.

A better measure of the incidence of birth than the crude rate is *the general fertility rate*, which is computed by dividing total live births occurring in one calendar year by the mid-year population of women aged 15 to 44 (or 15 to 49) years, thus:

$$\text{General fertility rate} = \frac{\text{Number of births occurring during one calendar year}}{\text{Mid-year population of women } 15\text{–}44 \text{ (or } 15\text{–}49\text{) years of age}} \times 1000.$$

In 1960 there were 4,257,850 live births in the United States and an estimated mid-year population of 36,079,000 women in the childbearing years 15 to 44, resulting in:

$$\text{General fertility rate} = \frac{4,257,850}{36,079,000} \times 1000 = \frac{118 \text{ births per } 1000}{\text{women of child-bearing age.}}$$

If more refined information is required about the fertility of *married* women, the population of women aged 15 to 44 years may be limited to the mid-year population of married women in those age groups.

Age-specific birth rates provide information about the distribution of a year's births by age of mother. In computing the rates, mothers are usually

---

* An "old" population is one having a relatively large percentage of its population 65 years of age and over.

TABLE 3-3 Live Birth Rate per 1000 Women in Each Category, by Age and Color of Mother, 1960

By Age of Mother	No. of Live Births per 1000 Women
10–14 years	0.8
15–19	89.1
20–24	258.1
25–29	197.4
30–34	112.7
35–39	56.2
40 and over	16.4
By Color of Mother, for Ages 15 to 44	
White	113.2
Nonwhite	153.6

Source: Adapted from U.S. Bureau of the Census, *Statistical Abstract of the United States, 1965* (p. 50).

classified in five-year age groups. Table 3-3 shows the birth rate in 1960 per age category of mothers; the table also presents birth rates specific for race, i.e., white and nonwhite.

For purposes of comparison among various populations at a given time and for the same population over time, the general fertility rate and the age-specific birth rate are preferable to the crude birth rate. If one assumes there is agreement about the definition of live birth, the specific birth rates are more comparable than crude rates because other influencing demographic characteristics have been eliminated.

Another useful vital rate employing data on number of births is *the infant mortality rate*. It may be defined as the number of deaths occurring among persons less than one year of age, divided by the number of births. Multiplied by 1000, this ratio gives the rate of infant deaths per 1000 live births, thus:

$$\text{Infant mortality rate} = \frac{\begin{array}{c}\text{Number of deaths occurring in one} \\ \text{calendar year among persons less than} \\ \text{one year of age}\end{array}}{\begin{array}{c}\text{Number of live births in one} \\ \text{calendar year}\end{array}} \times 1000;$$

$$\begin{array}{l}\text{Infant mortality rate} \\ \text{(U.S., 1960)}\end{array} = \frac{110,873}{4,257,850} \times 1000 = \begin{array}{l}26 \text{ infant deaths} \\ \text{per 1000 live} \\ \text{births in the} \\ \text{U.S., 1960.}\end{array}$$

The infant mortality rate has been relied upon a great deal as an indicator of health and well-being; changes in its size have been used to assess changes in the extent and effectiveness of medical care and public health programs. The relatively high risk of death in the first year of life has made the infant mortality rate sensitive to various circumstances, particularly to conditions of sanitation and other environmental factors, as well as to quality of medical care and to the level of general education and health education.

MORBIDITY STATISTICS

Statistical measures of morbidity, or the amount of illness in a population, are useful in public health in assessing the relative importance of a given illness or injury at a particular time or over a stated time period. They also provide measures of change over time in the occurrence of an illness or injury and in its relative importance to all other illnesses or injuries.

Two common measures of the amount of illness are the incidence rate and the prevalence rate. The difference between the two is that the prevalence rate counts all the cases of an illness or injury which exist during a time period, while the incidence rate counts only the new cases which occur. They differ from the rates and ratios described in preceding sections in that they do not use vital registration data in the numerator.

The Incidence Rate

The incidence rate for an illness is defined as the number of new cases that occur during a given time period, divided by the number of persons exposed to the risk of the illness (the number of persons at risk is often the total population of the relevant geographic area, and thus a "crude" incidence rate is produced). The resulting ratio is multiplied by a constant, 1000 or 100,000, as follows:

$$\text{Incidence rate} = \frac{\text{Number of newly reported cases of a stated disease or injury during a given time period}}{\text{Population living in stated area during that time period}} \times 1000 \text{ or } 100,000.$$

Thus, for example, there were 266,222 cases of measles reported in the United States in 1965.[6] These cases occurred among a population of about 194,204,000 persons, so that:

$$\text{Incidence rate for measles} = \frac{266,222}{194,204,000} \times 1000 = \frac{1.371 \text{ cases of measles}}{\text{per 1000 persons.}}$$

More refined rates of incidence may be computed by age, sex, race, or other demographic characteristics. For some injuries or illnesses it is important to define more specifically the population at risk. An example is the complications of pregnancy, to which only a fairly well-defined segment of the population is at risk.

The Prevalence Rate

The crude prevalence rate may be defined as the number of cases of an illness which exist at a particular time, divided by the number of persons living in the defined geographic area at that time, and multiplied by 1000 or 100,000. The prevalence rate indicates the relative number of persons who have a stated illness at a given time. For example, an estimated 3,300,-000 persons were afflicted with rheumatism or arthritis in the United States for the period July 1961–June 1963.[7] Using the 1962 population estimate of 185,-890,000 persons, the prevalence rate was 17.752. In other words, during the stated time period, an estimated 17.752 persons out of every 1000 had rheumatism or arthritis. More refined prevalence rates may be computed by age, sex, race, marital status, or some other characteristic which more precisely defines "population at risk" than does the total population estimate.

USES OF DEMOGRAPHIC DATA AND VITAL STATISTICS IN PUBLIC HEALTH

Utilization at the Local Level

In planning local health programs it is essential to know how many persons need a particular program and, in evaluating the program, how much benefit is being derived from it. In all its activities, the local public health agency must know the size, location, and characteristics of the population. Without this information it would be impossible to estimate personnel needs and to evaluate what proportion of the target population is taking advantage of public health services.

Census data are used to describe the density of various areas of a community, and information on characteristics of the population such as race, age, transiency, and income are used in program planning. Data collected from birth certificates are used to anticipate the need for postnatal care programs for mothers and their children, to plan vaccination and immunization programs, and to develop programs for the congenitally handicapped. Likewise, data derived from death certificates are used by the local public health agencies to plan control programs for specific communicable diseases (especially in countries where epidemics such as smallpox exist); to clear other records such as police, social security, and welfare status of deceased persons; and to plan public health programs for accident or suicide prevention and chronic disease.

Other local groups in schools, hospitals, and businesses use census and birth information in planning facilities and anticipating personnel needs. Voluntary agencies also use the vital statistics records in planning when and where to concentrate their efforts.

Utilization by the State

On the state level, public health personnel provide a continuing surveillance of reportable diseases in terms of morbidity statistics as an aid to local agencies. If unusually high values occur, action can be taken at the state and local level. These same morbidity and mortality statistics are used to plan campaigns by health educators in deciding when specific diseases peak, so that they can start their campaign at an appropriate time of the year.

Census, morbidity, and mortality information is used by the state for comparison purposes. The incidence rate of a disease such as measles could be plotted year by year to assess trends and compare them with public health program efforts and medical advances in prevention of these diseases. One may think that a disease such as tuberculosis is disappearing, only to find later that there is still considerable incidence among certain population groups. By checking the morbidity and mortality trends over time the public health programs can be kept up to date.

Census, mortality, and morbidity statistics are also used for in-service training programs, to pinpoint problem areas, and to make administrative decisions as to budgeting and personnel needs. Good planning requires a description of the needs of the various areas and population subgroups of the state. A particular subgroup such as migrant workers might need special health programs at certain times of the year. The need for special efforts in air pollution programs, vector control, inspection of fish or meat, or pesticide control can be evaluated.

Utilization at the National Level

At the national level, there is a greater emphasis on research, and demographic data and vital statistics are used for this purpose. The data reported by the National Center for Health Statistics are used as basic elements in public health and medical research. The census data are used to estimate the present population and to project the future population. These, combined with the morbidity and mortality statistics, form the guideposts for deciding where research efforts should be encouraged. Besides encouraging research by outside groups, special research teams are formed in the Public Health Service to tackle particular public health problems. As in the states, trends over time in morbidity and mortality statistics are useful in planning future research efforts.

In the future, it is anticipated that with the use of computers, data will be compiled much faster and users will have more current information. Furthermore, it will be possible to match records on the computer from various sources in the government for comparison purposes. If the problems of protection of the rights of the individual can be overcome, then these combined records will be even more useful planning tools for the development of public health programs.

SUMMARY

One component of *demographic data* is the size and characteristics of the population. The principal source of population information is the enumeration of the decennial Census, which is conducted by the Bureau of the Census, U.S. Department of Commerce. Data from census enumeration are utilized in the computation of a variety of distributions (e.g., age, income, and education), averages (e.g., median age and median income), and ratios (e.g., sex ratio and dependency ratio). A second component of demographic data is the vital events of births, deaths, marriages, and divorces. The main sources of information on vital events are records of vital registration which are maintained by official agencies through a variety of procedures. When vital registration information (used in the numerator) is combined with census enumeration information (used in the denominator), various *vital statistics* are generated, usually expressed as rates. Those most commonly used in public health are birth rates and death rates.

Morbidity statistics indicate the amount of illness in a population; the two most common measures, the incidence rate and the prevalence rate, utilize the number of cases of an illness or injury in the numerator and the size of the population at risk in the denominator. The prevalence rate takes account of all cases of an illness or injury existing during a time period; the incidence rate takes account only of the new cases which occur.

Demographic data, vital statistics, and morbidity statistics describe a population and indicate its general level of health and well-being. Such information is useful in assessing health needs, in identifying the existence and severity of health problems, in evaluating programs, and in conducting research on a variety of topics. Local, state, and national public health agencies, as well as a variety of other organizations, institutions, and individuals, make extensive use of these data and statistics.

REFERENCES

1. U.S. BUREAU OF THE CENSUS. *Statistical Abstract of the United States: 1965*, 86th ed. U.S. Government Printing Office, Washington, D.C.

2. U.S. BUREAU OF THE CENSUS. *1960 Census of Population*. Vol. 1, *Characteristics of the Population* (Part 3, Alaska; Part 23, Massachusetts). U.S. Government Printing Office, Washington, D.C.

3. UNITED NATIONS. *Handbook of Vital Statistics Methods*. The United Nations Statistical Office, New York, 1955.

4. NATIONAL OFFICE OF VITAL STATISTICS, Public Health Service, U.S. Department of Health, Education, and Welfare. *Physicians' Handbook on Death and Birth Registration*, 11th ed. U.S. Government Printing Office, Washington, D.C., 1958.

5. NATIONAL CENTER FOR HEALTH STATISTICS, Public Health Service, U.S. Department of Health, Education, and Welfare. *Vital Statistics: 1964*. Vol. 2, Part B. U.S. Government Printing Office, Washington, D.C.

6. NATIONAL CENTER FOR HEALTH STATISTICS, Public Health Service, U.S. Department of Health, Education, and Welfare. *Morbidity and Mortality*, **14**, January 1966.

7. NATIONAL CENTER FOR HEALTH STATISTICS, Public Health Service, U.S. Department of Health, Education, and Welfare. *Chronic Conditions and Activity Limitation, United States, July 1961–June 1963.* Vital and Health Statistics, Public Health Service Publication 1000, Series 10, No. 17. U.S. Government Printing Office, Washington, D.C.

ADDITIONAL READING

BARCLAY, GEORGE W. *Techniques of Population Analysis.* John Wiley and Sons, Inc., New York, 1958.

PETERSEN, WILLIAM. *Population.* The Macmillan Company, New York, 1961.

RODGERS, EDWARD S. *Human Ecology and Health.* The Macmillan Company, New York, 1960.

SPIEGELMAN, MORTIMER. *Introduction to Demography.* The Society of Actuaries, Chicago, 1955.

U.S. BUREAU OF THE CENSUS. *Fact Finder for the Nation.* U.S. Government Printing Office, Washington, D.C., 1965.

CHAPTER 4

EPIDEMIOLOGIC INVESTIGATION AND OTHER COMMUNITY HEALTH RESEARCH

Definition and scope of epidemiology

Basic epidemiologic elements

Scientific investigation and research: principles and procedures

Principal aspects of epidemiologic investigation

Other community health research

Summary

The concepts and methods of investigations in epidemiology and of research in other areas of community health are discussed in this chapter. By way of background, the first two sections of the chapter provide a general overview of epidemiology as a body of knowledge and a method of investigating the health-disease process. The next section reviews the various principles and procedures which characterize scientific investigation generally. The principal aspects and kinds of methods of epidemiological investigation are discussed in the fourth section. In the last section of the chapter, some of the major areas of other kinds of researches which have a health-related focus are described, and the disciplines which contribute to these researches are reviewed briefly.

DEFINITION AND SCOPE OF EPIDEMIOLOGY

Contemporary epidemiology describes the distribution of human health problems and seeks to establish the causes of these problems in order to discover and formulate effective preventive measures. Specific definitions of epidemiology vary somewhat, the differences being largely a matter of degree of inclusiveness. In certain definitions, the focus is on the investigation of disease; in others, disease is included as part of a broader spectrum of concern. Thus, epidemiology has been defined as "the study of the distribution and determinants of disease prevalence in man"; [1] or it has been viewed as being "concerned with measurements of the circumstances under which diseases occur, where diseases tend to flourish, and where they do not." [2] The circumstances referred to in the latter definition may be microbiologic or toxicologic, and they may be based on genetic, social, or environmental factors. In the more broadly based definitions, epidemiology is considered to include "the various factors and conditions that determine the occurrence and distribution of health, disease, defect, disability, and death among groups of individuals"; [3] or it is "concerned with the study of the processes which determine or influence the physical, mental, and social health of people." [4] In general, these definitions of epidemiology—whether the focus is on disease or on the total health-disease spectrum—share in common an emphasis on *process* and a recognition of the involvement of a *multiplicity of influencing factors.*

The most significant early contributions of epidemiology were in connection with the infectious diseases. These contributions, which have been described in Chapter 1, included the discovery of microorganisms as causative agents of disease (thus ushering in the bacteriologic era), the development of immunology, and the acquisition of new knowledge regarding the transmission of disease. Such discoveries did not, of course, occur as an uninterrupted chain of events. For example, in 1854 John Snow proved that cholera was transmitted in water and by personal contact, but the identification of the cholera organism was not made until 27 years later. Similarly, William Budd established the contagious nature of tuberculosis 15 years before the tubercle bacillus was identified.[5] Thus, the contributions of epidemiology have, historically, come about through a series of steps which have sometimes extended over a considerable period of time and in which important epidemiologic facts have sometimes been discovered before specific mechanisms have been identified.

In recent years, the scope of epidemiology has broadened considerably. As a consequence of its early concern with infectious diseases, the principal function of epidemiology for many years was to investigate epidemics of such diseases, including tracing their sources, controlling spread, and initiating measures to prevent recurrences. On the international health scene, there is still great concern with well-known communicable diseases that continue to wrack many regions of the world, including smallpox, typhoid, schistosomiasis, and trachoma. However, in the more developed industrial nations where infectious diseases have largely been brought under control, the concerns of epidemiology have tended to shift to the vast array of *noninfectious* diseases which have gained increasing prominence.

Epidemiologic activity in the noninfectious diseases is by no means new.

Even during the eighteenth and early nineteenth centuries, a number of epidemiologic achievements in the noninfectious diseases had occurred, for example, in nutritional disease and occupational disease through investigations of scurvy among merchant seamen and of scrotal cancer in chimney sweeps.[6] Today, the chronic and degenerative diseases such as cardiovascular disorders, cancer, and arthritis, as well as mental illness, nutritional disorders, congenital defects, and accidents, are all considered to be highly appropriate for epidemiologic study and investigation. Conditions in which social pathology is clearly present, such as alcoholism, drug addiction, divorce, delinquency, and suicide, also have aspects to which epidemiology is relevant.

Epidemiology provides both a body of knowledge and a formulation of methods for learning about health and disease status with the goal of ultimately finding solutions to health problems. It constitutes part of the scientific foundation of public health and a basis for public health action.[7] With respect to the distribution of disease, epidemiology provides information on the frequency of occurrence of disease in different populations and in different segments of the same population. This aspect is often referred to as *descriptive epidemiology*. It attempts to answer questions regarding "who," "where," and "when" in terms, for example, of age, sex, race, and various geographic and time dimensions. Such information enables the maintenance of general surveillance of the health status of a population and alerts health workers to outbreaks of infectious diseases and to increases in the occurrence of specific noninfectious diseases. Descriptive epidemiology also provides historical perspective regarding the prevalence of diseases in different epochs of time.

In addition, descriptive information underlies another major concern of epidemiology, namely, the search for causes of disease. Knowledge of the cause of disease, in turn, serves as the basis for preventive measures. In establishing disease causation, epidemiology attempts to answer questions regarding "how" and "why." To do this, two levels of investigative techniques may be employed. On one level, an effort is made to determine the statistical association between a specific factor and a given disease; for example, a great deal of evidence has been assembled that shows a strong statistical association between cigarette smoking and the incidence of lung cancer. This kind of investigation has been called *analytic epidemiology*.[1] On the other investigative level, an attempt is made to determine exact disease causation through controlled experiments using techniques which are also the basis for much clinical research. Such investigations have been referred to as *experimental epidemiology*.[1] The principles and methods of descriptive, analytic, and experimental epidemiology will be discussed in greater detail in a later section of this chapter.

In addition to generating its own knowledge and methods, epidemiology also utilizes those of certain other relevant and important disciplines. *Clinical medicine* and *pathology* contribute to the accurate description and classification of disease, which are important in determining disease frequency. *Biostatistics* provides methods for analyzing epidemiologic data, including the determination of whether variations in disease frequency within or between population groups are chance occurrences or form systematic patterns. Other disciplines such as *microbiology* and *biochemistry* contribute methods of experimental investigation. *Genetics* and the *behavioral sciences* provide information on the characteristics of persons and on the social and cultural characteristics of population groups, respectively, which may influence the occurrence of disease.

BASIC EPIDEMIOLOGIC ELEMENTS

The human population group constitutes a basic element of study in epidemiology. Epidemiologic investigations may involve many different kinds and sizes of groups depending on the nature of particular studies. Once a population group has been defined, however, attention is directed toward the total group, including both its sick and well members. This approach differs from that of clinical medicine and dentistry where the focus is on the individual case and in which the clinician deals with a discrete series of patients and their illnesses.[3, 8]

The concept of the natural history of disease, or the processes through which deviations from health occur and the course and outcome of the deviations, is another basic element in epidemiology. The natural history of a disease describes "its development from the first forces which create the disease stimulus in the environment or elsewhere, through the resulting response of man, to the changes which take place leading to recovery, disability, defect, or death."[9] This process involves the interaction of three different kinds of factors: the causative *agent*, the susceptible *host*, and the *environment*.[3, 7] Epidemiologic investigations are concerned with the assembly and analysis of information about these factors for the purpose of describing the occurrence, distribution, and cause of disease.

An agent is usually thought of as a factor whose *presence* causes disease, but it may also be a factor whose *absence* can cause disease. An example of the latter is insufficient intake of vitamin C, which may lead to scurvy. There are several general categories of causative agents. One category consists of *physical agents,* which include various kinds of mechanical forces or frictions that may be the source of injury and several different kinds of atmospheric abnormalities such as extremes of temperature or excessive radiation. A second category consists of *chemical agents,* which can occur in various forms such as dusts, gases, vapors, and fumes; such agents may be acquired by inhalation, ingestion, or contact. A third category consists of *nutrient agents,* which are also chemical in nature, but include the lack or the *over*abundance of one or more of the basic dietary elements. The final and historically most prominent category consists of *biologic agents,* which are living organisms, and include insects (arthropods), worms (helminths), protozoa, fungi, bacteria, rickettsiae, and viruses.

The human host's susceptibility or resistance to a disease agent, and hence the occurrence and distribution of disease in a population, are influenced by many factors. Habits, customs, and characteristic modes of living may serve either to encourage or to inhibit the disease process. Factors in this general category may range from matters of personal cleanliness and food habits to sanitation practices, extent of interpersonal contacts, and degree of crowding. Various population characteristics may also be important factors in determining the onset, type, and course of certain diseases. Such attributes include age, sex, ethnic origin, marital status, and socio-economic indicators such as occupation and income. The status of various general and specific mechanisms in the host which provide defenses against disease constitute another set of influencing factors in the disease process. These defenses include immunity as well as numerous anatomic structures (e.g., the skin, hair, nails, and secretions) and physiologic processes (e.g., coughing, temperature regulation, and tolerance development) which protect against disease and injury. Other host factors which may contribute to the disease process are heredity and general constitutional make-up.

The environment may, depending on its characteristics, help to suppress disease or assist it to flourish. The total environment consists of several components: physical, biologic, social, and economic. The most prominent aspect of the *physical environment* is geography, to which climate, season, and weather are closely allied. Health status may be directly or indirectly influenced by the topography, the nature of the soil, the availability of water, and the climatic conditions of a particular area. The *biologic environment* includes living animals and plants, some of which, as mentioned earlier, may be agents of disease. They may also harbor disease agents, or they may serve as transmitters of disease. Of the many aspects of the *social and economic environment* which may influence health and disease, economic status is among the most important. The economic status of a population as a whole, as reflected in its general standard of living, may have considerable impact on health level. The range of economic gradation within the population and the extent and severity of economic deprivations in particular population groups may also be of considerable importance. The social environment is characterized by many different kinds of attitudes, beliefs, and behavior, some of which may alleviate the threat of disease while others may foster it, for example, attitudes and beliefs which lead to the use of properly accredited medical practitioners and facilities as opposed to those that lead to the use of untested or quack remedies. In general, as a population develops socially and economically, ideology and practice tend increasingly to support the growth of environmental factors that promote health and minimize disease.

The nature of the interaction between agent, host, and environmental factors determine the relative health or disease status of a population. The process of interaction has been conceptualized as the degree of equilibrium of forces on a scale in which environmental factors are the fulcrum, and agent and host factors are the opposing balances.[3] If the balance is in favor of the host, disease occurrence decreases. However, if the balance shifts because of deleterious changes in environmental factors or the greater "weight" of agent factors, disease occurrence increases until equilibrium is again restored. At any time in a population, groups of individuals are in various phases of this interaction process; the function of some epidemiologic investigations is to identify these groups and analyze the process.

SCIENTIFIC INVESTIGATION AND RESEARCH: PRINCIPLES AND PROCEDURES

Epidemiologic investigations and various other kinds of related researches endeavor to adhere to the basic principles and orderly procedures which are embodied in the "scientific method." Information is assembled through systematic observations or measurements using techniques which will ensure as high a degree of accuracy and precision as possible. The data thus assembled are analyzed through a variety of appropriate statistical methods and give rise to conclusions which are tied to the observations and measurements. Throughout a scientific investigation, special efforts are made to reduce bias that may arise from a variety of sources such as subjective or preconceived ideas or from human, mechanical, or other kinds of error. Specific methods and techniques which help to accomplish these aims have, over the years, been contributed by statistics, biomathematics, and many other disciplines in the fields of the physical, biologic, and social sciences.

Definition of the Problem and Review of Existing Relevant Knowledge

The first step in the conduct of a scientific investigation is the definition of the problem to be studied and an assessment of the knowledge that already exists on the subject. Scientific knowledge is generally built up through a series of investigations, each new endeavor utilizing what has already been learned and in turn adding to the foundation for subsequent studies. Occasionally an investigation is undertaken to replicate or retest the findings of a preceding study, and this, too, adds to the total body of knowledge. In any case, careful and thorough review of relevant, accumulated information aids in defining the problem, objectives, and methods of the investigation being undertaken. In connection with studies of diseases for which adequate therapies or preventives are as yet only partly known, such review of past work is sometimes a sizable intellectual task.

An important part of the initial stage of a study is the determination of the nature of the problem to be investigated, as well as its extent and significance. At this time, also, questions are formulated for which answers will be sought during the course of the investigation. These considerations provide inklings as to the nature of subsequent steps in the study and give some indication of the possible contributions to knowledge that could be expected to accrue from the effort.

Design of the Investigation

As the body of sound knowledge on a subject grows, it becomes possible to formulate statements of relationships that might reasonably be expected to occur between particular phenomena. Such statements, or *hypotheses,* may postulate an association between phenomena, or they may even postulate a chain of causation. If the status of accumulated knowledge permits, hypotheses are formulated during the planning stage of an investigation, and the means for testing them thoroughly are then provided through appropriate study design. Hypotheses may also be generated during the course of an investigation or as an end product. If existing knowledge is not sufficient to enable formulating hypotheses at the outset, the investigation should be designed to maximize the possibility of obtaining information that will lead to such formulations.

In addition to provisions for testing or developing hypotheses, there are also several other considerations in the design of an investigation; all are closely related to one another. One of the first has to do with the nature of the population that will be studied. The population may consist of individuals from a particular group (e.g., members of a health insurance plan), a particular setting (e.g., patients in a hospital), or a particular locality (e.g., residents of a city block). There are also countless additional ways in which a population may be defined, such as persons with or without a certain disease or with some other attribute. Once the population has been designated, the *universe* of the investigation has been established.

This leads to another consideration in design, namely, the proportion of the universe that is to be investigated. Since only rarely will it be possible to investigate the entire population, some smaller element, i.e., a *sample,* must be established according to optimally useful sampling design. A sample usually must be representative of the universe from which it is drawn in order for the results of the investigation to be applicable to the total population as it has been defined. One of the most common sampling procedures is the random sample in which every individual in the defined population has an equal chance of being chosen. Other sampling procedures (all requiring technical competence for best use) include probability sampling, which often involves several steps or stages, as well as stratified sampling, systematic sampling (e.g., one in n), etc.

Other considerations in the design of an investigation have to do with the sources and methods of data collection. These may include clinical examinations, personal interviews, diaries, laboratory tests, clinical case records, or various kinds of official records. In some investigations, more than one source and method of data collection are used. Appropriate instruments are required, such as forms for recording the results of diagnosis, observations, or measurements; questionnaires or interview guides, etc. Other instruments, often derived from the social sciences, help to measure important attributes of the patients or other study subjects, e.g., social position, economic status, psychological state, and social stress. Such instruments must be carefully designed and pretested—or tried out—on a population that resembles the one which will ultimately be studied. Pretest results are analyzed, preferably statistically, and modifications are made in the instruments as needed. Appropriate and detailed instructions for the use of the instruments are also required.

The frequency with which data are to be collected is a further consideration in the design of an investigation. Measurements or observations may be made at one point in time only, or they may be made repeatedly over a period of time. These elements of design are generally referred to as cross-sectional and longitudinal methods, respectively. If an investigation uses the longitudinal method, the number of times observations or measurements are to be made and the length of the time intervals between them are established as part of the design.

Collection of the Data

The data collection phase of an investigation consists of the implementation of all aspects of the basic study design. Data collection, of course, involves whatever labor that is needed to obtain the required observations or measurements. However, it also requires special efforts to minimize as much as possible the amount of human error that otherwise can be introduced at this stage of an investigation (although, of course, it can be introduced at other stages as well). In addition, special efforts need to be made to obtain *all* of the observations or measurements that have been established as the goal of the study, i.e., a sample or a specified universe. A large proportion of missing observations or measurements at best limits the usefulness of the data, and at worst may invalidate the investigation. The goals of reducing human error and maximizing completeness of data collection pertain uniformly whether the investigation is small and has a relatively simple design, or whether it is large and complex.

The selection and training of appropriate personnel to make the observations or measurements required by the study design are important preliminaries to the actual data collection task. Once the collection of data has begun, careful and continuous supervision of personnel is required in order to ensure that instructions are being followed and that uniform practices and procedures are being maintained. Checks on the quality and reliability of the information that is being obtained should be initiated at the outset and continued systematically. The objective of such procedures is to test for uniformity of judgments by comparing the observations and measurements that have been made independently by different individuals. Corrective action can be taken if the results of these reliability checks show anything other than inconsequential differences. Such procedures help considerably to ensure the soundness of the resulting data.

Data Processing and Analysis

Careful organization and complete analysis of the observations or measurements obtained are additional major tasks in the conduct of an investigation. The purpose of this phase of a study is to gain a thorough understanding of the information so that sound conclusions can be formulated. Analysis involves the assessment of data which have been quantified by classifying and tabulating the observations and measurements that have been made. Appropriate statistical computations and tests of the data are then performed, and the results are carefully reviewed and interpreted. The nature of this entire process should be outlined during the early planning stages of the investigation. A study is likely to encounter serious difficulty if information is collected without considerable planning at the outset as to how it will ultimately be classified, tabulated, and analyzed.

Analysis consists, in effect, of asking various relevant questions of the data. Depending, of course, on the nature of the study, such questions might include: How many persons have different diseases at a particular point in time? Is one age group more likely than another to have a particular disease? Is a particular disease more likely to be found in one geographic area than another, and if so, what factors account for its occurrence? If an investigation has set out to test hypotheses, the question asked is: Do the data confirm or reject the hypotheses? The ways in which the data are classified and the kinds of tabulations made are governed by the nature of the questions that are posed.

The actual appraisal of data is made through the application of various appropriate statistical tests which are used to assess the significance or importance of differences, associations, or trends. For example, if the data indicate a relationship between two phenomena, the strength of the association can be tested statistically. If a universe has been sampled, it is important to know how much the results could be expected to vary from additional samples, if the latter were to be made. This can be estimated statistically, and the result provides an indication of the reliability of the data, or the extent to which the results may be generalized to the entire universe. If the investigation set out to make observations or measurements of a specified universe but some were missed, the seriousness of the omissions can be determined and perhaps even compensated for statistically. Biostatistics, by applying the principles and methods of statistics to the health sciences, provides the techniques for making these and other kinds of assessments.[10, 11]

PRINCIPAL ASPECTS OF
EPIDEMIOLOGIC INVESTIGATION

As indicated earlier in this chapter, epidemiology may be viewed as
having descriptive, analytic, and experimental aspects which, in effect,
represent progressions along a continuum that ranges from an account of
disease occurrence and distribution to the establishment of disease causation. At present, the status of knowledge along this continuum varies among
diseases. For some diseases such as cancer and heart disease, epidemiologic
investigation has provided some knowledge of their distribution in the
population, but exact causes are yet to be determined. For others, such as
certain kinds of mental illness, neither the exact distribution nor the causes
are known. Epidemiologists seek continuously to close these gaps in knowledge in order further to extend the breadth of disease prevention.

Descriptive Epidemiology

In investigating and describing the occurrence and distribution of disease
in a population, epidemiology customarily deals with three classes of characteristics: those pertaining to the *time* and the *place* in which persons are
found affected, and those pertaining to the affected *persons* themselves.[1, 12]

Characteristics Describing Time. Time, as one element in the description of disease distribution, may be defined in many different ways, such
as year, season, or day. Disease frequency may be measured over a long
period of time and observed for changes in its pattern of occurrence. The
change occurring over a period of years is known as *secular change* and is
illustrated by Figure 4-1, which shows death rates for tuberculosis and
malignant neoplasms over a 60-year period. Death certificates for cause of
death and autopsy reports for incidental pathology have traditionally been
the best means of measuring secular change. Data on morbidity that are
appropriate for such measurement are at present limited mainly, first, to
the infectious diseases that are reportable to health departments and,
second, to the cases of mental illness in mental hospitals. In recent years,
at least two other sources of epidemiologic information have come into use
in the United States and are sometimes found in other parts of the world.
These are *registries* (e.g., cancer registries), which attempt to assemble
information on incidence and prevalence of a few particular diseases of
interest, and *morbidity surveys* (e.g., the U.S. National Health Survey),
which systematically screen defined populations for prevalence of illness.

Seasonal fluctuations, cyclic fluctuations, and "point" epidemics are additional ways to describe the time characteristics of disease distribution.
In measuring *seasonal fluctuations,* cases are plotted by time of onset using
units—hours, days, weeks, or months—that are small enough to show suc-

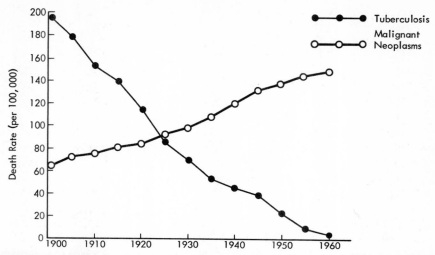

FIGURE 4-1. Secular change: tuberculosis and malignant neoplasms, 1900–1960. (All forms of tuberculosis. Includes neoplasms of lymphatic and hematopoietic tissues.) (Source: Adapted from U.S. Bureau of the Census. *Historical Statistics of the United States, Colonial Times to 1957.* Washington, D.C., 1960, p. 26. Also, *Statistical Abstract of the United States, 1965,* p. 59.)

cessive variations in the occurrence of the particular disease being investigated. Seasonal fluctuations in acute diseases, especially those of an infectious nature, have received considerable attention in epidemiologic investigations. However, most chronic diseases have not been studied for periodicity of occurrence, partly because of the difficulty in defining the date of onset and partly because the induction period is likely to be prolonged and variable and thus not apt to be related to a periodic factor such as season. Seasonal fluctuation of disease may reflect changes in weather conditions (e.g., cold-induced frostbite), the presence of plants (e.g., pollen, causing hay fever), the presence of insects (e.g., mosquito-borne encephalitis), or the influence of any one of a number of other kinds of environmental factors. Human host factors may also play a role in seasonal fluctuations, such as increased drownings and exposure to diseases from infected waters as the result of swimming during summer months.

Cyclic fluctuations, or cycles of disease, may be related to the seasons, but they are not limited to annual occurrences. For example, cyclic epidemics of measles every third year are almost predictable in some stable communities. *"Point" epidemics* refer to large but temporary excesses in disease frequency, usually occurring over a period of a few days. Figure 4-2 illustrates a "point" epidemic of cholera in London as identified by John Snow from data which he assembled in 1848.

The time relation between exposure and onset of disease provides valuable epidemiologic information in the search for means to prevent disease. A clustering of cases following a medically connectable event often suggests

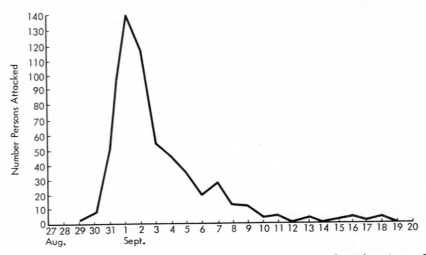

FIGURE 4-2. "Point" epidemic of cholera, Golden Square area of London, August-September, 1848. (Source: Adapted from Snow, John. *On the Mode of Communication of Cholera.* John Churchill, London, 1855.)

hypotheses of causation, a good case in point being the large number of children born with congenital defects following the use of thalidomide by their mothers during pregnancy. The detection of clustering depends on precise measurement of the time elapsed between the presumed causative event and the onset of disease or other manifestation of pathology. The time relationship is most readily apparent in the infectious diseases (e.g., food poisoning due to salmonella), but it should not be overlooked in those diseases having a long, variable induction period (e.g., myocardial infarction due to arteriosclerosis) or in those diseases occurring only after prolonged exposure (e.g., lung cancer due to smoking).

Characteristics Describing Place. Place, as another element in the description of the distribution of disease, is defined in terms of geographic units, which may vary in size ranging from an entire nation, state, or county to relatively smaller units, including a city or other urban area, a rural area, or a local community. Data on morbidity and mortality are assembled by these geographic units from routinely available sources such as vital records (as described in Chap. 3) and official records of reportable diseases. Occasionally, information is also obtained through special surveys. There are certain limitations in the use of the routinely available data, one of which stems from the differences that occur from place to place in standards of medical care and in the reporting of diseases. Another difficulty arises from the fact that boundaries of geographic units are, of course, established for administrative or political purposes, and these demarcations may obscure rather than differentiate the geographic factors which could influence the distribution of disease.

In some parts of the world, a good deal is known about the existence of certain infectious diseases from gross epidemiologic observations despite the fact that precise data are often missing. Thus, sometimes not even such basic information as births and deaths is routinely and accurately recorded. For example, the most accurate epidemiologic information in India derives from routine statistics only in "registration" areas surrounding large cities; information elsewhere in India is sometimes reliable only if collected as part of a special "survey."

Geographic units are often compared in order to ascertain variations in disease distribution. The comparisons customarily made are between or among nations, and within countries. It is often desirable to use special techniques in making such comparisons. For example, in state-to-state comparisons, industrial or agricultural areas of one state may be compared to similar areas in the other state. This helps to ensure that the geographic units being compared are generally similar to one another except for the factor being measured, namely, the occurrence of disease. Disease frequency is often compared between urban and rural areas within a state, although variations in standards of medical care between these two kinds of geographic units often make the results difficult to interpret.

In local communities, the distribution of disease is sometimes ascertained by plotting cases on a spot map. This technique is especially likely to be used in the investigation of an outbreak of a disease. In interpreting a spot map, the number of persons in the area must be taken into account since, for example, relatively few cases in a segment of the map may mean only that there are few inhabitants. This problem is overcome by the computation of rates (as explained in Chap. 3), and such computations are desirable if the population at risk in the area is sufficiently large.

Characteristics Describing Person. Several attributes of the persons affected are of particular importance in investigating and describing the distribution of disease. Age is perhaps the most important attribute of all. It has been found to be associated with variations in disease frequency more often and more strongly than has any other single factor. As explained in Chapter 3, this attribute is used in computing age-specific rates, which measure the association between disease occurrence and age. The association may be measured at one point in time, or it may be measured over a period of time among the members of a specified age group. A special instance of the latter is known as the cohort method, which consists of starting with a group of individuals who were all born in a specified period and subsequently observing the members of the same group at stated time intervals as they grow older.

Sex and race or ethnic group are other important population attributes in describing the distribution of disease. As with age, sex-specific rates or race-specific rates measure the association between disease occurrence and the attribute. Differences between males and females and between white and Negro populations have been demonstrated with respect to the occurrence of certain specific diseases. For example, heart disease and lung cancer are more likely to be found among males than among females. In the United States, mortality rates of arteriosclerotic heart disease and suicide are considerably higher among whites than among Negroes, whereas death rates from hypertensive heart disease, pneumonia, and tuberculosis are higher among Negroes than among whites.

Additional population attributes which are commonly investigated for possible association with disease frequency include occupation, socioeconomic status, and marital status. The first two are to some extent related to one another, but there are problems of definition and measurement in connection with both, and the information is sometimes difficult to obtain or is not available at all. Marital status, on the other hand, has fewer problems of definition and the information is generally more readily available.

Analytic and Experimental Epidemiology

As indicated in the foregoing discussion, data describing the occurrence and distribution of disease are analyzed for possible relationships between various phenomena in the disease process, such as the association between season and disease, age and disease, or locale and disease. In the analytic and experimental phases of epidemiology, investigation of the disease process is carried forward in greater depth, with the ultimate aim of understanding the determinants and mechanisms of disease. This kind of investigation involves the testing of hypotheses, which are often suggested by descriptive information.

Although information which serves as a basis for the description of disease generally comes from readily available sources, data for more intensive investigations usually must be obtained through special studies. In seeking to ascertain relationships between health-disease states and human and/or environmental factors, two kinds of study designs are commonly used: one design is referred to as a prospective study; the other as a retrospective study.[1, 5]

In a *prospective study*, a population group initially free of a disease about which there is concern is generally followed up over a period of time. Particular interest is shown in the disease experience of portions of the population exposed and not exposed to a suspected noxious agent or element in the environment. For example, radiation due to atomic fallout may be suspected of giving rise to leukemia. Communities or other subpopulations initially generally free of the disease are identified as having been exposed to radiation from fallout and are compared with other communities not having been so exposed. If exposure to radiation causes leukemia, the exposed group will contract the disease and the nonexposed group will not. It may turn out that only slightly more of the exposed than of the nonexposed group ultimately contracts the disease, which then leads to hypothesizing about possible factors which, along with exposure to radiation, may serve as codeterminants of incidence of the disease (e.g., age or sex). In some investigations, efforts have been made to rule out at least a few possible influencing factors by initially matching the groups on several measurable attributes. However, there still may remain unmatched a multiplicity of factors, both human host and environmental, which may be influential. Moreover, matching of attributes often is not feasible for very large groups.

In a *retrospective study*, a series of cases of a specified disease is compared to a series which is free of the disease for the purpose of ascertaining the factors that are responsible for the two disease statuses. This method generally utilizes what is known as the case-control technique, in which each case is matched to a control on several characteristics such as age, sex, race, and marital status. In order to test hypotheses regarding factors leading to the disease under investigation, information is sought for both groups concerning the frequency of *past* exposure to the suspected cause. Since such information usually must be obtained from the individual members of the two groups, problems of accuracy and completeness of recall become important considerations. The sources of both cases and controls are also of prime importance in a retrospective study. For example, if the cases under study consist of a representative sample of all cases of the disease in the community, the controls should also provide a representative sample of the locale. Similarly, if the cases are drawn from a hospital population, it is usually desirable to draw the controls from the same setting. If two or more hospitals separately provide cases and controls, it must be established in advance that the hospitals are comparable with respect to admission policies or other factors that might serve as a source of bias.

Prospective and retrospective studies utilize what are known as *observational methods*, meaning that a series of measurements are made and conclusions or inferences are derived through a process of reasoning from the evidence. By this means a statistical association may be demonstrated between a specific phenomenon and a specific disease, and it is sometimes possible to infer whether or not the association is causal. However, the most stringent test of an association and sometimes the only way in which it is possible to establish true causality (i.e., the exact determinants and mechanisms of disease) is through an *experiment*.[1, 5] Experimental epidemiology was originally developed in the context of colonies of laboratory animals into which disease was introduced and its spread observed in relation to various controlled conditions such as crowding and size of colony.[2, 5] In human populations, experiments usually have been undertaken in clinical or institutional settings, but a few experiments have also been conducted on a community basis. The experiments may involve, for example, the testing of the efficacy of a therapeutic drug or of a preventive measure such as a vaccine.

An experiment tests a clearly defined hypothesis stating, for example, that the incidence of a disease will be reduced by the introduction of a specific experimental condition, the latter perhaps consisting of a deliberate alteration of the environment, or the introduction of some preventive measure, or the use of some therapeutic agent. The hypothesis is tested by instituting the experimental condition in one group of individuals (or in a community), but not in a comparable group (or community), and observing the effects over a period of time; an experiment, therefore, is a special kind of prospective study. Those subject to the experimental condition are known as the experimental, or test, group; their counterparts are known as the control group. Such groups may be established by alternate or random assignment of individuals to one group or another or by pairing test subjects to control subjects through strict matching procedures. Ideally, neither those who make the observations nor the subjects themselves know to which group, test or control, any individual belongs. An investigation which adheres to this condition is known as a "double-blind" experiment. The most massive "double-blind" experiment undertaken to date consisted of the field trials conducted in the United States in 1954 to test the effectiveness of the Salk vaccine in preventing paralytic poliomyelitis. More than 400,000 children six to eight years of age received either vaccine or non-vaccine (placebo) inoculations, and neither the observers, the children, nor their parents knew the nature of the inoculation.

There are several instances in which epidemiologic investigations have gone through the entire process of observational and experimental methods.[6] A classic illustration is Joseph Goldberger's studies of pellagra beginning in 1914. Prior to his work, it was generally believed that pellagra was an infectious disease. Goldberger, however, noted that the disease was essentially rural, that it was associated with poverty, and that when it occurred in institutional settings, it was not found among the nurses and attendants. These considerations led him to hypothesize that the disease was caused by a dietary deficiency and that it could be prevented by increasing protein intake. Goldberger first tested the hypothesis *observationally* by demonstrating an association between pellagra and protein-deficient diet in seven cotton mill villages in South Carolina. He next proved the hypothesis *experimentally* by preventing pellagra in institutional patients through an adequate diet and by inducing pellagra in prison volunteers through a protein-deficient diet.

OTHER COMMUNITY HEALTH RESEARCH

Public health research has traditionally had a strong epidemiologic emphasis appropriate to the state of knowledge of the cause, cure, and prevention of the world's diseases. In recent decades, particularly in economically and technologically well-developed nations, interest has also turned to research activities that may be grouped under the heading of "community health research." In this type of research, the focus is principally on those factors that inhibit or promote optimal delivery of health services to populations that need them.

In this connection, there are three basic elements that are studied, some studies involving all three in the same research. First, there is focus on populations or subpopulations, their health requirements, health-related behavior, and health attitudes. Second, there is focus on the medical and public health armamentarium (manpower, preventives and therapeutics, etc.) pertinent to the health needs and requirements of study populations. Third, there is the administration of procedures designed to bring medical and public health care to populations needing it, in appropriate quality and cost.

Thus, reference is particularly to the broad fields of community health programs and services and of medical care administration. In some community health researches, data from routinely maintained records are assembled and analyzed; in a great many others, data are obtained through field studies in the general community or in particular settings such as health agencies or hospitals. Such researches utilize the principles and procedures that characterize scientific investigation generally (as described in an earlier section of this chapter), and some in particular rely on the knowledge and methods of epidemiology.

Areas of Community Health Research

In *planning community health services*, a first essential is knowledge of the occurrence and distribution of disease—a contribution of descriptive epidemiology. Such information might then be supplemented by research to determine how many and what kinds of persons would be likely to utilize a proposed service and the means of getting those who need the service actually to use it. The kinds of health services for which research-based planning is required range from the establishment of clinics to the provision of hospital beds, often for specific categories of diseases or for particular segments of the population.

The *organization and delivery of services* is another area of concern in community health research. On the broadest level, the problem of how to integrate the total complex of community health services constitutes an important research subject. Related considerations include the effect of existing patterns of local government on health services and the relative merits of narrowly based versus broadly based regional health jurisdictions. Knowledge gained through research on various aspects of professional-lay relationships, patient expectations regarding services, and the roles and responsibilities of administrative and professional staffs in various settings also aids in improving the organization and delivery of services. Program evaluation studies measure the effectiveness of existing services and provide clues that assist in future planning.

The *costs, financing, and utilization of health services* constitute a third broad area toward which research efforts are directed. The costs of medical care both to consumers and to producers are important elements in this category of research, as are the assembly and analysis of information on various payment and financing mechanisms. Research on the utilization of health services helps to improve the development and allocation of health resources, and such data also have implications for medical education and for the development of new forms of medical practice.

Research on *health services manpower* is concerned with the supply, distribution, recruitment, and training of health workers. The impact of changing patterns of health services on the requirements for health personnel, including new types of personnel, is an important aspect of this area of research. Some specific topics of investigation include the factors that affect the current distribution of health workers and the choice of field or health specialty. Professional training programs are the subject of research on topics such as methods of training and the relationship between training programs and subsequent professional performance. Research on methods of continuing education of health practitioners and the effects of such programs contributes to the goal of improving the quality of performance of health workers.

Disciplines Contributing to
Community Health Research

Many disciplines are involved in the conduct of community health research, and the nature of an increasing number of studies requires utilizing an interdisciplinary team approach. The fields traditionally associated with research in community health and medical care include epidemiology, preventive medicine, public health administration, and medical care administration. However, the increasing scope and complexity of the health services have led to the recognition that the knowledge and methods of several other disciplines are also particularly appropriate.

Economics has obvious relevancy in research on the problems of the costs and financing of health services. Researchers from political science, law, and metropolitan and community planning are gradually becoming involved in the sociopolitical aspects of the organization and administration of community health services and medical care. Studies of the structure and process of governmental decision making are also within the area of these latter disciplines, and such topics are of considerable importance in the field of community health.

The behavioral sciences, i.e., anthropology, social psychology, and particularly sociology, are important in the emerging community health research picture. Within the last decade, social scientists from these disciplines have undertaken a wide variety of studies in the health field, pertaining to the social, psychological, and cultural aspects of health problems. A review of more than 500 such researches being conducted during a recent five-year period revealed that the studies were fairly evenly divided into two general categories.[13] The first category had to do with disease or impairment and health and included studies of the relationship of social factors to disease etiology, incidence, prevalence, and distribution. This category also included the study of problems concerning patient response and adjustment to disease and to the therapeutic process. The second category of researches was concerned with the organization of medical care and included investigations of social factors relating to the utilization of services and facilities. Health personnel was also the subject of study in this category, as was the nature of the social structure and relationships within organizational settings.

Potentially, payoff is great for improvement of services from studies of the elements of health systems of nations and their regional subdivisions. However, research progress is complicated by the fact that the analysis of the delivery of community health services must sooner or later involve itself with society's larger social values in a way that pure epidemiology does only rarely. This often gives rise to resistance or apathy regarding the conduct of such research. Health delivery systems characteristically involve vested cultural, professional, and organizational interests at all levels, with these interests not always being congruent with public good.

There is also the fact of the sheer size and complexity of modern society, making difficult the development of appropriate methodologies for the study of community health phenomena. Moreover, much community health research—largely descriptive in nature—has tended to document the facts of unequal distribution of health and medical care services. Certain innovations have taken place in recent decades (e.g., the emergence of home care services and prepaid health insurance plans), and it has been possible to assess their impact. However, community health research will only reach maturity when serious alternatives of appropriate magnitude are presented for appraisal of their impact on the public's health.

SUMMARY

Epidemiology is both a body of knowledge and a method of investigating the occurrence, distribution, and causes of disease in human populations. Broadly defined, it deals with the entire health-disease spectrum, and its ultimate goal is the prevention of disease. Although during early stages of its development epidemiology was concerned mainly with the infectious diseases, in more recent years its scope has broadened to include all diseases.

Epidemiology seeks to add to the knowledge of the natural history of disease, which describes the health-disease process in terms of the interaction among numerous specific agent, human host, and environmental factors. The interaction between agent, host, and environmental factors determines the relative health or disease status of a population. Through epidemiologic investigations, information about these factors is assembled and analyzed for the purpose of describing the occurrence, distribution, and cause of disease.

The conduct of epidemiologic investigations and various other kinds of related researches requires the utilization of the basic principles and orderly procedures which characterize the "scientific method." Accuracy and precision of observations and measurements, reduction of bias that may originate from a variety of sources, and formulation of data-substantiated conclusions are among the goals of scientific investigations of all kinds. The orderly procedures of scientific investigation and research generally involve several steps: the definition of the problem to be investigated; review of existing knowledge on the subject; several considerations in connection with the design of the investigation, including provisions for testing hypotheses; collection of the data through observations and measurements; and classification, tabulation, and statistical analysis of the data.

The descriptive, analytic, and experimental aspects of epidemiology may be viewed as representing a continuum that ranges from an account of disease occurrence and distribution to the establishment of disease causation. The descriptive phase involves ascertaining the frequency and distribution of disease in a population in terms of the characteristics of the time and the place in which persons are found affected and in terms of the attributes of the affected persons themselves. Analytic and experimental investigations are designed to test hypotheses regarding the determinants and mechanisms of disease; such hypotheses are often suggested by descriptive information. Analytic investigations, which commonly involve the conduct of prospective or retrospective studies, seek to determine the statistical association between a specific factor and a given disease. Experimental investigations provide a rigorous test of an association by introducing an experimental condition in a test group, but not in a comparable control group, and observing the effect over a period of time. Ideally, an experiment is conducted under "double-blind" conditions.

In addition to epidemiologic investigations, there are also many other kinds of research that have a health-related focus. There are countless specific topics which constitute the subject of research within the broad areas of planning, organizing, and delivering health services. Costs, financing, and utilization of services, as well as health services manpower, are other areas of community health research. Numerous different disciplines are involved in the conduct of these researches, often on an interdisciplinary basis. The social sciences, political science, law, and economics are among the disciplines that particularly contribute to community health research.

REFERENCES

1. MacMahon, B., Pugh, T. F., and Ipsen, J. *Epidemiologic Methods*. Little, Brown and Company, Boston, 1960.

2. Paul, John R. *Clinical Epidemiology*, revised ed. The University of Chicago Press, Chicago, 1966.

3. Clark, E. G. The epidemiologic approach and contributions to preventive medicine. In: Leavell, H. R., and Clark, E. G., eds. *Preventive Medicine for the Doctor in His Community*, 3rd ed. McGraw-Hill Book Company, New York, 1965.

4. Cassel, John M. Potentialities and limitations of epidemiology. In: Katz, A. H., and Felton, J. S., eds. *Health and the Community*. The Free Press, New York, 1965.

5. SARTWELL, PHILIP E. Epidemiology. In: Sartwell, P. E., ed. *Maxcy-Rosenau Preventive Medicine and Public Health*, 9th ed. Appleton-Century-Crofts, New York, 1965.

6. TERRIS, MILTON. The scope and methods of epidemiology. *Amer J Public Health*, **52**:1371–76, September 1962.

7. ROGERS, FRED B., ed. *Studies in Epidemiology: Selected Papers of Morris Greenberg, M.D.* G. P. Putnam's Sons, New York, 1965.

8. MORRIS, J. N. *Uses of Epidemiology*, 2nd ed. The Williams and Wilkins Company, Baltimore, 1964.

9. CLARK, E. G., and LEAVELL, H. R. Levels of application of preventive medicine. In: Leavell, H. R., and Clark, E. G., eds. *Preventive Medicine for the Doctor in His Community*, 3rd ed. McGraw-Hill Book Company, New York, 1965.

10. DENSEN, PAUL M. Statistical reasoning. In: Sartwell, P. E., ed. *Maxcy-Rosenau Preventive Medicine and Public Health*, 9th ed. Appleton-Century-Crofts, New York, 1965.

11. GREENBERG, BERNARD G. Biostatistics. In: Leavell, H. R., and Clark, E. G., eds. *Preventive Medicine for the Doctor in His Community*, 3rd ed. McGraw-Hill Book Company, New York, 1965.

12. TAYLOR, I., and KNOWELDEN, J. *Principles of Epidemiology*. Little, Brown and Company, Boston, 1958.

13. WELLIN, E., and SEACAT, M. S. Social science in the health field—a review of research (1954–1959). *Amer J Public Health*, **52**:1465–72, September 1962.

SECTION III

CONCEPTS, NATURE, AND SCOPE OF PUBLIC HEALTH PROGRAMS

CHAPTER 5

MEDICAL CARE

The various aspects of medical care organization in the United States are discussed in this chapter, and current needs, aspiration, and challenges in the field of medical care are reviewed. Following the presentation of a general definition of medical care in the first section of the chapter, the second section describes the responsibilities which the different levels of government—local, state, and federal—have assumed for medical care over the years. The factors that have led in recent years to a broadened point of view regarding government's role in medical care are discussed in the third section. The next two sections are devoted to a description and evaluation of various contemporary, specific modes of providing and financing medical care. The last section of the chapter reviews the outlook for the future regarding the attainment of a desirable partnership between public and private efforts in the provision of medical care for the American people.

THE SCOPE OF MEDICAL CARE

Medical care consists of the provision of services to the individual with the intention of preventing illness or of aborting or mitigating the course of illness once it has begun. From a community vantage point, medical care services are all the personal health services, including the care of sick and disabled persons, which are rendered by individual physicians, nurses, and related personnel and by private and public agencies.

It is generally recognized that to be effective, medical care must extend well beyond the provision of treatment to the sick and, indeed, must cover the entire range of services: preventive, curative, and rehabilitative. It is therefore understandable that, with such a gamut of varied needs to be met, there has developed over time a vast complex of individuals and institutions laboring in the field of medical care.

THE HISTORIC ROLE OF GOVERNMENT IN PROVIDING MEDICAL CARE IN THE UNITED STATES

Government involvement in the direct provision of medical care in the United States is a phenomenon as old as the country itself. Over the years, the various levels of government—local, state, and federal—have each undertaken different kinds of responsibilities in generating programs in medical care.

The Role of State and Local Governments

The provision of medical care for the poor was one of the earliest responsibilities of state and local governments. It was a direct outgrowth of the Elizabethan Poor Laws, which were in force in England at the time the colonies were settled. The so-called "poor doctors" appointed by colonial town governments were certainly no examples of providers of high-quality medical care, and neither were the almshouses set up to get the sick poor off the streets. However, many of these latter institutions, of which the Bellevue Almshouse in colonial New York is but one example, developed into charity hospitals where the greatest men in American medicine subsequently taught and practiced.

The control of communicable diseases likewise was largely taken on by state and municipal governments as part of the powers reserved to the states by the United States Constitution. The more enlightened states early introduced such measures as compulsory vaccination of school children and built sanitaria where infectious tuberculosis could be isolated and treated. Local governments set up clinics, as well, for the control of venereal diseases and, in the course of time, frequently developed programs providing services at the preventive end of the medical care scale, such as screening for glaucoma, diabetes, and cancer of the cervix—all filling an unmet need in their communities.

The Role of the Federal Government

Despite the general consensus that public health matters largely belonged within the purview of state and local government, the federal government, almost from its inception, became involved in the direct provision of medical care services. Thus, the federal government assumed responsibilities for the care of merchant seamen in special marine hospitals which were operative by 1798. This program was the origin of the U.S. Public Health Service, which today, among its other duties, operates a clinical center to which patients are referred for specialized care. The federal government likewise undertook to establish and operate a national leprosarium, a hospital for drug addiction, and two special hospitals in Washington, D.C., one for Negroes and one for the mentally ill.

Another responsibility the national government assumed was the rendering of medical care to the American Indians. This obligation began informally when U.S. Army doctors sought to control smallpox and other contagious diseases among the Indians living near military posts. Subsequently, as the tribes were pushed back onto reservations, the federal government entered into numerous treaties with the tribes. Of the 400 treaties written between 1778 and 1871, 24 contained provisions by which the government promised to render medical care to the Indians—including, occasionally, hospital care. While most of these medical clauses were written to cover only a period of less than 20 years, the medical care was in fact continued by so-called "gratuity appropriations" which Congress allotted year by year. After being shifted from the War Department to the Department of the Interior and finally, in 1955, to the Department of Health, Education, and Welfare, the health care of the Indians became the responsibility of the U.S. Public Health Service. Today the Indian Health Service of the Public Health Service provides direct medical care from the federal government to approximately 380,000 people through a system of 50 hospitals, 26 health centers, and several hundred field clinics. Largely through the efforts of this program, the health standards of the American Indian, which up to now have been a national disgrace, have begun to improve in the last ten years.

Along with its obligations to protect the nation's safety by maintaining a military force, the federal government assumed the responsibility of assuring the health of military personnel. In a civilian nation such as the United States, the military is of necessity at a disadvantage in competing for career medical officers. Despite the limitations imposed by this circumstance, however, the American military medical system has managed not only to maintain world renowned medical facilities, such as Walter Reed Army Hospital, in which United States presidents and other dignitaries are often treated, but also has introduced throughout its facilities such well-accepted guarantees of high-quality care as the requirement that all surgery be done by specialists. This is no small feat in a country where fully one half of surgery is performed by general practitioners. The federal government also has taken major responsibility for the medical care of retired military personnel and of military dependents. The number of military dependents now exceeds 3,360,000.

American service veterans constitute a final, large group for whom the federal government has, over the years, assumed responsibility for pro-

tality; an increasing demand for more and better medical services, which has been outstripping the ability of the private sector to meet the demand; and an increasing social consciousness among the population, which has motivated efforts to make society's benefits available to all and not merely to a privileged few.

The ascendancy of chronic diseases was a by-product of the introduction of the "wonder drugs," such as the sulfas, penicillin, and the broad-spectrum antibiotics, and the new vaccines, such as those for the prevention of polio and measles. As these and other pharmaceutical innovations brought under control infectious diseases which had once been major killers, the United States population, already receiving the benefits of modern environmental sanitation, began to live to more advanced age and to fall prey to chronic diseases which tend to run their course in prolonged and costly fashion. These chronic diseases, afflicting largely people who were beyond their prime earning years, created a large pool of patients who could not readily afford to purchase care from the private sector and who, therefore, looked to government for assistance.

The increasing demand for more and better medical services, which has been termed a "revolution of rising expectation in consumer demand," was brought about in part by World War II, when many Americans experienced for the first time in their lives the benefits of comprehensive medical care for themselves and their dependents as a by-product of military service. Another factor in the drastically increased demand was the advance in medical technology, which affected a host of techniques, from blood banking to operative surgery, and gave medicine capabilities that were undreamed of only a few years before. The revolutionary advances in communication which paralleled these gains in medical technology created an expanded awareness of, and demand for, the new type of medical care. The dimensions of this demand were so great, and the cost of making the benefits of the new medical technology generally available were so prohibitive, that again people looked to government to provide what was wanted.

The increasing social awareness in the United States has led to a recognition of the existence of great pockets of unmet medical needs within a generally affluent society. The benefits to be derived from the advances of medical technology have been particularly unattainable for the segments of the population who are in impoverished circumstances. These segments include minority groups, the elderly, migrant workers, and numerous other groups who are at or near the poverty level. In such groups are found the most urgent medical needs, often compounded by a complex of health and social problems. The American people have become unwilling to tolerate inequities in the distribution of medical and social benefits, but the complexity of rectifying the problems of some groups of the population are too great for the private sector to solve without substantial government help.

As a consequence of the influence of the various factors just described, there is in the United States the beginning of a partnership between government and the private sector, seeking together to provide fully comprehensive medical care for everyone. The goal is not yet in sight, and even the first tentative beginnings of the partnership have been fraught with major problems, although there also have been some notable gains. The scope of medical care services in which the government is involved is today already broad, and continues to broaden. Still, for many reasons, the great task of bringing order to the field of medical care has not been assumed by government in this country. Without government to play the role of leader and coordinator in the area of medical care, the American health story is one of inequities, rising costs, and widely disparate standards of quality. There is still an enormous gap separating technical know-how and the ability to apply the benefits of this know-how to the population at large. The American people tolerate this situation partly through fear of the deleterious consequences of government involvement and partly through ignorance of the potential benefits which organization offers in the field of medical care.

ORGANIZING THE PROVISION OF MEDICAL CARE

The health agency complex, that is, the portion of society, both public and private, involved in rendering medical care or otherwise protecting the health of the population, is a vast array of individuals and agencies. Only a portion of the health agency complex is engaged in the direct provision of health services. The "direct providers" of services include, among others, physicians, nurses, technicians, hospitals, nursing homes, and home care programs. These are surrounded by, and increasingly dependent on, a large network of "indirect providers" consisting of individuals, institutions, and agencies that constitute a sizable segment of the health agency complex. The functions of the "indirect providers" cover a broad spectrum. Some are involved with the financing of health services, and these include the insurance companies, welfare agencies, and certain charitable foundations. Some are involved in research and evaluation activities and include certain divisions within universities and some national voluntary agencies. Still others are educational, such as the professional schools and national professional associations; or regulatory, such as the federal Food and Drug Administration or the professional licensing boards. The ratio of total health workers to physicians has been steadily increasing.

Physician's Services

Private Practice. The system of private medical practice is rooted in the American tradition of individualism and free enterprise which gained prominence at the turn of the century. Most private practice is conducted on a solo, fee-for-service basis. In receiving medical care under private practice, the patient employs whatever physician he wishes or is able to employ, at such times and in such circumstances as the patient may feel the need of service and is able to pay for it. The physician attends the patient for as long as the arrangement is mutually satisfactory, has responsibility to no authority other than the patient, and looks to him and him alone for payment.

Government does not at all enter into this private arrangement, except that the physician must be duly licensed to practice medicine in the state in which he is located and must, of course, observe the laws of the state regarding medical practice. Should he exhibit what the patient regards as carelessness or neglect or incompetence, the patient may attempt to recover through the courts on a malpractice charge. Should the patient prove unable or unwilling to pay for services rendered, the physician may follow the usual civil procedure of creditor versus debtor in an attempt to collect. It may be said that malpractice suits are relatively unusual, as is court action by the physician in an attempt to collect a bill.

Group Practice. With regard to the provision of medical care, the medical profession in the United States traditionally has been individualistically and entrepreneurially oriented. In its struggle to defeat "socialized medicine," the profession, through its official spokesmen, has viewed high-quality care and fee-for-service reimbursement of physicians as dual concepts. However, there are numerous instances to be found—for example, the Mayo Clinic and the best university teaching hospitals—in which physicians receive a salary and yet, by common consensus, deliver some of the highest quality of care available today in the United States and perhaps in the world. In addition, most of the great recent advances in American medicine are the product of salaried, university-based physicians, aided by government research grants. Yet solo, fee-for-service practice still persists as an ideal.

In spite of counterpressures, however, increasing numbers of physicians are electing other than a solo, fee-for-service practice, including salaried positions and group practice. The term *group practice* is confusing, because if group practice is considered as being the opposite of solo practice, then the large number of physicians who fall into the group category are in a variety of practice settings covering a broad spectrum. At one end of this spectrum is the physician who is actually in solo practice, but who is located in a setting, such as a medical arts buildings, in which he habitually refers patients to a small group of colleagues located in his proximity. At the other end of the spectrum are the physicians organized into closed-panel, multispecialty groups, with some formalized arrangement for sharing of income and expenses. Even in this latter extreme of the spectrum, the number of physicians has been increasing, and in fact has more than tripled since 1946.

The key factor in the shift toward group practice has been the increasing specialization of physicians, which in turn was the offshoot of the rapid advances in medical technology of recent years. As technology brought rapid change to every aspect of medical practice, specialization and sub-specialization became the only mechanism by which a physician could manage to keep abreast of the latest developments in the field in which he was working. It soon became apparent to the specialists, however, that they were not treating the *entire* patient in the way the general practitioner traditionally had done. By forming into groups no matter how loosely orga-nized, the specialists restored among themselves the ability to treat the whole patient by the provision of ready mechanisms for consultation in case a patient happened to cross specialty lines in his symptom complex.

From the standpoint of quality of medical care rendered, groups offer several distinct advantages over solo practice. First, the close collaboration among several physicians tends to establish an atmosphere of peer review of each person's professional activity. Second, each physician has easy access to consultation when he is in an area of uncertainty and has no fear of losing his patient to the consultant. Third, many groups have sufficient income and volume of patients to permit the purchase of superior, expensive equip-ment and to justify a laboratory on the premises. Both these measures aid the physician in improving the quality of care he delivers. Fourth, many group practice agreements specify that the physicians may take time each year to attend medical conferences and refresher courses, thus again increas-ing the potential for betterment of quality of care.

For the consumer likewise, there are many benefits from receiving care through a group practice. First, in a well-developed group, he is offered the benefits of an entire array of specialists, each ready to consult as his case may require. Second, many groups offer patients preventive care of a kind that is not readily available from solo practitioners. Some groups effect a cost saving to patients by stressing the use of out-of-hospital treatment wherever possible. Finally, groups offer the patient continuity of care and coverage that is available every hour of every day.

Comprehensive group practices are still very few in number in the United States, and many of those that exist are understaffed and overworked, with resultant patient complaints about long waiting lines and depersonalized care. Few patients, however, complain about the quality of care they re-ceive, and the statistics on group practices seem to confirm the impression that quality of care delivered is better than average. Also, few patients complain about the cost of care from a group. Those defects that exist in group practices today are mostly not inherent in the group practice con-cept and can be corrected. The concept is sound and, if intelligently applied, offers many advantages over individual, solo practice.

Institutions: Hospitals

Changing Role of the Hospital.   The place of the hospital in American medical care has undergone dramatic change in recent years. Not long ago, the hospital was a place where the very poor and the hopelessly sick languished in their misery. Today all this has changed.

One reason for the change in the status of the American hospital stems from advances in medical technology. Pharmaceutical advances and intricate, new machinery have provided modern medicine with previously undreamed-of potential for altering the course of disease. Other technologic advances have enormously extended the diagnostic acumen of medicine. Because the new technology is often dependent on expensive machinery and large numbers of personnel, the locus for application of its innovations has come to be the hospital. Patients today come to the hospital expecting to be improved, rather than to die, and physicians look upon the hospital as their workshop—a place where they can do more for their patients than is possible in a home or office setting. The trend is illustrated in Figure 5-1, which shows that, over the past three decades, more and more people

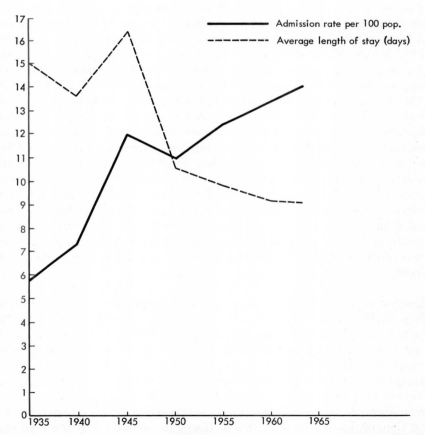

FIGURE 5-1. General hospital use: 1935–1963. (Source: Adapted from Public Health Service, U.S. Department of Health, Education, and Welfare. *Health, Education, and Welfare Trends.* 1964 Edition, Part I, p. 28.)

have been admitted to the hospital annually, while length of stay per admission has been concurrently declining.

A second reason for the changing role of the hospital in America today is related to the physician specialization which has already been mentioned. The strong, current trend toward physician specialization is resulting in a scarcity of general practitioners. Additionally, many of the practicing physicians are reluctant to make house calls or to see patients at odd hours. As a result, the hospital emergency room and outpatient department are replacing the family physician to a large extent. It is estimated that as few as one half of the patients seen in the emergency room of today's hospital are genuine emergency cases, or even in need of urgent attention. While admissions to hospitals have increased markedly since 1945, increases in the volume of patients seen in the emergency rooms and in the outpatient department are even more pronounced.

Factors in the Cost of Hospital Care.   The cost of hospitalization has been rising extremely rapidly for a number of reasons. Much of the increase can be traced to the change in content of a day in hospital. The new medical technology, often relying on the employment of many personnel in order to be properly applied, is expensive; and the hospital patient, as the beneficiary of the medical advances, must pay the cost. One need only think of the modern intensive-care unit, with its complex of machines and around-the-clock personnel, to appreciate the heavy cost of one aspect of modern hospitalization. To a less dramatic degree almost every phase of hospital operation has been affected by the same cost-increasing phenomena. Salaries of hospital employees, which have traditionally been held at substandard levels, have been forced upward by shortages in the labor market in recent years. The need to hire additional personnel also has helped to increase hospital costs. Finally, the percentage of unpaid bills is much greater among outpatients and emergency clinic patients than among inpatients, and so the expansion of the former services results in an enlarged deficit which must be added to the inpatient's bill if the hospital is to remain solvent.

Quality of Hospital Care.   There are 7127 hospitals in the United States today. Eighty-six per cent of these are run as nonprofit institutions; the remaining 14 per cent are run for profit.[1] The latter group consists mostly of smaller institutions, and these are the cause of most of the concern regarding the quality of American hospital care.

Hospitals in the United States operate with a fair degree of autonomy in regard to quality of care delivered. The major effort to achieve quality care is through the mechanism of *accreditation,* which is granted by the Joint Commission on Accreditation of Hospitals, sponsored by the American Hospital Association, the American Medical Association, the American College of Physicians, and the American College of Surgeons. Only hospitals having approved intern and residency training are required to be accredited; for other hospitals, accreditation is voluntary. Eleven per cent of hospitals are approved for intern training, and 18 per cent are approved for residency training (only 6 per cent are affiliated with a medical school). Altogether, 63 per cent of hospitals are currently accredited, but they contain over 80 per cent of the nation's hospital beds.[1]

The standards set for accreditation are not excessive. Many of the regulations refer to proper record keeping. In addition, an accredited hospital must have at least 25 beds, a proper system for dispensing of drugs, clinical and pathology laboratories, and an x-ray department. The hospital staff must be organized into committees, including a tissue committee to review surgical practices at the institution. Since the passage of the new federal Medicare legislation,* accredited hospitals are also required to have utilization review committees to examine bed occupancy in terms of admitting diagnosis, length of stay, and treatment prescribed. Many of the better hospitals have long maintained standards far in excess of these rather minimal requirements, but the existence of the accreditation process has helped motivate institutions to achieve at least minimal quality standards.

The Role of Government in the Provision of Hospitals. Government at the local, state, or federal level is a major force in American hospital care. In 1946, under the provisions of the Hospital Survey and Construction Act (Hill-Burton), federal matching funds were made available to the states for hospital construction. The purpose of the Act was to improve the distribution of hospitals, particularly in the many rural areas which were far removed from adequate facilities. In order to qualify under the program, the states had to develop a statewide priority list for hospital construction, so that the majority of construction under the joint program would take place in areas of greatest need. Rural facilities were of necessity stressed, because population-to-bed ratios were the basis for setting statewide priorities. In the 20 years that the Hill-Burton program has been in operation, the states, with federal participation, have invested over $6 billion for hospital construction, providing over 300,000 beds and over 2000 laboratories, diagnostic and treatment centers, and other health facilities.[2]

The net effect of the Hill-Burton program has been perhaps an overbuilding of rural facilities, since in the same 20 years, the population of the United States has shifted markedly into urban centers. The plight of urban hospitals, many of them old and overcrowded, was not alleviated by the Hill-Burton Act. Very recent amendments to the Act, however, now make it possible to modernize urban hospitals with what are currently called Hill-Harris funds.

Despite the efforts of the Hill-Burton program to achieve statewide plans for hospital construction, a true national effort at areawide hospital planning

---

* Medicare, which provides government-sponsored health insurance for persons aged 65 and older, is discussed in a later section of this chapter.

has not materialized. The reason for this lies largely in the fact that Hill-Burton funds represent but a fraction of the monies put into hospital construction annually. Since the government program does not really control the purse strings of hospital construction, its attempts at control have been predestined to failure. In the absence of consistent areawide planning, hospitals have tended to grow in an unplanned manner. More often than not, the final decision to add costly equipment or beds has been based on local pride rather than demonstrated need. This has resulted in much duplication of effort, waste of funds, and construction of facilities that were not subsequently fully utilized. This is the picture by and large across the nation today. There are a few exceptions in places such as Rochester, New York, where hospital planning on an areawide basis has been successfully achieved. Almost invariably, however, such success is predicated on the fact that one major economic power has been present and has used its influence to help achieve the desired end. In most places, where sources of funds for hospital construction are diffuse, the pressure to achieve areawide planning has been notably lacking.

The need to establish a network of hospital facilities which would bring the benefits of the most up-to-date medicine from the large medical centers to the smallest rural facility has been apparent to the federal government for some time. Aside from duplication of effort and waste of funds, the absence of such a network has prolonged the gap between advances in medicine and their general availability to the public. It was to remedy this situation that Congress, in 1965, enacted legislation creating a "Heart Disease, Cancer, and Stroke" program. Under the rubric of fighting the three major killer diseases affecting the United States, the program established grants to assist areas in planning and demonstrating the feasibility of developing regional complexes for diagnosis and treatment of disease. This program is still in its infancy but promises to become of major significance. The government hopes that, within the new regional complexes, an interchange will occur leading to continuing education of physicians and health personnel who are currently remote from the great medical centers. Hopefully, also, the new complexes will educate the communities they serve to the advantages of areawide planning and allocation of resources. The potential for upgrading quality of care through such complexes is apparent. In addition, some real cost savings should be possible as facilities are drawn into a cooperative network in which, ideally, each will operate at maximum efficiency without wasteful interinstitutional rivalry.

Institutions: Nursing Homes

The American network of nursing homes, which today includes over 13,000 institutions, is largely an unexpected offshoot of the Social Security Act passed by the federal government in 1935. The original Act, which has often been amended in the intervening years, contained not only sections setting up old-age and unemployment insurance programs, but also provisions for federal matching funds to be given to states in order to provide public assistance to the aged and to needy children. Mindful of the existence of public poorhouses however, and anxious to empty these out, the federal legislators specified that recipients of public assistance under this program could not be residents in public institutions. Residents in private institutions were not similarly excluded, however.

The net result was that nursing homes, privately owned and catering primarily to old people eligible for public assistance money, sprang up all over the country. Although the Social Security Act subsequently was amended to allow payment for medical care in public institutions, the proprietary nursing homes, many owned by physicians, continued to dominate the scene. In contrast to hospitals, about 90 per cent of nursing homes in the United States today are run for profit. Approximately half of the patients in nursing homes are recipients of public assistance benefits, mostly in the category of Old Age Assistance.[3]

Nursing homes generally are depressing places and, again in contrast to the majority of American hospitals, are no credit to the general system of medical care. The patients in these institutions, average age around 80, offer little challenge to the medical and nursing professions and have been gladly ignored as much as possible by the medical care system of the average American community. Often the physical plant of a nursing home is antiquated and even hazardous. Even newer nursing home construction, while geared to better standards of hygiene and nursing staff convenience, often ignores the fact that nursing homes are not hospitals and that the requirements of the two patient populations are widely disparate. Certain countries in Europe have recognized this difference and are far ahead of the United States in almost every aspect of nursing home care today.

Quality of care within nursing homes has been largely inadequate, with absence of even such minimal measures as a nurse in attendance around the clock, a physician on call at all times, and acceptable maintenance of patient records. The new federal Medicare legislation, in its provision for extended care, has sought to bring some improvements in the quality of care provided by nursing homes.

The Medicare law specifies that, in order to qualify for treating Medicare beneficiaries, a nursing home must have an arrangement with a hospital for an orderly transfer back and forth of both patients and records. In addition, to qualify, a nursing home must have round-the-clock nursing services, with at least one registered nurse employed full time; a physician available to handle emergencies; appropriate medical policies governing the facility's skilled nursing care and related services; specified methods and procedures for the handling of drugs; and utilization review procedures similar to those required of hospitals participating in the Medicare program.[4] It was estimated that, at the time of the passage of the Medicare legislation, only a very small percentage of American nursing homes met even these rather minimal standards, and therefore, the beginning of the extended care benefits under the law was delayed six months beyond the start of the rest of the program in order to allow a reasonable number of nursing home beds to come into compliance. The Medicare legislation has also stimulated the formation of a Joint Committee on Accreditation of Nursing Homes, similar in sponsorship and purpose to the body that has for years been successfully handling the hospital accreditation program.

The ultimate hope of most responsible people in the medical care field is to see nursing homes become predominantly nonproprietary and closely linked with nonproprietary hospitals to the benefit of patient care in both types of institution. At the moment, with the extreme shortage of available nonproprietary nursing home beds relative to the need for extended care, the outlook is for continued preponderance of the proprietary nursing home. With the advent of emphasis on improved quality of nursing home care, however, as illustrated by the new federal legislation and efforts from the private sector as well, the ability to turn a profit in the ownership of a nursing home may diminish, and the balance may shift to nonprofit ownership in time.

There still remains, also, the problem of redefining the function of nursing homes, so that they may be organized to suit more closely the needs of the patients themselves. Within the nursing home population there are those whose primary needs are for nursing care and those whose primary needs are for custodial care. These two groups would benefit from widely differing institutions, and ultimately one would hope that nursing homes, in their architecture and staffing, would reflect a recognition of this divergence in patient needs.

Auxiliary Services: Home Care Programs

In view of the rising cost of hospital care, it would seem desirable to handle as much of medical care as possible on a nonhospital basis, and home care, when feasible, offers an attractive alternative to hospitalization. Although the cost of a day in a hospital may average $50 or more, a day of home care will cost about $5. Furthermore, for the patient with a satisfactory home environment, many comforts are available that no institution can provide. It is important, however, to emphasize that home care is a desirable alternative to hospitalization only when the home itself is adequate. There are many patients whose home situation precludes rest or proper attention, and for these, care in an institution is preferable even though more expensive.

It is estimated that only about 60 of the nation's hospitals have home care programs today, and few health departments and private agencies have alleviated this deficiency. Again, the new federal Medicare legislation is stimulating progress in this area. The law provides funds for home care, in addition to care in institutions, and it is widely recognized as being to the taxpayer's ultimate advantage to develop this alternative maximally. The federal law requires that Medicare patients on home care be under a treatment plan established by a physician within 14 days of discharge from a hospital or extended care facility. In addition, home health agencies, in order to qualify, must be either publicly owned or nonprofit; or, if they are proprietary, they must meet specified staffing and quality regulations.

Many local health departments have viewed the development of comprehensive home care programs as one of the chief roles that they can fulfill under the Medicare program, and their multidisciplinary staffing would appear particularly well suited for this. Various ancillary programs devoted primarily to other than the medical aspects of home care, such as meals-on-wheels and the homemaker programs, need to be expanded and integrated with the newly developing programs of home medical care. The over-all problem is partly one of current personnel shortage and partly one of redefinition of goals for existing programs. The problems are great but not insurmountable, and there are significant potential benefits to be derived from successful development of home care programs on a large scale.

Auxiliary Services: Community Projects

There are many other areas of problems and promise in the organization for provision of medical care, one of them being community projects which have medical care components. In recent years there have been a number of major programs, funded federally and implemented locally, such as Project Headstart, which is a program to overcome the cultural deprivation of preschool-age children from the slums, and the Job Corps, which seeks to redirect deprived young people into economically productive channels. These programs are not primarily health oriented, but in attempting the total rehabilitation of victims of poverty they soon find themselves embarked on a health program in addition to their other activities, and not infrequently the health component of the program mushrooms, adding scope and cost at an alarming rate. The organizational difficulties that ensue are often equally alarming. The problems that these projects encounter in attempting to render medical care to a defined population are, in miniature, the same problems that are encountered in seeking to provide medical care to the community at large.

The first difficulty comes in trying to estimate the extent of need for care in the target group. Usually there is some commitment to do a thorough physical examination in order to screen the program participants for health defects right at the outset. These initial examinations present logistic problems in themselves, but the real problems relate to what will be uncovered at the examinations and what should be done in the nature of follow-up on these initial diagnoses. It soon becomes apparent that if the goal is to achieve perfect health for every member of the target group, the size of the demand for medical care services is close to infinity, as is the cost.

The second problem, therefore, is that of establishing a cutoff point beyond which the project will not attempt to provide care. There generally develops a consensus that all acute conditions diagnosed, that is, all life-endangering conditions, should be remedied if at all possible, and likewise that physical barriers to work or learning (depending on the emphasis of the over-all project) should be corrected as much as possible. This still leaves a large gray area, however. A frequent thorny problem that arises is dental care—whether or not, for example, everyone in the project should have a full mouth x-ray, receive total mouth restoration, and perhaps even have orthodontia. There is also the issue of the provision of psychiatric service for the majority of the group, who will probably have identifiable, if not totally disabling, mental disease. Still other dilemmas arise concerning the provision of elective surgery, expensive diagnostic work-ups of borderline abnormalities, and prophylactic drug therapy.

The third problem is the determination of the best method for obtaining whatever care is thought to be required. Some will argue that all available monies should go on a fee-for-service basis to physicians in the community and that the physicians should see the patients only in their private offices. Others will try to get the target group accepted as one more group by a comprehensive prepayment plan that is tied in with a group practice arrangement. Still others will try to hire personnel to staff a special clinic for the sole use of the project.

Finally, the recruitment of necessary physician time tends to be a problem in community projects, and good referral for follow-up treatment is especially difficult to obtain. Often, the best specialists are too busy to get involved at all, or, if involved, they lose interest as the project continues over time. Quite often it is found that funding for the medical care portion of the project, determined on the basis of inadequate or spurious data, is insufficient to do all that the project personnel consider to be necessary for rendering adequate medical care. At that point the preventive and rehabilitative aspects of the medical care program generally give way before the pressing demand for curative services, and the entire program slips out of balance.

These problems, while easy to describe, are not easy to solve. What is required most of all is a cadre of people trained in the disciplines of medical care organization, able to foresee the needs and pitfalls of medical care programs, and able to take the requisite administrative steps to carry out a successful program. At present, the medical care aspect of community projects is often appended as an afterthought, and the medical program itself is subsequently put together under much pressure by individuals who are not adequately trained to organize a highly complex operation in medical care. The result is frustration and much wasted time, effort, and money.

It is necessary to recognize that the organization of medical care, whether in a community project or in an entire community, is a difficult task requiring special knowledge spanning the fields of medical care, economics, education, administration, and the social sciences. Currently, some schools of public health are attempting to train this type of specialist, but the number of graduates is still very small relative to the number of tasks requiring their skills.

Problems in Organizing the Provision of Medical Care

The preceding discussion has pointed out particular problems in connection with various specific kinds of medical care provisions. For the field of medical care as a whole, there are two important issues pertaining to the organization and provision of services, namely, the maintenance of quality of care and the availability and distribution of medical personnel.

Maintenance of Quality of Medical Care. The maintenance of quality in medical care is a difficult problem, partly because there are no really reliable measures and partly because quality of care is a communitywide phenomenon, extending well beyond the care rendered to an individual patient by an individual practitioner. On a communitywide basis, quality of care is related to the range of services available; the range of medical need in the population; the extent of coverage of the population by the services available (including the appropriateness of the services to the needs of the patients); the cost of care in both money and personnel; and the relation between cost and benefits. One can reasonably hope with effort to gauge all of these factors, but the actual problem of assessing the quality of the medical care services rendered to an *individual* can only be approached by indirect measures.

Probably the best of the indirect measures of quality is peer judgment, that is, an assessment of competence by acknowledged experts in the field of specialization of a professional person or in the area of operation of an institution. Licensure, accreditation, and specialty certification are all variants of peer judgment, and have come into increasing use as mass means for trying to assure quality of care. It is still quite common, however, to see an unaccredited hospital or extended care facility in operation, and many professional services requiring the skill of a specialist are still rendered by physicians who lack specialty certification. In many instances, licensing requirements for facilities and personnel are likewise not sufficiently stringent to ensure high-quality care.

Tissue committees and bed occupancy committees have long been features of the staff organization of better hospitals. The tissue committees have focused on the elimination of unnecessary surgery and have had a high degree of success in many institutions. Bed occupancy committees have so far focused largely on the fiscal aspects of under- or overutilization of hospital beds. However, with the advent of the Medicare program, these committees, renamed utilization review committees, are focusing on the appropriateness of bed use in relation to admitting diagnosis, length of stay, and treatment prescribed.

The technique of medical audit provides procedures in which an institution's practices are continuously assessed against standards derived from comparable institutions. It involves an evaluation of total performance from the audit of multiple, individual operations within the particular institution being examined. Medical audit is still in its infancy, but gives promise of developing into a most useful measure of quality.

Continuing postgraduate education for all levels of professional personnel involved in medical care also predisposes to improved quality. The advance of medical knowledge and technology today is so rapid that it is difficult to avoid obsolescence after leaving school. Professional associations, the universities, and government and private organizations are all developing programs to provide continuing education opportunities on a broad scale.

Government, while constituting a large and increasingly dominant force in the provision of medical services, has been loathe, because of its traditional role, to assert itself in questions regarding quality of care. Too often attempts by government to enforce quality controls have been fearfully rejected as steps leading toward "socialized medicine," a system in which it was asserted doctors and patients alike would lose freedom of action, with consequent disastrous effects on quality of medical care. In the recent Medicare legislation, the federal government has begun to move into the area of quality control by insisting that utilization review be carried out regularly at participating institutions. Some state governments also have attempted to establish quality controls by various measures, including strenthening the functions and authority of regional hospital planning councils. Such steps are the exception, however, and by and large, government has not been active in the area of providing quality controls in medical care.

Availability and Distribution of Medical Personnel.   Many studies in the past sought to assess the adequacy of physician supply in the United States. The study by Roger I. Lee and Lewis W. Jones, conducted for the National Committee on the Costs of Medical Care in 1933, was the first to conclude that a shortage of physicians existed nationally. However, serious action on a national scale to improve the supply of physicians was not undertaken until 1959, after the Surgeon General of the United States had appointed a consultant group which discovered a need for an increase in the yearly output of American medical schools from 8250 to 11,000. Since the lag between planning new medical school facilities and graduating physicians can be as long as ten years, the need for better, ongoing projections of future physician need continues to be very great.

The shortage of nursing personnel in the United States is as great as or greater than the shortage of physicians and is compounded by much confusion regarding educational requirements and the proper role of the nurse on the health team. A report made to the Surgeon General in 1961 found an acute nursing shortage and stated that a tripling of annual nursing school output by 1966 (from 30,000 to 100,000) would be desirable, though clearly not achievable.[5]

Certain groups of health professionals have been much more successful than others in developing cadres of auxiliaries to augment the ranks of the fully trained practitioners. Nurses, dentists, and mental health professionals can be cited as leaders in this area. However, it is quite clear that there is still a noticeable personnel shortage in every sector of American medical care. This shortage is due to increased demand for service and simultaneously increased complexity of the services rendered. Both these factors will become more pronounced in time and will continue to result in an ever-increasing shortage of personnel. It is unrealistic to think of expanding the corps of top professionals indefinitely at a time when, for example, fully 6 per cent of budgeted full-time faculty teaching positions in medical schools are unfilled.[2] The need today is to expand the capabilities of a numerically limited group of professionals. To do this, it is necessary to develop and expand the supply of auxiliaries in every health field. Such a plan would assist immeasurably in forestalling a decline in the quality of medical care offered, a decline which is almost inevitable if the too few trained professionals are forced to carry increasingly excessive work loads.

In addition to general shortages, the various categories of medical personnel are not equally available to all the people or to all geographic parts of the country. Physicians, increasingly specialized in their training, are choosing to work at, or in close proximity to, large modern medical centers, where they can find the latest technologic devices at their disposal, and where they can find a full complement of highly trained colleagues for consultation and referrals. The medical centers are almost invariably located in cities, where the concentration of population is sufficient to carry the high cost of operation. Areas of lesser population density are finding it increasingly difficult to attract the better trained young physicians.

The problems of physician distribution are compounded by problems in the distribution of other highly trained personnel. Nurses in particular tend to congregate with physicians at medical centers and appear reluctant to extend their authority in areas where acute shortage of physicians has produced total gaps in medical care coverage.

ORGANIZING THE FINANCING OF MEDICAL CARE

The Influence of Economic Status on Health

The long-standing provision of free medical care to charity patients gave rise to the popular misconception that, in the United States, the very poor —and, of course, the very rich—got excellent medical care, while those neglected were only the lower middle class who were too poor to pay for the best and not poor enough to qualify for free care. Health statistics do not bear out this myth. On closer examination it becomes clear that the best quality of American medical care is not available to all, and the ones who suffer most are those possessing the least means.

The relation between income and medical care is indicated by Figure 5-2, which shows that, in a recent year, there was a definite correlation

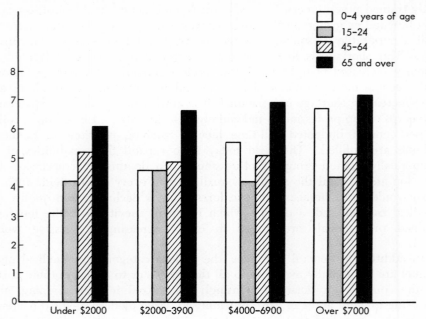

FIGURE 5-2. Physician visits per year, by age and income: 1963–1964. (Source: Adapted from Public Health Service, U.S. Department of Health, Education, and Welfare. *Vital and Health Statistics.* Series 10, No. 19, June, 1965.)

between income and amount of physician services received. Especially dramatic is the effect of income on care received by young children, whose neglect in the early years may lead to irreversible impairments in adult life. Figure 5-2 also shows that the elderly—the typical patients in a charity ward—in reality received more physician services as income increased. The unpleasant truth is that, for many years, priority for care in the United States has been assigned largely in accordance with the patient's ability to pay, and statistics on morbidity and mortality show a strong correlation between level of income and health and longevity at all ages.

An indication of the relationship between economic status and longevity is provided by Figure 5-3, which compares the average life expectancy at birth of white and nonwhite (predominantly Negro) males for the past 60 years. Nonwhite minority groups, because of economic deprivation, have had much more limited access to good care than have white Americans. In 1900, this fact undoubtedly underlay the large discrepancy in white and nonwhite life expectancy noted in Figure 5-3, and the discrepancy still persists, although it has been diminishing over the years.

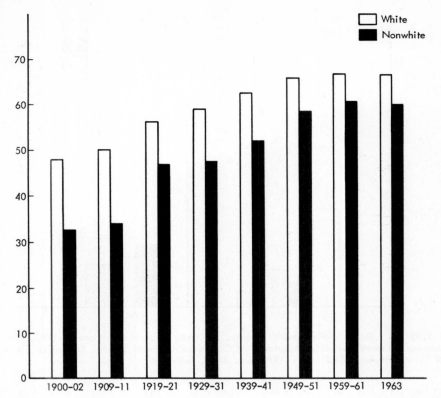

FIGURE 5-3. Average expectation of life in years at birth (males), selected years: 1900–1963. (Source: Adapted from U.S. Bureau of the Census. *Statistical Abstract of the United States, 1965*.)

Income is also related to education, and it is clear that there is wide variation in the United States not only in the people's ability to pay for care, but also in their understanding of the benefits and limitations of presently available care. Those who are less well informed tend to underutilize existing available services and facilities. Nor is this merely a matter of lack of factual information. In many instances, ignorance is accompanied by lack of motivation to seek help—partly due to distrust and partly due to lack of hope, both of which are not uncommon among those whose lives are spent in the shadow of unending, severe poverty.

Costs of Medical Care and Sources of Financing

The cost of providing medical care has been rising steadily and at a rate far in excess of the rise in general price levels. Not all elements of medical care have risen in cost at the same rate, however. Figure 5-4 illustrates the dramatic over-all increase in family expenditures for medical care

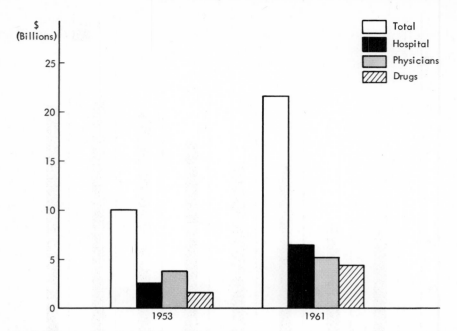

FIGURE 5-4.   Gross family medical charges, by types of services or goods: 1953, 1961. (Source: Adapted from U.S. Department of Commerce, Office of Business Economics. *Survey of Current Business*, 37:21, July, 1957, and 42:14, July, 1962.)

in the past decade. It also shows that expenditures to meet hospital costs and drug costs have had the greatest percentage increase, while expenditures for physician costs have risen much more modestly.

The funds for meeting the cost of medical care come from multiple sources, as was indicated in Chapter 2. The main source is *the consumer* himself, who makes over 70 per cent of the expenditures for health and medical care in the United States today. *Government agencies* are the next largest spenders, paying out over 20 per cent of the total, annually.[6] Much of this government money goes for medical care of the poor, both in clinics, such as well-child centers, and in several state-federal programs of public assistance medical care. Other federal government money goes to programs such as the Veterans Administration and the Indian Health Service, as described earlier. Local governments also make up part of the 20 per cent spent by government agencies. Local governments provide general assistance medical care, which is usually limited to hospitalization and is available only to extreme indigents who are not otherwise eligible for public assistance medical care financed by state and federal monies. The *philanthropic organizations* of the United States provide most of the rest of the funds expended annually for health and medical care, but their overall contribution is small, comprising just over 2 per cent of the total.[6]

Health Insurance: Privately Sponsored

Health insurance emerged as one solution to the problem of providing medical care in the face of rising costs, increasing demand, and declining ability of the consumer to pay his own way. Several types of voluntary health insurance plans, including Blue Cross and Blue Shield, have been in operation since around 1930, but growth was slow until after World War II. In the immediate postwar period, however, there was a major effort to bring government-sponsored health insurance to the country, and strong national forces who saw in this a threat to the traditional American way of life gave their support to the promotion of voluntary health insurance as a preferable method for providing health care financing. The resultant growth was dramatic. In 1940, about 12 million Americans had hospitalization insurance; in 1950, almost 77 million; and by 1963, 145 million persons were covered.[7]

Types and Provisions of Privately Sponsored Health Insurance. There are three principal types of privately sponsored health insurance: provider-sponsored *hospital* insurance (Blue Cross); provider-sponsored *physician's care* insurance (Blue Shield); and commercial health care insurance issued by a variety of commercial insurance companies. A fourth type is the "independent" health insurance plans, which account for about 5 per cent of the total health insurance coverage in force.

In Europe, where government had long operated most of the hospitals, there was no need for hospital insurance, and the advocates of health insurance concentrated on providing coverage for the cost of out-of-hospital physician services. By contrast, in the United States, general hospitals are mostly nongovernment owned and the first effort, of necessity, was an attempt to underwrite hospital costs. Hospitalization insurance has remained the most prevalent type of health insurance policy. Next most prevalent is insurance coverage for surgical expenses, followed rather closely by coverage for nonsurgical physician expenses.

The most recent innovation in health insurance provisions, and still much less prevalent than the other kinds, is the "major medical" plan, which was pioneered by the commercial insurance companies. This covers many items, including hospitalization, physician services, drugs, and nursing care in the event of expensive illness. "Major medical" insurance may be supplementary to basic health insurance or may represent the only coverage that the patient has. In either case, it is typically characterized by a deductible amount of expense which the patient must pay before the policy begins to reimburse his expenses. Furthermore, there is usually a coinsurance feature whereby the patient pays about 20 per cent of all expenses beyond the deductible and a large but definite maximum sum beyond which the insurance policy will not be liable. "Major medical" plans have recently become a feature of Blue Cross and Blue Shield policies.

Blue Cross Plans. Blue Cross was generated by the American Hospital Association, and the Association's Blue Cross Commission must approve any plan that wishes to use the Blue Cross symbol. There are currently 77 plans in the 50 states. The plans operate with a great deal of autonomy. Almost all are enabled, by special state legislation, to operate outside of the confines of state insurance laws. The Blue Cross Commission originally required of each approved plan that it be nonprofit, be organized as a public service, be financially sound, have an advisory board containing hospital trustees and physicians, allow all recognized hospitals to participate in benefits, grant the subscriber free choice of hospital, and allow responsibility for services to rest with the hospitals. These criteria were widely interpreted as endorsing the *community rating system of premiums,* which involves uniform premium rates for all persons regardless of differing risks of illness. The criteria were also interpreted as endorsing *service benefits* (such as coverage for stated number of days in hospital) rather than *indemnity benefits* (such as a fixed dollar sum per day in hospital regardless of charges incurred).

The Blue Cross principle, while laudable in theory, proved very difficult in practice, partly owing to rapidly rising hospital costs and partly owing to competition from the commercial insurance companies. Younger, healthier workers were offered "package deals" by the commercial insurance companies, which included life insurance, disability insurance, and various other benefits in addition to low-cost health insurance. In these "packages," the profitable policies, such as life insurance, covered losses incurred through the health benefit being offered at low premium rates. Blue Cross suffered under this competition and was left with a progressively larger percentage of poor-risk clients attracted by the community rating system of premiums. In 1950, Blue Cross plans paid out in benefits, or put into reserves for future payments, about 88 cents on the dollar, leaving 12 cents to cover administration costs. By 1958, about 97 cents on the dollar were being paid out in benefits, leaving only 3 cents for administration. Soon the plans were dipping into reserves or asking for sizable premium increases. Premium increases, as might be expected, were strongly opposed by the public. The net result has been that Blue Cross, while managing to keep up with the commercial companies in expanded benefits and more flexible contracts for groups, has done so only at the expense of largely abandoning the principle of service benefits.

Commercial Health Care Plans. The commercial companies, arriving on the health insurance scene after the Blue Cross plans and the "independent" plans, soon acquired the dominant position. The "package deals," including health insurance which the commercial companies offered labor groups, as already described, were one reason for their ascendancy. Another reason stemmed from the fact that the commercial companies had no commitment to the ideals of the community rating system of premiums or to service benefits. Using the *experience rating system of premiums*—where the premiums are determined by the actual loss experience in past years of the group at risk—the commercial companies could offer broad health insurance coverage to the better health risks at reduced rates. By paying indemnity benefits rather than service benefits, the companies limited their risk even further.

Blue Shield Plans. Blue Shield, while often working closely with Blue Cross plans, and identified with them in the minds of many people, has had a different history from Blue Cross. The origin of the Blue Shield idea was in the "medical bureaus" set up by local medical societies in the states of Washington and Oregon as an alternative to the closed-panel medical plans provided by the lumber companies. Only gradually were statewide plans formed, and not until 1948 did the American Medical Association consolidate the idea nationally. Blue Shield plans were then required to operate with approval and under responsibility of the state and local medical society; to provide free choice of physician to subscribers; to be nonprofit; and, if possible, to provide service benefits rather than indemnity benefits.

There are today 71 Blue Shield plans in the country. In 30 states they operate outside of the insurance laws, under special enabling legislation which differs, however, from the Blue Cross enabling legislation in the same states. In the remaining 20 states, regular insurance laws cover the Blue Shield plans as well.

Unlike Blue Cross, which has had fairly smooth relations with the hospitals that gave it origin, the relations between Blue Shield and its parent —the medical profession—have been more troubled. There has been much debate about whether physicians should be allowed to charge patients with higher incomes a surcharge beyond the established Blue Shield schedule of fees, thus in effect converting the service benefit of Blue Shield policies into an indemnity benefit for one category of patients. The general rule adopted has been to surcharge patients earning more than a specified amount, or at least to allow the physician freedom to do so. Blue Shield has been more expensive to administer than Blue Cross but still has managed to pay out benefits of around 90 cents on the premium dollar.

"Independent" Health Insurance Plans. The "independent" health insurance plans, although providing only a very small percentage of the coverage nationally, have pioneered the principle of combining prepayment for medical care with group practice and have shown the combination to be workable. The "independents" cover a broad spectrum, from small fraternal programs and consumer cooperatives to giant operations such as the Kaiser Foundation Health Plans and the Health Insurance Plan of

Greater New York. Some plans own their own hospitals, some are closely affiliated with one hospital although they do not own it, and some use a variety of totally unaffiliated community hospitals. The "independents," unlike the Blue Cross and Blue Shield plans or the commercial insurance plans, have always kept close watch on the type of medical care rendered to purchasers of their insurance and have found that, as a result, they are often able to counter the trend toward increased use of hospitalization which has helped to inflate the costs of other types of insurance plans.

Because of their dependence on closed-panel group practices, and also because of much opposition from the medical profession, the "independents" have not shared the phenomenal growth which has characterized the rest of the health insurance industry in the decades since World War II. For years the "independents" were also hampered by lack of an effective voice. In 1959, however, two groups that had represented different factions among the "independents" merged to form the Group Health Association of America, which ever since has worked hard and effectively to unite and represent the diverse organizations that constitute the "independent" category of health insurance plans.

Problems in Privately Sponsored Health Insurance. The various types of privately sponsored health insurance combined are said to provide some coverage for over 70 per cent of the population. This coverage is not uniform in scope, however, and the most comprehensive policies by and large are available to those possessing the least likelihood of being sick. Figure 5-5 shows that the percentage of the population covered by hospital insurance increases with increasing levels of family income. However, increased family income is also related to better nutrition, clothing, and housing and more frequent visits to a physician—all conducive to better over-all health status. Figure 5-5 also indicates that, while all age groups have a larger percentage of insured as income increases, the increment of increase lags far behind for those age 65 and over. This again reflects the fact that health insurance is less available to persons with increased risk of illness. Furthermore, for the aged and infirm who do manage to obtain insurance, the comprehensiveness of coverage is markedly diminished.

Rural families have far less health insurance coverage than do urban families, largely because rural people are less likely to work in a setting where group enrollment is possible. In 1963, the National Health Survey found that only 51 per cent of the rural population in the United States had some kind of insurance for hospitalization.

On a national average, only about one quarter of all individual consumer expenditures for health and medical care are covered by health insurance.[6] Part of the reason for this discrepancy is, again, the patchy coverage of health insurance, which leaves many of those with highest medical care expenses totally uninsured because they have disqualifying "pre-existing conditions" or because they simply cannot afford to pay the premiums.

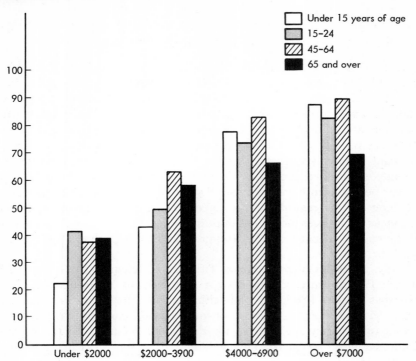

FIGURE 5-5. Percentage of U.S. population with hospital insurance, by age and family income: 1962–1963. (Source: Adapted from Public Health Service, U.S. Department of Health, Education, and Welfare. *Vital and Health Statistics.* Series 10, No. 9, May, 1964.)

Part is also due to the fact that even those people who have health insurance do not have comprehensive coverage. For the fortunate individuals who are properly insured, of course, a very high percentage of medical expenses (up to 80 or 90 per cent) is paid by the insurance policies.[8]

The insurance companies, in the provision of health care plans, have tended to see themselves more as fiscal agents than as spokesmen for improvement of the product that their money is buying. This unwillingness to use the fiscal power at their command to effect changes toward better quality of care has characterized not only the commercial insurance companies who write health insurance as a side line, but also most Blue Cross plans nationally. A few Blue Cross plans, especially recently, have begun to change in this regard and have sought to become spokesmen for the consumer's interest, but to date the potential force for good inherent in the insurance company's great fiscal power has not been sufficiently exerted.

The over-all health insurance picture in the United States has not been satisfactory. The wealthiest nation in the world tends to have a system of health insurance that is patchy with regard to population coverage, less than comprehensive in the range of services covered, and in great measure indifferent to the quality of care rendered to the insured.

Health Insurance: Government Sponsored (Medicare)

The burden of providing elderly persons with comprehensive health insurance is clearly more than the private sector can bear as long as the better health risks are selectively withdrawn from the community-risk pool. As a result, the aged in the United States have lived under the constant threat of pauperization due to medical care costs. They are likely to be burdened with excessive ills whose costs can only be insured against, if at all, at exorbitant premium rates, and at the same time they are likely to have markedly diminished incomes. This same threat has also hung over the younger people who have responsibility for older relatives. The need to do something in this regard for the aged has long been apparent, but the decision as to the best means to adopt in rendering aid was not an easy one, and the ensuing debate raged in Congress and through the nation for many years.

Finally, in 1965, Congress passed Title XVIII, amending the Social Security Act. This measure became known, popularly, as Medicare. Title XVIII establishes a federal program of health insurance for almost all Americans of age 65 and over, regardless of means and, currently, regardless of whether or not they are eligible for the Social Security old-age pensions. Within the next few years, however, eligibility for Medicare and Social Security old-age pensions will become identical. The Medicare program is divided into two parts: *Part A,* which is financed largely from the Social Security tax, and *Part B,* which is voluntary, requires a monthly payment of $3 from the beneficiary, and, as far as the government's portion is concerned, is financed from general revenues.

Medicare, Part A, provides hospitalization up to 90 days per spell of illness; posthospitalization care in an extended care facility for up to 100 days; posthospitalization home health care services; and outpatient hospital diagnostic services. Part B provides physician's and surgeon's services; home health visits even with no prior hospitalization; many diagnostic tests; dressings, splints, casts, rental of durable medical equipment, and many other ancillary services; and limited out-of-hospital treatment for psychiatric disorders. Many of the services in Part A and all services in Part B require the payment of deductibles and coinsurance charges by the beneficiaries.[4]

The coverage under Medicare, while a great advance over that previously available to most of the aged, is by no means comprehensive. Major items of medical care expenses not covered under either Part A or Part B include the cost of out-of-hospital drugs, private-duty nurses, any custodial or domiciliary care in nursing homes, immunizations, routine physical examinations, eyeglasses, hearing aids, and almost all dental work. It is estimated that between 40 and 60 per cent of the medical care bill of the aged still remains unpaid for those having only Medicare coverage.

The gaps in the Medicare coverage are disturbing, but so are the needs of other "uninsurables" in the population who are not 65 years old and therefore do not qualify for Medicare's benefits. While Medicare represents a step forward, it still by no means has put the United States in a position of parity with the great European social insurance plans. Under present circumstances, the federal government still must seek to achieve a cooperative arrangement with the private sector, wherein the private sector will supplement the present government health insurance program by extending comprehensive health insurance coverage to as many of the people as possible who are not covered by government insurance.

No one knows what will eventuate in the future and whether Medicare is the first step to national health insurance for all Americans. Many would welcome this development, while others, equally thoughtful and concerned, would not. The answer may well be determined by the speed and eagerness with which the commercial insurance companies, the Blue Cross and Blue Shield plans, and the "independents" move to extend comprehensive health insurance to all those who need it.

Public Assistance Medical Care

The philosophy underlying the new federal Medicare program is that of social insurance. This means that the benefits are in large measure paid for through some method of prepayment, in this case Social Security taxes which individuals pay while they are young and working. Benefits are made available to the recipients as a right rather than as some type of charity, so that eligibility is not contingent upon poverty of the beneficiary.

Another, and far more long-standing, philosophy concerning the financing of medical care is that government assistance should be made available only to those who are poor and willing to prove it by undergoing a procedure called a *means test*. A means test consists of a review of all the recipient's assets. It may be perfunctory or thorough, harsh or lenient, but its presence invariably marks public assistance programs, and it is almost universally resented by the applicants for aid.

The categorical programs of public assistance, in which the federal and state governments jointly share financial responsibility, date back to the Social Security Act of 1935. Over the years, four categories of persons were singled out for assistance under the provisions of the Social Security Act. These four were the aged (Old Age Assistance), the blind (Aid to the Blind), needy children and their families (Aid to Families with Dependent Children), and the permanently and totally disabled (Aid to the Totally and Permanently Disabled). All these categories were given assistance under programs which, while authorized federally, were individually designed and operated by the various states. No uniformity existed in benefits or eligibility requirements for similar categories of recipients from state to state.

Before 1950, public assistance was guided by the *cash grant* rule, which had two principal characteristics. First, in an effort to uphold the beneficiary's dignity, payments for all benefits, including those for medical assistance, were made in cash directly to the public assistance recipients. Significant disadvantages of this provision were that a welfare recipient might not seek medical aid with the few extra dollars he received for this purpose; or he might not get the best care available, partly because of the meager sums at his disposal and partly because lack of health information might lead him to misspend the funds. The second characteristic of the cash grant rule was that the federal government, while donating matching funds for public assistance, did not contribute money toward medical care for the recipients. Rather, medical care for public assistance beneficiaries was paid out of a separate fund containing only state and local monies. There was thus every incentive to the states to hold down the medical care part of their public assistance programs.

In 1950, the cash grant rule was changed, and states could then receive federal matching funds, up to a specified maximum, for direct medical care given to public assistance recipients. Furthermore, such care was to be financed by *vendor payments,* with public assistance funds being paid directly to physicians and other providers of medical care, while the patient, who was certified as eligible for treatment, would not directly receive or disburse the funds necessary for his care. The level of maximum expenditure specified under the 1950 program for federal matching funds was so low, however, that wealthier states, who were already expending far more for welfare medical assistance through cash grants, had no incentive to change their practice. This situation persisted until 1956, when the federal government began making supplementary grants. Although the supplementary grants still had to be matched by state funds according to a formula, they were of sufficient size to motivate the larger wealthier states to set up vendor payment programs for public assistance medical care. It was still left with each state, however, to decide whether it wanted to have a public assistance program at all, what categories of public assistance were wanted, and, for each desired program of public assistance, what level of medical benefits would be provided.

Medical Assistance to the Aged (MAA) was written into law in 1960, when the Kerr-Mills bill provided a further amendment to the Social Security Act. This measure was offered as an alternate to government-sponsored health insurance for the elderly, which was gaining momentum at that time. Medical Assistance to the Aged provided funds for those older individuals who were not sufficiently impoverished to require assistance for their every subsistence need, but who nonetheless were unable to pay for their own medical care. The term *medical indigency* was used to describe this financial bracket. Not all states saw fit to develop an MAA program, though most eventually did. It was later found on closer inspection that many of the beneficiaries of this new program of medical care assistance were not newcomers to the public assistance rolls, but were really people confined to nursing homes who had been carried previously under the Old Age Assistance program and who were now transferred to the MAA category to take advantage of its more liberal federal matching funds.

The public assistance medical care program, serving as it does approximately 4 per cent of the nation's population yearly, has received much public scrutiny and criticism in recent years. In 1965, because of this, the Social Security Act besides being amended to include Medicare also had Title XIX added as an amendment. This Title, which became known as Medicaid, establishes a *single* and separate medical care program to consolidate and expand the care for all those declared eligible for public assistance by the individual states. Medicaid is financed through federal and state matching funds determined by a formula, but the financial arrangement is in all cases more favorable, from the state's point of view, than the matching formula which governed its public assistance medical care program. Thus, the Medicaid formula is different for the various states, with the federal government's share ranging from a minimum of 50 per cent to a maximum of 83 per cent. Furthermore, there is currently no ceiling on the *amount* of state funds which the federal government will match, although this provision may be modified in the future.

At the end of 1969, MAA and the other four programs of categorical public assistance medical care under the Social Security Act will stop. States not having a Medicaid program at that time will get no further federal matching funds for public assistance medical care. Those states that elect to establish a Medicaid program must, by July 1967, have provided at least the following to all public assistance recipients in all categories of any program which that state may have: (1) inpatient hospital services; (2) outpatient hospital services; (3) other laboratory and x-ray services; (4) skilled nursing home services for individuals over 21 years old; and (5) physician services. Coverage of other items of medical service is optional with the states. However, any medical benefit offered to one category or subgroup of public assistance recipients must be offered in identical amount, duration, and scope to every other person or group receiving public assistance support.[4] Thus, the new law seeks to establish, at least *within* each state, uniformity of medical care benefits available to public assistance recipients in all categories. Furthermore, medical indigency is recognized by Medicaid to exist not only among the aged, but among every other group for whom categorical assistance is provided. A means test is still required in order to establish both indigency and medical indigency.

Despite the advances embodied in recent legislation, the problem of the poor and their medical care is by no means solved. The deterioration of health which results through the fact that large segments of the population are denied access to adequate care has far-reaching implications for the economy of the nation. The prevalence of expensive, long-term illnesses is definitely greater among the lower income groups. Much of this illness could have been treated at great saving had it been brought to proper care at an early stage. The greater cost of treating the advanced illnesses must come from the taxpayers. Thus, society is forced ultimately to pay for the social inequities that it permits, often in the name of economy.

Workmen's Compensation

Just as industrial accidents are the inevitable companion of industrialization, so programs for treating and rehabilitating workers injured on the job have been generated in almost every country with any degree of industrialization. In some *developing* countries which have a minimum of industrialization and a severe general scarcity of medical care resources, the care available under workmen's compensation is actually superior to that available for the remainder of the population's health needs.[9]

Workmen's compensation is based on an understanding by both the worker and his employer that work injuries are predominantly related to the intrinsic nature of work itself rather than to negligence on anyone's part. In line with this understanding, all work-related injuries are considered to be compensable, and the amount of the award, covering both loss of wages and necessary medical care, is related to the degree of injury, the age of the worker, his occupation, and the number of his dependents. The award is determined without having reference to the courts, and this results in substantial savings to the worker, who is spared the cost of legal fees. In the early years of this century, prior to the enactment of workmen's compensation laws, it was estimated that only one in eight industrial accidents resulted in compensation to the injured workers. In cases where compensation was awarded, legal costs ran as high as 50 per cent of recovery. In New York, Pennsylvania, and Minnesota, fully one third of on-the-job fatalities received no compensation, while another 24 per cent received less than $100.

Another problem which workmen's compensation tries to solve is that of lapsed time between injury and compensation. When the worker must resort to the courts, the time interval is likely to be long. Meanwhile the injured worker's bills, medical and otherwise, continue to pile up. Under workmen's compensation, this time lapse is reduced to a minimum so that the worker can begin, soon after injury, to receive payments which help meet his household expenses and enable him to pay his medical care bills as they arise.

In the United States, workmen's compensation is administered through autonomous programs set up by the individual states, with the insurance carried mainly by commercial insurance companies. Injured workers are treated by private physicians in the community and are hospitalized in community hospitals. This contrasts with many other countries, where injured workers receive care in government-sponsored hospitals and health centers.

A great advantage inherent in the American system of workmen's compensation is that it provides incentive to employers to reduce any hazardous work conditions that may exist. Since, as in most insurance, the premium under workmen's compensation varies with the loss experience, employers benefit when the number of work accidents is reduced.

One major task of the workmen's compensation program is to arouse sufficient interest in the rehabilitation aspect of medical care in all parties concerned. Employers, facing no great labor shortage, have not fully felt the need to rehabilitate the injured individual worker. They and the insurance companies have found it less troublesome to make a cash settlement than to get involved in the intricacies of a rehabilitation program. The worker, blinded by the temporary windfall of a sizable sum of cash, has also often missed the point that, in the long run, the cash offered has little value in comparison to what a full rehabilitation effort would offer him. From a moral point of view, and from the point of view of the over-all good of the community, it is important to concentrate a workmen's compensation program on restoring the individual's work capacity rather than on the payment of compensatory cash awards, for in time, the individual who cannot be productive must become a burden on himself and society. Workmen's compensation represents a major step forward in extending the worker's rights, but until the program is primarily focused on restoring the worker to maximal productivity, it has not yet met the full challenge of its mission.

FUTURE ROLES OF THE PUBLIC AND PRIVATE SECTORS IN PROVIDING MEDICAL CARE

Certain trends in medical care organization in the United States during the past decades stand out clearly. Giant strides in medical technology and in consumer demand for medical care have gone hand in hand. Medical care costs have soared. The ability to distribute the fruits of improved medical technology equitably throughout the population has not kept pace with the technologic advances themselves. Few, if any, component parts of the health agency complex have defined their mission as broadly as that of providing the entire range of preventive, curative, and rehabilitative services for a target population. Rather, most tend to work in a limited area, concentrating on one medical care function or on one diagnostic category of patient. Government, by default, has taken on responsibilities for assuring adequate medical care for many who would not otherwise receive it. As government sees it, this responsibility needs to be further extended, for inequity in the provision of medical care still exists. From the point of view of the private sector, there is a threat in this of government encroachment on activities that could and should be left in private hands. The current situation is actually an uneasy equilibrium, and it poses a challenge to government and the private sector alike.

For government, there is the challenge of clarifying the definition of its mission in the medical care field. It is widely apparent today that government's proper role in medical care should not be at the bedside, delimiting or in any way intruding on the therapeutic relationship between patient and doctor. Government is clearly needed, however, to provide coordination and quality control for the community's medical care system. No other agency, individual, or institution of society can do equally well this job of making certain that all segments of the population are getting adequate care, and that barriers—financial or otherwise—are not permitted to be placed between the sick and the care that they require.

A second challenge to government is to mobilize for the defined task. This means introducing new ways of thinking and functioning into agencies that have become stagnant through excessive adherence to traditional task fulfillment. It means training, and introducing into the government hierarchy, new types of personnel whose educational qualifications are unorthodox by standards of the past. It means learning to understand, and use to advantage, computers and complex analysis systems that alone can monitor the medical care of an entire population and that can help in researching and solving problems of future resource allocation.

Once government has redefined its role in medical care and has geared up for fulfilling this role, it must then seek out the areas in which the medical care system of the community is insufficiently large or of too low quality and attempt to stimulate the private sector to provide the needed care in these areas. In rare instances, the government might fail in this effort and be required to go about actually giving care itself, but this should not happen often. By various incentives which can be brought to bear and by the use of the contract mechanism, it should be possible for the great bulk of care to be rendered by the private sector. The major barriers to equitable distribution of medical care—poverty, ignorance, and geographic isolation—can all be attacked directly by government. Indeed, such attack is part of the coordinating role that government should play in medical care. The need for government to render direct care, however, is largely illusory and, with use of imaginative administration, can probably be largely ended.

The challenge to the private sector in medical care is to demonstrate the full extent of its ability to provide needed care at high levels of quality. The perceived threat of government to the private sector—both providers of service and providers of financing—is the threat to replace inaction or inadequate action with government action. If government is not to be the answer to satisfying the unmet demands for medical care that have become apparent, then the private sector must demonstrate that it can perform in a new way which will meet more of the demand than it is currently doing. The American people are becoming unwilling to settle for less than equitable medical care for all segments of society. In face of this, it is too late for the private sector to get by on mere pronouncements concerning the dangers of government encroachment.

If both government and the private sector recognize the challenges which the present medical care situation holds for them, and if they can adequately meet these challenges, then there is hope for the development of a fruitful partnership between the two sectors, each performing the task for which it is best suited without detriment to the other. The net result will be improved medical care for the nation as a whole, and thus, as in every measure that works for the betterment of society, each individual in the population will ultimately be benefited.

SUMMARY

Medical care covers a wide range of preventive, curative, and rehabilitative services which are delivered by a vast network of individuals and institutions in both private and public settings.

Historically, government at all levels in the United States—local, state, and federal—has undertaken medical care activities primarily for special purposes and in connection with special groups of the population. However, since World War II, several factors have caused an expansion of the role of government in medical care. These factors include the ascendancy of financially costly, chronic diseases as the principal causes of morbidity and mortality; a generally increasing demand for more and better medical services; and an increasing social awareness of inequities in the availability of high-quality medical care to numerous segments of the population, such as low-income families, the elderly, minority groups, migrant workers, and rural families.

In the provision of medical care, key *individuals* include physicians, dentists, nurses, and many other professional persons; principal *institutions* include hospitals and nursing homes; and sources of *auxiliary services* include home care programs and various community projects that have medical care components. Most physicians are in private, solo practice, but some are in group practice and in public settings; they are usually reimbursed on a fee-for-service basis, but some are employed on a salaried basis. Over the years, the number of persons admitted to hospitals has increased, the average length of stay has declined, and the costs of hospitalization have risen rapidly. Accreditation is the principal device for establishing and maintaining the quality of care in hospitals. Although nonprofit operation characterizes a majority of hospitals, most nursing homes are operated for profit. In general, the quality of care in nursing homes has been less than satisfactory in the past, but it is anticipated that the new Medicare requirements will result in considerable improvement. However, there still remains a need to clarify and redefine the function of nursing homes. Principal problems in the over-all organization of the provision of medical care include the maintenance of quality of care and the quantity of medical personnel; the prevailing somewhat uneven distribution of medical personnel is also of concern.

In the financing of medical care in the United States, several methods attempt to alleviate the problems associated with rising costs, increasing demands, and declining ability of the consumer to pay his own way. One method is through privately sponsored health insurance, which includes Blue Cross hospital insurance, Blue Shield physician's care insurance, health insurance plans offered by commercial insurance companies, and the "independent" health insurance plans.

A second method is government-sponsored health insurance for persons aged 65 and over through Medicare (Title XVIII of the Social Security Act). A third method is public assistance medical care, which consists of jointly sponsored, federal-state medical aid to several categories of needy persons; recent Medicaid legislation (Title XIX of the Social Security Act) establishes uniform benefits within, although not among, states. A fourth method is through workmen's compensation, which makes legal provision for treating and rehabilitating workers injured on the job. In spite of these and various other existing methods for financing medical care, there are still segments of the population in the United States for whom there is *no* provision, and for many of those who receive *any* benefits, only a portion of the total cost of medical care is covered.

The numerous problems which remain to be solved in connection with organizing the provision and financing of medical care present a variety of challenges to both the public and private sectors. In meeting the challenges, there is a potential for the development of a fruitful partnership between the sectors.

REFERENCES

1. SLOAN, RAYMOND P. *Today's Hospital.* Harper and Row, New York, 1966.
2. COGGESHALL, LOWELL T. "Progress and Paradox on the Medical Scene." (The 1966 Michael M. Davis Lecture.) Center for Health Administration Studies, Graduate School of Business, University of Chicago.
3. TUNLEY, ROUL. *The American Health Scandal.* Harper and Row, New York, 1966.
4. COHEN, WILBUR J., and BALL, ROBERT M. Social Security amendments of 1965: summary and legislative history. *Social Security Bull*, 28:3–21, September 1965.
5. U.S. DEPARTMENT OF HEALTH, EDUCATION, AND WELFARE. *Toward Quality in Nursing—Needs and Goals.* Report of the Surgeon General's Consultant Group on Nursing, 1963.
6. UNIVERSITY OF MICHIGAN SCHOOL OF PUBLIC HEALTH, Bureau of Public Health Economics. *Medical Care Chart Book*, 2nd ed. University of Michigan, Ann Arbor, 1964.
7. HEALTH INSURANCE INSTITUTE. *Source Book of Health Insurance Data, 1965.* The Institute, New York.
8. U.S. BUREAU OF THE CENSUS. *Statistical Abstract of the United States: 1965*, 86th ed. U.S. Government Printing Office, Washington, D.C.
9. ROEMER, MILTON I. Workmen's compensation and national health insurance programs abroad. *Amer J Public Health*, 55:209–14, February 1965.

ADDITIONAL READING

BURNS, EVELINE M. Policy decisions facing the United States in financing and organizing health care. *Public Health Rep*, 81:675–83, August 1966.
MULLER, CHARLOTTE. Income and receipt of medical care. *Amer J Public Health*, 55:510–21, April 1965.

RUSSELL, JOHN M. New federal regional medical programs. *New Eng J Med*, **275**:309–12, August 1966.

SHEPS, CECIL G., and DROSNESS, DANIEL L. Prepayment for medical care. *New Eng J Med*, **264**:390–96, 444–48, 494–99, February and March 1961.

SOMERS, HERMAN MILES, and SOMERS, ANNE RAMSAY. *Doctors, Patients and Health Insurance*. The Brookings Institute, Washington, D.C., 1962.

U.S. DEPARTMENT OF HEALTH, EDUCATION, AND WELFARE, Public Health Service. Agencies using public health personnel. In: Appendix B, Conference Working Paper: *Education and Training for the Changing Role of Public Health in Society*. Second National Conference on Public Health Training, August 19–22, 1963.

U.S. DEPARTMENT OF HEALTH, EDUCATION, AND WELFARE. *Health Manpower Source Book*. U.S. Government Printing Office, Washington, D.C., 1964.

U.S. DEPARTMENT OF HEALTH, EDUCATION, AND WELFARE, Public Health Service. *Medical Care in Transition*, 2 vols. U.S. Government Printing Office, Washington, D.C., 1964.

COMMUNITY MENTAL HEALTH

The background and current development of the relatively new and rapidly growing field of community mental health are described in this chapter. The first section reviews briefly the concepts, practices, and areas of knowledge underlying community mental health activities. The next section discusses various early and contemporary concepts of what constitutes mental health and illness. The third section presents some estimates of the extent of mental illness and discusses several problems in connection with its measurement. In the next three sections, a general description of mental illnesses and a system for their classification are presented; some of the known and presumed causes of mental illness are discussed; and several examples of the many topics involved in current research in mental health and illness are reviewed. The next major section of the chapter describes the principal historical developments in the care of mental illness and discusses contemporary national, state, and community provisions for the prevention, treatment, and rehabilitation of mental illness and for the general promotion of mental health. The last section reviews the nature, extent, and causes of mental retardation and describes several new approaches to the problem.

THE BASIS OF COMMUNITY MENTAL HEALTH

Mental health problems have existed throughout history; they may, today, be the most pressing and complex of all health disorders. Community mental health concepts and practices are very recent developments in the effort to cope with these burgeoning problems. The concepts of community mental health involve the recognition that mental health and illness are community responsibilities, and that attention must be directed not only toward overt and severe manifestations of mental illness but also toward prevention, treatment of incipient conditions, and rehabilitation. Community mental health practices involve the translation of these concepts into a variety of programs and services which ultimately are of sufficient magnitude to meet the needs of all segments of the population.

Several areas of knowledge provide the background for community mental health activity. These include knowledge of the *extent* of mental disturbances and knowledge of the *causes* of mental disorders, which in turn influences concepts of *what constitutes mental health and illness.* At present, there is a considerable deficit of knowledge in these areas, but the number and variety of scientific investigations under way provide hope for overcoming this deficit in the future.

CONCEPTS OF MENTAL HEALTH AND ILLNESS

Concepts of mental health and illness have changed appreciably throughout history. At one time, the mentally ill were considered to be "possessed," and witch hunting and exorcism of demons were integral parts of a community's approach to mental health problems. A book entitled *Malleus Maleficarum (Hammer Against Witches),* which was published in 1489, contained instructions for the recognition of a witch. Many of the listed criteria are those now associated with mental illness. This book was used for nearly 300 years as the standard guide for handling the "mentally afflicted," and "handling" frequently resulted in violence and death to the "handled."

The early organicists maintained that disease could not exist without some organic defect or injury. Therefore, if no lesion could be found, "insanity" (which is a legal rather than a scientific term, in modern usage) could not be regarded as disease, nor the patient as sick; rather, he was simply immoral or criminal.

In recent times, many attempts have been made to define what might be considered to be mental good health. It has been conceptualized in general terms as emotional stability and intellectual efficiency involving individuals who are psychologically effective in relationships with others. More specifically, good mental health has come to have several connotations, including: normal behavior, absence of mental disease, environmental adjustment, perception of reality as it is, and personality integration. Adequate criteria for measuring any of these components are subject to considerable debate.

Any consideration of *normal behavior* is relative to many considerations, such as general health, intelligence, the community in which one lives, and the groups with which one associates. Economic, religious, ethnic, and social factors may play a role in determining "normality." The *absence of mental disease* may be difficult if not impossible to determine because there is no clear-cut demarcation between the so-called mentally healthy and the mentally unhealthy. Most individuals at some time or other during their lifetime experience some degree of maladjustment or emotional impairment. Few persons, for example, escape some frustration and hostility resulting from environmental obstacles. *Environmental adjustment* as a measure of mental health is also difficult to evaluate. Conformity and adaptation are insufficient evidence of the absence of mental disease. Some maintain that adapting to or accepting degrading, dehumanizing, or humiliating experiences associated with one's environment may be an index of poor, rather than good, mental health. Conforming to an unstable social world, accepting impersonal relationships, and feeling powerless to participate in determining one's own destiny may be indicative of an unhealthy passivity. *Perception of reality* may be related to physiologic, psychologic, and sociocultural determinants. For example, the Navajos may perceive senility as neither illness nor deviance, but merely as behavior to be expected of older people.[1] Measurement of *personality integration* as an index of mental health involves still further difficulty. For example, evaluating self-sufficiency, sympathy, or sociability may be open to subjective determinations. The psychologically well-integrated person is judged by his ability to accept the need for delayed rewards, and his self-control lessens his need for external authority. Thus, the integratively adjusted person may "conform" because of the long-range consequences for him. If he should rebel against authority or custom, it will be because of considered judgment.

The social determinants of what constitutes sickness vary from one culture to another.[2, 3] However, in most cultures mental illness is markedly differentiated from physical illness. It is usually disruptive and socially intolerable. It seldom arouses sympathy, but, on the contrary, frequently produces anxiety and isolation. Many find it difficult to recognize mental illness as illness, or to see sickness as having psychological forms. The mentally ill as a group lack the capacity to evoke sympathy. The mentally ill person often presents himself as "stubbornly ill" or as an "uncooperative patient" whose behavior has reached a point where people no longer can stand him. It is not so much that he physically endangers them, although they may also fear this.[4, 5] (Actually, violence is the *exception* rather than the rule among the mentally ill.) The mentally ill tend to require *other* people to adjust to *them* at every point in their illness from onset to recovery. They often resist change for the better, and are difficult to work with in an efficient manner.

EXTENT OF THE PROBLEM OF MENTAL ILLNESS

Problems in Measuring the Extent of Mental Illness

As might be expected, the extent of mental illness detected in the population depends, first, on which one or more of the various possible components of mental health are being measured and, second, on the particular criteria used in defining each component. At one time, estimates of the extent of mental illness were based on the number of persons who were hospitalized in psychiatric or mental institutions. Although an enumeration of the hospitalized population is relatively accurate and easy to make, for a number of reasons it does not reflect the extent of mental illness in the population as a whole. First, in some cases, circumstances rather than the individual's mental or emotional condition may determine whether or not he is hospitalized. Thus, for one person the circumstances in the home may be such that he is able to be cared for outside the hospital, while another individual with a similar condition must be hospitalized because appropriate home care is lacking. Second, increased outpatient clinic and private psychiatric treatment arrangements have enabled some persons to remain in the community who might otherwise have had to be hospitalized. Third, a count of hospitalized cases does not include the vast remaining range of mental and emotional disturbances existing in the population which, according to certain criteria, should be considered as manifesting some degree of mental illness. Thus, included in this category are the many persons with conditions ranging from mild personality or behavioral disorders to those with feelings of excessive apprehension, tension, or insecurity. Furthermore, these conditions may be long-lasting or they may be associated with some stressful occurrence in the individual's life and thus be relatively transient.

Adding to the hospitalized population the number of persons receiving psychiatric treatment in the community improves the estimate of mental illness in the population, but still is by no means inclusive. The most obvious omissions, of course, are those persons who should be receiving treatment but are not. In addition, nonhospitalization treatment for some individuals may be intensive and extend over a period of years, while for others it may be of very short duration and consist essentially of guidance or counseling.

Thus, measuring the prevalence of mental illness is complex and difficult, and measuring the incidence is even more beset with problems. It has been said that reliable incidence data can be obtained only for those mental impairments which can be diagnosed at birth and reported on birth certificates;[6] incidence data for mental illnesses of later onset are less reliable because the disorders may develop slowly and go undetected for a long period of time. The diagnostic acumen of the physician in the recognition of disorders at birth as well as of incipient mental illness which may develop later influences the reliability of the incidence of mental disorders and illnesses.

Extent of Mental Illness in the General Population

Depending on the criteria used and the range of severity included, estimates of the number of persons in the United States with mental health problems have varied from 1 per cent of the population to 81.5 per cent. The latter finding was from one of the few epidemiologic studies of this problem.[7] In the population sampled, 2.7 per cent were considered incapacitated because of extreme mental disturbance, another 7.5 were considered to have severe disturbances, 13.2 had marked symptoms, 21.8 moderate and 36.3 mild symptoms. Thus, in this particular study only 18.5 per cent were *without* some degree of mental disturbance.

Size and Characteristics of the Mental Hospital Population

A census conducted in 1963 showed that there were slightly over one-half million patients in 284 state and county mental hospitals in the United States. The patients were about equally divided between males and females (approximately 254,000 males and 262,000 females). Almost 60 per cent of the patients were diagnosed as psychotic and 85 per cent of these were suffering from schizophrenic reactions. Over 29,000 children and young adults had been admitted for the first time for a serious mental disorder. Of these, 3734 were under 15 years of age, and over 25,000 were between 15 and 24. In spite of the seemingly high number of admissions to mental hospitals, it has been estimated that actually one-half million children are psychotic or borderline, and that most, as in the case of adults, have schizophrenic reactions.[8]

However, in spite of these large numbers, recent data indicate some progress. As shown by Figure 6-1, for the period between 1955 and 1964 the resident patient population in state and county mental hospitals decreased—moderately but steadily. This was in spite of the fact that the general population was increasing during the same period. However, Figure 6-1 also shows that total admissions have increased steadily, and in 1964 exceeded 300,000. This represented 164 patients admitted per 100,000 civilian population (compared to 110 in 1955). Thus, more patients are being admitted but are staying for shorter periods. Further information on admissions is provided in Table 6-1, which shows that, of the total patients admitted to state and county mental hospitals in 1964, slightly more than half were readmissions. This was in contrast to 1960, for example, when first admissions exceeded readmissions.

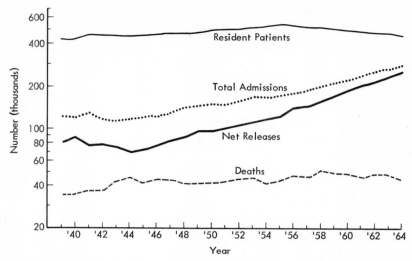

FIGURE 6-1. Trends in number of resident patients, total admissions, net releases, and deaths, state and county mental hospitals, United States, 1939–1964. (Source: National Clearinghouse for Mental Health Information, National Institute of Mental Health, U.S. Department of Health, Education, and Welfare. *Mental Health Statistics, Current Reports.* Series MHB-H-9, January 1965, p. 6.)

TABLE 6-1   Admissions and Net Releases, State and County Mental Hospitals, United States, Selected Years

Year	Total Admitted	First Admissions	Readmissions	Net Releases
1950	152,286	114,054	38,232	99,659
1955	178,003	122,284	55,719	126,498
1960	234,791	140,015	94,776	191,386
1964	302,946	139,250	163,696	271,506

Source: Adapted from Long, Luman H., ed. *The World Almanac and Book of Facts for 1966,* 81st ed. New York World-Telegram and The Sun, New York, p. 304.

PRINCIPAL TYPES OF MENTAL ILLNESS

General Description of Mental Illness

Psychological impairment may affect any person, at any age, at any time. However, it is usually long-standing, and can range along a continuum from feelings of inferiority or guilt, through psychosomatic disorders and psychoneuroses, to the organic and functional psychoses.

Personality disorders include *neuroses,* which may be relatively mild conditions. The neurotic or psychoneurotic suffers from unreasonable fears, obsessions, compulsions, and unwarranted exhaustion and is frequently very depressed. Although able to interpret his environment, he has reduced personal satisfactions.

Psychoses are more serious disturbances. The most common of the latter is *schizophrenia.* The psychotic is considered suffering from a major mental illness and has great difficulty interpreting the world around him. His behavior may be bizarre. Occasionally, he is dangerous to himself or others and usually requires some hospitalization.

Mental health is not just a function of the mind (psyche). Rather, the body (soma) interacts with the mind, thus giving rise to the term *"psychosomatic."* Stress on either may be reflected in the functioning of the other. Many individuals seek the services of physicians because of what are basically psychosomatic problems.

Another group of the mentally ill suffer from *character disorders*; this group includes sexual deviants, criminals, drug addicts, and alcoholics. Theirs is immature, impulsive, frequently antisocial behavior.

Finally, there are those children considered *emotionally ill,* many with incipient symptoms of the conditions listed above. This last group includes the school and home discipline problems and many of the so-called juvenile delinquents.

Classification of Mental Illness

A corollary to the difficulties in defining and measuring mental health is the equally difficult task of categorizing mental disorders. The present trend in treatment and in attempting to understand mental illness is away from pigeonholing mental diseases, but for diagnostic and statistical purposes some system of categorization is needed. In addition, a certain amount of confusion arose over the years in connection with the use of psychiatric terms, and it became apparent that some standardization of usage was in order. To serve these various purposes, the American Psychiatric Association developed a system of classification of mental disorders, the details of which are presented in a manual.[9]

The classification system of the American Psychiatric Association makes a basic distinction among three categories of conditions: those mental disturbances which result from, or are precipitated by, lesions of the brain; those in which brain damage is secondary, absent, or not demonstrated; and mental deficiency. Briefly, the classification covers:

1. Disorders caused by or associated with impairment of brain tissue function. This general category includes: acute versus chronic brain disorders associated with infection; intoxication; trauma; circulatory disturbances; convulsive disorders; disturbance of metabolism, growth, or nutrition; neoplasms; or uncertain causes.
2. Mental deficiency of a familial, or hereditary, and idiopathic nature.
3. Disorders of psychogenic origin, or without clearly defined physical cause or structural change in the brain. This general category includes:
   a. Psychotic disorders such as *schizophrenia,* which may be manifested by delusions, hallucinations, and inappropriate reactions including

showing unsuitable emotion in a given cultural context (e.g., laughing when sadness is more appropriate); and *paranoid states*, which may express themselves in delusions of persecution and/or grandeur, hostility toward others, and depressive and manic states.

b. Psychophysiologic disorders such as peptic ulcer, colitis, asthma, hypertension, or skin eruptions.

c. Psychoneurotic disorders such as anxiety reactions, depression, dissociative reactions including amnesia, phobias about objects or situations, and obsessive-compulsive reactions.

d. Personality disorders such as general emotional instability (e.g., a tendency to go to pieces under ordinary conditions), passivity, hostility, aggression, dissocial functioning represented by amoral disregard for the norms of society, antisocial behavior, and addiction to chemicals or drugs.

CAUSES OF MENTAL ILLNESS

Since one essential in understanding and treating or controlling any disease is a knowledge of its cause, establishing the etiology of mental disease is a major concern in the field of mental health. It is a complex matter partly because of the number of diverse conditions involved, and partly because of the difficulties of conducting scientific investigations of the kind that, for example, have been successful in pinpointing the specific causes of infectious diseases.

Physical causes of certain mental disturbances have been established slowly, and over time some conditions believed to have no physical cause have been shown, in part, to have such bases. An example is paresis, a mental disorder in which the individual is disturbed, irresponsible, and perhaps even violent. At one time there was no known cause of this condition, but it is now recognized as being due to syphilis. Similarly, it has been established that certain mental disturbances are caused by pellagra, a nutritional disease. It is possible that, as new scientific knowledge is accumulated, certain other biochemical or physiologic deficits or pathologies may be found to cause or at least to predispose individuals to the development of particular mental illnesses.

The vast, remaining array of mental disorders—those that have no known physical cause and thus are considered psychogenic in origin—constitutes the principal problem with regard to establishing etiology. Theories as to the causes of psychogenic disorders have existed for many years and serve as hypotheses in research and as guides in treating the sick. However, there are as yet only meager scientific demonstrations of causal relationships between specific factors in the individual's history and/or environment and the development of a particular mental disorder.

The concept of multiple factors in the cause of psychogenic disorders has become generally accepted; the factors are considered to involve the individual, his family, and the community. The role of heredity is open to question. It may play some part in schizophrenia although the evidence to date is not too persuasive. It is possible that a disturbing pattern of behavior in a family may be conducive to the development of psychotic behavior in other family members.[10]

It is also possible that certain mental disorders may be associated with socioeconomic factors, environmental stress, deprivation,[11, 12] and other phenomena which characterize modern life. Thus, the mass migration from simple, rural or small-town social systems to large, impersonal, automated, urban environments has contributed to individual conflict, group conflict, and frustration, which often lead to psychological disturbances and feelings of alienation and isolation.[13] Rapid social change has caused tension and conflict among adults, and this creates disturbed and problem children. Some children, deprived of normal affectional ties and stable families, go through a passive childhood only to break down later when confronted by the responsibilities of adult life.

RESEARCH IN MENTAL HEALTH AND ILLNESS

Through many and varied avenues of research, efforts are being made to understand the nature of mental health and illness, to determine the factors associated with a wide range of mental and emotional states from "general adjustment" to severe pathologies, and ultimately to shed light on the causes of mental disorders. The subject of a particular research investigation may be any one or several of the psychological or mental states along the broad mental health-mental illness continuum; its approach may be biologic, environmental, or social; and it may include the general population or some special segment of the population.

Investigations of abnormalities of the biologic system which may play a role in mental illness are designed to lead to a better understanding of the chemical substances affecting the central nervous system and of the structure, function, and mode of operation of the brain and its relationship to the body as expressed in psychosomatic illness. Also under study are the effects of stress on glandular systems: how they react to messages from the brain, and the part played by hormones known as the corticosteroids, which help mobilize the body's resources. Studies under way in genetics may answer some of the puzzling and conflicting findings on heredity and mental disease.

Studies of factors related to juvenile delinquency, which brings over 500,000 antisocial children before the courts each year, indicate that good family communication existed in homes of normal adolescents, whereas this factor was lacking in families having one disturbed child. Studies of broken homes do not confirm a strong association with mental disorder. Factors in childhood that have been found to pose the greatest risk to mental health were negative perception of parents' character, poor physical health, and parents' quarrels.

Some preliminary studies of factors related to living space and the need for privacy and maintenance of some distance from one's fellowmen may have direct relationships with stress. Studies on animals have shown that overcrowding leads to stress, which is reflected in disturbed behavior.

Investigations have been made of the relationship between social class and mental illness, and other demographic and epidemiologic studies are assembling information on the socioeconomic and cultural characteristics of communities; the extent to which mental disorders occur in the population, and the conditions which bring about their development; the factors which lead persons with specific mental disorders to seek psychiatric care; and the characteristics which distinguish those who seek psychiatric care from those who do not. Additional research on the relationship between mental health and social and cultural factors, including child-rearing patterns, is under way in other countries.

The foregoing are but a few examples of the concerted efforts being made through a wide range of research to attempt to understand human behavior and characteristics in general and to discover the circumstances that account for or contribute to mental health and illness in particular. Increased knowledge along these lines will help to provide the basis for planning the kind of mental health programs and services that will more effectively meet the needs of the entire population.

THE PROVISION OF MENTAL HEALTH SERVICES

Over a long period of history, attitudes toward the mentally ill and provisions for their care passed through several stages. Attitudes toward mentally disturbed persons changed from viewing them as criminals, to regarding them as objects of curiosity, and finally to recognizing them as being ill and subject to the same humanitarian treatment as that accorded to persons suffering from physical illness.

The evolution of provisions for the care of the mentally ill has reflected not only the attitudes toward mental disorders that prevailed at a given time, but also society's general sense of responsibility for those afflicted. Thus, at one time it was considered essential to confine the mentally ill and to segregate them from the rest of society; today the goal is to maintain as many of the mentally ill in their own communities as possible. Similarly, in earlier periods of history, no treatment was afforded to any sufferer from mental illness; now the goals of mental health programs include not only the provision of appropriate treatment for all who need it, but also the provision of preventive and rehabilitative measures in order to forestall the onset of illness and to ensure as complete restoration of functioning as possible. Finally, at one time only the mentally ill who were destitute were considered to be public responsibilities; today public responsibility is defined much more broadly and is expressed through the agency of government at local, state, and national levels.

Historical Developments in the Care of Mental Illness

In early periods of history, the well-to-do kept mentally ill family members at home or, if they were troublesome, chained or locked them in attics or cellars. They were of legal concern only insofar as their property was affected. The poor and homeless "insane" were public responsibilities and were incarcerated as felons or paupers.

"Madhouses" were established about the thirteenth century. Their purpose was merely to incarcerate the insane, and no treatment was provided. Bethlehem Hospital (Bedlam) in London was one of the earliest of such institutions. Its system of manacles, chains, locks and keys, and stocks was standard equipment for the inmates. For centuries a visit to Bedlam to watch the antics of the inmates was one of the sights of London.

In 1793, Philippe Pinel was appointed physician to Paris' notorious Bicêtre, where the lunatics were incarcerated. Shocked by what he saw, he freed those in chains. One man had been incarcerated for 40 years; another had been in chains for 36. The permission of the Revolutionary Commune for Pinel's actions was reluctantly given, and he was strongly criticized both by the public and by other physicians. In an essay on mania published after the French Revolution, Pinel outlined his theories on the humane treatment of the mentally ill. Subsequent writings laid the foundation for the French School of psychiatry, which was important throughout the nineteenth century.

In 1791, William Tuke, a merchant in England, noted that a Quaker died in the York County Asylum under circumstances indicative of mistreatment. The following year he proposed to the Yorkshire Society of Friends that a humane institution be established, and when this was accomplished, a revolution in the treatment of the mentally ill had begun. The new institution curtailed the use of restraint, and patients had considerable freedom and engaged in regular employment.

Despite the efforts of Pinel in Paris and Tuke in England, however, conditions remained essentially unchanged in most of the institutions for the insane. Dirt, filth, ignorant keepers, and cruel, inhumane treatment remained the order of the day. Attempts to bring about change continued, however, and in England, John Conolly became one of the nineteenth-century reformers. In 1828, Conolly was appointed professor of medicine at University College, where he tried, unsuccessfully, to inaugurate a course of clinical instruction in mental illness. Unhappy at his failure he left the College and, in 1839, became resident physician at the Middlesex Asylum, the largest mental hospital in England. He at once abolished all forms of mechanical restraint and later wrote that there was no place in the world this could not be done with safety. But the nonrestraint movement spread slowly against strong opposition. Its first successful use was by Benjamin Rush (1745–1813) and

Thomas Kirkbride (1809–1883). The fetters slowly gave way to the padded cell, which, in turn, has only recently been rendered unnecessary.

In the United States in the mid-1800's, Dorothea Lynde Dix, who was a retired Boston schoolteacher, became interested in various kinds of institutions and made personal investigations of their conditions. Traveling thousands of miles, addressing state legislatures, and reporting directly to Congress, she was responsible for the establishment of 32 new state institutions for the mentally ill. As they were built, local authorities very willingly transferred their mentally ill to these institutions because this saved local tax expense. Soon the institutions were overburdened with chronic patients many of whom were soon forgotten in back wards. The enormous foreign immigration during the latter half of the nineteenth century brought additional persons with physical, emotional, and social problems who further overtaxed various health and welfare institutions. It was not the intent of those who established state mental hospitals to have them become human warehouses, but over the years they did, and overcrowding became a way of life which has persisted to this day.

Early in the twentieth century, another social reformer renewed public interest in the mentally ill. Clifford W. Beers, who was a graduate of Yale University, became a patient in private and state mental hospitals between 1900 and 1903. Gathering first-hand evidence of the inhumane treatment methods, he was later discharged and wrote a book entitled *A Mind That Found Itself*. This led directly to the establishment of the National Committe for Mental Hygiene, a voluntary association, with Beers as secretary and prominent physicians and laymen as officers. This Committee was the forerunner of the present National Association for Mental Health.

Like Dix, Beers was concerned with the improvement of the *care* of the mentally ill. Others wanted to *prevent* mental illness similar to the prevention of epidemic diseases. However, equivalent techniques such as immunization were not applicable, but public education in the form of child guidance and early treatment of emotional disturbances were encouraged. The National Association for Mental Health established state and local chapters, which pressed for wider public understanding and support of legislation and programs promoting child guidance services and other psychiatrically oriented services. Their efforts were frequently hampered by public apathy and inadequate financial support. Despite this, the Association played an important part in obtaining legislative support for necessary programs.

Numerous other developments in the present century have also helped to promote understanding and action in the field of mental health. The World Health Organization focused world attention on mental health when it included *emotional* and *social* well-being of the individual as part of its general definition of health. The experiences gained during World War II in the treatment of psychiatric casualties encouraged radically new treatment methods. In the 1950's, newer drugs helped reverse the usual pattern of prolonged, institutional treatment. Interest and activity in mental health matters increased among public health, welfare, and education workers, and thus contributed to the general advancement of mental health goals.[14, 15]

The Federal Government in Mental Health

Traditionally, the United States government has provided extensive, direct mental health services for veterans of the Armed Forces through a system of clinics and hospitals. In addition, in 1855 it established the Government Hospital for the Insane in Washington, D.C., which became Saint Elizabeths Hospital in 1916. Saint Elizabeths maintains therapeutic, rehabilitative, and protective programs for approximately 7000 patients; provides a professional training and educational program; and conducts research on a number of mental health-related topics. The federal government also maintains hospitals for narcotics addicts; these are primarily for federal prisoners, but they also have provisions for a limited number of persons from the general population who enter on a voluntary basis. In recent decades, two significant federal legislative acts have given strong impetus to mental health programs and services in the United States: one was the National Mental Health Act of 1946; the other was the Community Mental Health Centers Act of 1963. The principal agency of the federal government in mental health matters is the National Institute of Mental Health of the Public Health Service.

The National Mental Health Act of 1946. The federal government, through the National Mental Health Act of 1946, provides grants-in-aid to the states for the development of state and local programs in mental health. Emphasis is on the development of community mental health programs, particularly for the prevention and early treatment of mental disorders. The law also provides funds for training and for research. Under the grant-in-aid arrangement, a state provides two dollars from state and local sources for each dollar of federal funds it receives.

The Community Mental Health Centers Act of 1963. A significant step was taken by the United States government in 1955, when Congress created a Joint Commission on Mental Illness and Health, which was charged with studying and making recommendations for combating the increasing mental health problems in this country. In a final, ten-volume report, the Commission recommended a broad, comprehensive attack on mental illness.[16] Following this report, President John F. Kennedy early in 1963 delivered to Congress a Special Message on Mental Illness and Mental Retardation, proposing "a bold new approach . . . designed . . . to use Federal resources to stimulate state, local and private action." He urged the search for, and eradication of, the causes of mental illness and mental retardation; the strengthening of knowledge and skilled manpower; and the improvement of programs and facilities. He stated that "when this approach is carried out, reliance on the cold mercy of custodial isolation will be supplanted by the open warmth of community concern and capability."

In response to the President's request, Congress enacted the Community Mental Health Centers Act, which authorized the appropriation of $150 million to finance up to two thirds of the cost of construction of community mental health centers. In 1964, Congress amended the Act, authorizing support for staffing by professional and technical personnel during the first 51 months of a center's operation. The ultimate goal is to establish 2000 community mental health centers throughout the United States.

The basic intention of the community mental health center is to provide *comprehensive treatment* for all who need it. Furthermore, the treatment is to be provided *in the community,* so that patients can stay at home, be treated at home, and become well at home, thus avoiding the harmful effects of isolated institutional residence in long-stay mental hospitals. Under the new plan, a patient's own family physician may continue to see him and to participate in his treatment. Some patients will not even need to give up their jobs during treatment; rather, they may need to be absent from work for periods ranging from only a few days to a month, and such absence can be handled as regular sick leave. The breakup of families can be forestalled because mentally disturbed fathers or mothers will be able to continue to assume at least a part of their family responsibilities while receiving treatment at a center. Finally, the vast number of professional persons in the community whose work entails contact with disturbed persons or any handling of mental health problems will be able to receive guidance through consultation with the center's professional staff and by attending formal and informal classes and meetings conducted by the center's staff.

There are ten component services that are considered requisites for a community mental health center if it is to be genuinely comprehensive: inpatient services for limited time periods; outpatient services; partial hospitalization (i.e., day care and night care); emergency services 24 hours per day; community services (i.e., consultation to professional personnel and agencies in the community); diagnostic services; rehabilitative services; precare and aftercare services (i.e., home visiting and placement of patients in foster homes and halfway houses); training of mental health personnel; and research and evaluation. These components need not be under one roof, but the administration of the various elements must be such that the goal of *continuity of care* is achieved.

The National Institute of Mental Health. The National Mental Health Act of 1946 was instrumental in establishing the National Institute of Mental Health, which came into being in 1949. The Institute, it will be recalled from Chapter 2, is now one of the five operating bureaus of the Public Health Service. The Institute conducts and supports interdisciplinary basic, clinical, and developmental research in the causes, prevention, and treatment of mental illness and the improvement of mental health. It also supports training of mental health and related personnel; conducts and supports demonstration projects in new and improved methods of caring for the mentally ill; provides consultation and technical services to states and communities; and collects, evaluates, and disseminates information germane to the mental health field. The Institute has established several centers for special mental health programs, such as the National Center for the Prevention and Control of Alcoholism and the Center for Studies of Narcotics and Drug Abuse. Under the Community Mental Health Centers Act of 1963, the National Institute of Mental Health is responsible for the administration of grants for the construction and staffing of community mental health centers. The budget for the Institute was $18 million in 1956 and more than $225 million in 1967.

The Role of the States in Mental Health

Organization of State Mental Health Services. In most states in this country, the public agency which is responsible for mental health services is a separate department reporting directly to the governor of the state. There are variations, however. In a few states, mental health services are provided through the state social welfare departments. Sometimes mental health is combined in a department with other institutional services such as prisons and specialized hospitals, or mental health and public health services may be grouped in a single governmental unit. Figure 6-2 illustrates how one state has organized its various mental health programs and services into a separate, independent department.

One of the most difficult problems confronting a state mental health agency is coordination of planning and activities with the large numbers of other agencies which also have some responsibility for or interest in mental health. Since mental health problems are not only prominent but also pervasive, it is not surprising that many agencies devote all or part of their efforts to one or more aspects of mental health service. One solution to the problem of coordination is the formation of joint commissions consisting of agency representatives and/or prominent citizens. In order to be effective, of course, such bodies must have sufficient prestige and be granted enough authority to permit their proper functioning.

State Mental Health Programs and Functions. The official mental health agency on the state level optimally has responsibility for general planning and coordination and for the provision of several kinds of services and programs. These include hospital services, psychiatric outpatient services, consultation, personnel training programs, public education programs, and research.[6]

Although the trend is away from the large state mental hospitals as a

State of California Department of Mental Hygiene

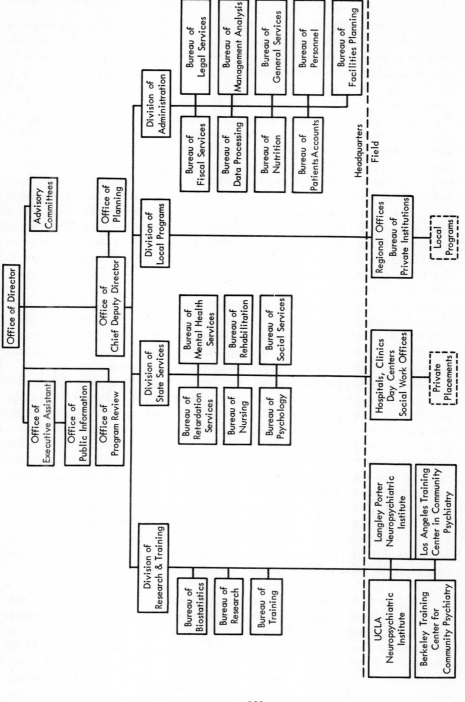

FIGURE 6-2.

method of treatment for mental illness and the number of such hospitals has declined in some states, this category of institution undoubtedly will need to remain in existence for some time to come. The state mental health department or other agency responsible for the administration of these hospitals is in a key position to improve the quality of care provided, and considerable effort has been made in this direction in recent years. Thus, the organization of hospital treatment in some states includes placing all patients from one area in the same unit so they can maintain community identity. Other hospitals have been established as "therapeutic communities" with open wards and free movement of patients and staff.[17] Rehabilitation of elderly patients has resulted in the discharge of some who had been forgotten in back wards. Further advances along these lines are expected to be stimulated by provisions of the Community Mental Health Centers Act, whereby funds are made available to state mental hospitals for the improvement of their treatment programs. Anticipated beneficial results include the earlier discharge of many more patients and new solutions to the treatment of patients who in the past have been considered chronically and hopelessly ill.

Over the past years, many states, in exercising their prerogatives with respect to delegating authority to local governments, have adopted legislation which permitted the establishment of a local mental health authority or board with the power to develop extensive programs of case finding, diagnosis, treatment, education, consultation, and rehabilitation.

With the passage of the Community Mental Health Centers Act, the states acquired new responsibilities. As a prerequisite for participating in the program, a state was required to develop a comprehensive, long-range, interagency, mental health plan. All 50 states have developed such plans. In implementing the provisions of the Community Mental Health Centers Act, a state must designate a single state agency to administer the plan for centers or to supervise administration of the plan. The designated agency must then review and approve all proposals for centers that are advanced by any community within the state. Finally, each state must designate a state advisory council, composed of representatives of nongovernmental groups, other state agencies concerned with any facet of mental health center operation or administration, and citizens' groups representing consumers of the services to be provided by the centers.

State Laws Governing Commitments to Mental Hospitals.

A traditional function of the states has been the provision of laws regarding commitments of patients to mental hospitals. The laws of the different states vary as to commitment procedures, but in general the admission of a mentally ill person to a hospital is on one of four bases.

The first is *involuntary commitment*, a long-standing and formal practice which involves petition to the courts (by relatives or others), medical certification, a court hearing, and final disposition. In some states, formal notice must be served on the mentally ill person, and sometimes arrest on a warrant is the required procedure. Practically all states provide that there may be a jury trial if requested by the person concerned or by someone else.

The second method is *emergency commitment*, which is provided if an individual becomes suddenly and seriously disturbed. In these cases the judicial process is waived temporarily, and patients may be admitted to hospitals on the formal certification of the health officer. Such patients can be held only for a few days, pending action for more formal court commitment procedures, if needed.

The third method is *observational commitment*, which is for a period of from one to three months and is for the purpose of diagnosis and planning future care and treatment.

The fourth method is *voluntary admission*, which may also have the concomitant of voluntary release: when such a patient requests release, he must be freed within a specified period—not more than two weeks in most states. In order to detain him longer, formal involuntary commitment procedures must be initiated. Since voluntary admission does not involve court action, the stigma of a legal record of the patient's mental illness is avoided.

In general, there is a growing public and professional concern regarding state laws and procedures involving commitments to mental hospitals. Some view the processes as too legalistic. On the other hand, since the individual is deprived of liberty perhaps for an indefinite period and since he is usually unable to handle his own affairs, definite legal issues are involved, and some means of providing protection through due process of law seems indicated. In an effort to assist the states in revising their laws, the National Institute of Mental Health has provided guidelines that embody the more modern concepts of commitment laws and procedures.

Community Mental Health Programs and Services

The gradual shift in emphasis from treatment for mental illness in large, long-term hospitals to treatment in the patient's own community has been accompanied by a broadened point of view as to what the concerns of mental health should be within the community. Thus, treatment remains a major concern, but there is a growing focus on *early treatment*, and in addition, attention is being directed increasingly toward *prevention* and *rehabilitation*. Prevention and early treatment of mental and emotional disturbances are the basis for the newly developing subspecialties of *community and social psychiatry*. New kinds of facilities have also been increasing as part of the community effort in the prevention, early treatment, and rehabilitation of mental illness.

Social and Community Psychiatry in the Prevention of Mental Illness. In recent years, psychiatrists have become less concerned about abnormal behavior and have been giving more attention to conditions governing those who are *not* ill. This has given birth to the new subspecialties of social and community psychiatry. Social psychiatry attempts to provide for the mentally ill, and for those in danger of becoming so, opportunities for making contact with forces which are favorable to the maintenance or reestablishment of social adequacy.[18]

Emphasis is placed on trying to understand what has reduced a person's effectiveness, and efforts are directed toward early intervention and mitigation of the destructive influences. As part of this process, an attempt is made to establish mechanisms for "crisis intervention." This involves enlisting the understanding and support of those persons in the community who are most likely to have contacts with individuals experiencing an emotional crisis, and who therefore can be providers of aid at the earliest possible stage in mental health problems. Such persons constitute the community's caretaker and caregiver groups and include ministers, counselors, probation and parole officers, public health workers, social agency personnel, teachers, and physicians in fields of medicine other than psychiatry.[15] Community psychiatry focuses on providing consultation to these caregiver and caretaker groups in order to increase their effectiveness in handling persons who come to them with problems of living.

The new concept of treatment may also take the form of environmental manipulation. Thus, a "war on poverty" may be an attack on incipient mental illness. Promoting mental health in a community may require the improvement of community schools. Individual therapy may involve shifting the patient's personal relationships or reducing reactions by the use of sedatives or tranquilizers. Such chemical agents, effective for the overexcited as well as depressed psychotic, permit the stabilizing of many patients outside an institutional setting.

The general shift in treatment philosophy which has given rise to community psychiatry has been stimulated by several factors, including studies by social scientists pointing up the poor therapeutic value inherent in mammoth institutional settings; the gradual acceptance of the fact that increasing numbers of the community population are, or may become, mentally ill; the developing acceptance of health insurance coverage for mental illness (an example is the coverage effective late in 1966 of the United Auto Workers 2.5 million members and their families); research indicating that brief therapy may be as effective as other methods; and the gradual acceptance of appropriately trained personnel—other than psychiatrists—as therapists, including clinical psychologists, social workers, nurses, and rehabilitation specialists.

Community psychiatry has been gaining worldwide acceptance. Many pioneering developments have taken place in other countries. The first International Congress concerned with community psychiatric problems met in London in 1964 and attracted psychiatrists, behavioral scientists, and other specialists from 40 countries. Topics discussed included the training of community psychiatrists, family therapy, and techniques of mental health consultation.

Facilities for Prevention, Treatment, and Rehabilitation. For many years, the chief sources of aid to the mentally ill within the community were psychiatrists in private practice and a few clinics. Under such circumstances, there was minimal possibility of prevention of mental illness through measures such as early treatment of incipient conditions, since most patients who sought help were already likely to be acutely ill. As mental health problems became more pressing, the gap between available resources and needs widened increasingly even with respect to treatment, alone. Communities were thus impelled to action, and as a result, several different kinds of mental health facilities have developed. These include the psychiatric services of general hospitals, outpatient clinics, emergency services, and modified residential services.

In an effort to detect mental illness at an early stage and to increase the treatment of patients closer to home, an increasing number of *general hospitals* have been adding psychiatric screening and acute treatment facilities. In 1962, only 585 general hospitals were known to admit psychiatric patients, but two years later the number had risen to over 1000. In 1963, general hospitals and private mental hospitals admitted and discharged more psychiatric patients than did state and county mental hospitals.

The number of psychiatric *outpatient clinics* and the number of patients served also have been increasing. In 1955, about 379,000 patients were treated in outpatient clinics; by 1962 the number of patients had risen to 741,000 and there were 1683 clinics involved in the provision of treatment. One of the main problems encountered by outpatient clinics is that of excessive case loads which necessitate long waiting lists and hence delays in treatment.

In an effort to provide immediate psychiatric help to individuals experiencing a sudden emotional crisis, *emergency services* usually in the form of walk-in clinics have come into being, although as yet in limited numbers. The walk-in clinic provides 24-hour, low-cost service with no waiting period. In addition to the initial emergency visit, several subsequent visits are possible, usually up to a total of seven. If the patient needs additional treatment, appropriate referrals are made by the clinic staff. In addition to the walk-in clinics which provide general psychiatric service, a similar but more specialized emergency service is also provided by suicide prevention centers.

There are several kinds of *modified residential services.* One consists of *day care and night care centers and hospitals.* Day care offers a full program of therapy, activity, and rehabilitation for patients who are able to return home at night. Night care is designed for those who are able to work or attend school during daytime hours but need treatment and a place to sleep at night. Prior to 1960, there were only 37 day and night services available; by 1963 the number had grown to 114. *Halfway houses* are a second form of modified residential service. These are institutions in which patients live together after being discharged from a mental hospital and while they are readapting to the community. The patients receive some supervision and gradually resume their life in the community through employment and social activity. *Foster homes* constitute a third kind of provision and are available in situations in which the patient is able to return to the community from a mental hospital but has no home to go to.

Today by no means all communities have all these facilities; some may have only a few and these may be on a minimal basis, while others still have none at all. The provisions of the Community Mental Health Centers Act should, however, help considerably to overcome these deficits since, as pointed out earlier in this chapter, such facilities are among the several component services of a center's total program.

Other Contributions to Prevention, Treatment, and Rehabilitation. Specific methods used in the prevention, treatment, and rehabilitation of mental illness have been changing and have helped to contribute to general advancements in the mental health field. Thus, new drugs have replaced surgical procedures, and various kinds of shock treatment are used less frequently. Group psychotherapy is being used increasingly, and there is greater emphasis on the treatment of the family as a unit. Counseling programs, vocational rehabilitation services, and educational programs dealing with subjects ranging from attitudes toward the mentally ill to principles of personal and family mental health are being offered increasingly.

Mental health is coming more and more to be viewed as an integral part of community public health programs. Public health nurses and social workers are being utilized in a variety of case-finding, preventive, and rehabilitative programs, including the follow-up supervision of former hospitalized patients.[15] Public health educators are involved in community education programs which focus on mental health needs and services.

Future Needs in the Provision of Mental Health Services

Solutions to the Problem of Cost of Care. Although the number of resident patients in state and county mental hospitals has been declining, maintenance expenditures have been increasing. This is illustrated by Table 6-2, which shows that in 1964, the cost of care in these institutions had risen to over $1 billion. The cost per patient per day was $6.23 compared to $3.06 in 1955. These increasing costs have been due not only to factors contributing to the general cost spiral in the United States but also to the increasingly greater numbers of personnel employed in mental hospitals. The upward trend in personnel is also illustrated by Table 6-2, which shows that in 1964, there were almost 200,000 full-time employees in state and county mental hospitals, compared to about 146,000 in 1955.

Indications are that at least part of the solution to the problem of mounting costs may lie in the further development of community-based psychiatric facilities of the kind described in the preceding section. For example, in psychiatric units of general hospitals, although the *daily cost*

TABLE 6-2 Number of Resident Patients, Number of Personnel, and Maintenance Expenditures, State and County Mental Hospitals, United States, Selected Years

	1955	1960	1964
Resident patients, at end of year	558,922	535,540	490,754
Personnel (full time), at end of year	146,392	179,162	199,600
Maintenance expenditures	$618,087,247	$916,236,166	$1,133,015,675
Per resident patient			
Per year	1,116.59	1,702.41	2,281.27
Per day	3.06	4.65	6.23
Per patient under treatment			
Per year	849.31	1,177.75	1,403.28
Per day	2.33	3.22	3.83

Source: Adapted from National Clearinghouse for Mental Health Information, National Institute of Mental Health, U.S. Department of Health, Education, and Welfare. *Mental Health Statistics, Current Reports.* Series MHB-H-9, January 1965, p. 6.

per patient is much greater than in state and county mental hospitals, the *total cost per patient* is much less because the treatment period in the community hospital is much shorter. Also, there is evidence that the cost of psychiatric care in modified residential service facilities is even less than in general hospitals. In one community, when the cost of care in a 24-hour psychiatric unit of a general hospital was compared to that of a day/night care unit, it was found that the fee per unit of time in the day/night unit was considerably lower. This was because approximately twice as many patients could be treated in a day or night unit as in a 24-hour unit of similar size and staffing.

Solutions to the Problem of Personnel Shortages. Some increase in the availability of the most highly skilled professional personnel has occurred. For example, in 1966 there were 18,740 psychiatrists in the United States, which was an 11 per cent increase over 1964. However, state and county mental hospitals still remain understaffed in spite of the increasing total number of personnel. Thus, in California, there is only one physician for every 150 patients, although the American Psychiatric Association recommends a minimum of one for every 90. In all areas of mental health activity, increasing numbers of mental health professionals are required, including clinical psychologists; social workers; psychiatrically trained nurses; health educators; occupational, physical, and recreational therapists; vocational counselors; and psychiatric aides and technicians.

It is apparent that for the foreseeable future there will not be sufficient professional mental health personnel available to meet the increasing problems of mental illness. One promising solution is the further development of the "crisis intervention" technique of community psychiatry mentioned earlier, in which mental health professionals, who are scarce in number, teach principles of handling mental health problems to the caretakers of society, who are greater in number. A second solution consists of the more extensive participation in mental health activities by private physicians. As in any kind of community health program, the private physician, who is in the front line of service to persons who are ill, can make an invaluable contribution to the prevention, diagnosis, treatment, and rehabilitation effort. This requires, however, a change in emphasis from the more apparent problems of physical illness to the more subtle problems of mental and emotional illness, as well as an orientation not only to the individual but to society as a whole. A third solution is inherent in the various mental health training programs which are being financed by the federal government. These programs include in-service training and also the support of academic work leading to advanced degrees.

The Development of New Knowledge.   Great strides have been made in improving the care and treatment of the mentally ill, but much more is unknown than known about the cause, diagnosis, and cure of mental disease. A critical need is sound knowledge on which to base the development of programs related to prevention. The Joint Commission on Mental Illness and Health has outlined two courses of action which are considered to be of primary importance. One is the intensification of the search for new knowledge on preventive measures or treatment methods that are faster working and better adapted to mass application. The second consists of the better use of the already available knowledge and experience in the treatment of mental illness.

MENTAL RETARDATION

Mental retardation is one of the most handicapping of all childhood disorders. Until recently, the problems of the mentally retarded child and his family received very little public attention. With the exception of the provision of large, overcrowded residential institutions and special classes for the more educable, little else was done for many years. In the late 1940's and early 1950's, interest in the handicapped increased greatly, and parents of mentally retarded children began to demand that attention be given to their problems. Increasing research, programs, and facilities gradually appeared, and in 1962, the attack on all phases of the problem of mental retardation accelerated markedly.

The Nature of Mental Retardation

A mentally retarded child may be defined as one whose intelligence is so limited that it interferes seriously with his functioning as an independent person in society, either because he cannot become economically independent or because his behavior is not socially acceptable.[19] Retardation varies greatly among individuals. In severe cases protective care throughout life is required. In milder cases many tasks can be learned which make some independence possible, and, with some help, afflicted persons can become self-supporting.

The degree of retardation as determined by one or more standardized testing techniques is commonly classified as follows:

Approximate I.Q. Range	Estimated Maximum Mental Capacity	Description	Probable Educational Potential
70–84	10–12 years	Borderline	Educable
50–69	6– 9	Mild (moron)	Educable
20–49	3– 8	Moderate (imbecile)	Trainable
0–19	0– 4	Severe (idiot)	Totally dependent

Extent of the Problem of Mental Retardation

Most nationally standardized tests show that persons with I.Q.'s of around 70 have significant difficulties in adapting to the modern environment. About 3 per cent of the population score below this level, and it is estimated that there are approximately 5.5 million mentally retarded persons in the United States. In addition to the cost of some $550 million a year to care for the mentally retarded, several billion dollars are lost in economic output because of their nonproductivity.[20]

Of the approximately 4.2 million children born each year in the United States, more than 126,000 are, or will be, classed as mentally retarded. Among the retarded, some 4200 (0.1 per cent of all births) will be *severely* retarded and helpless, and another 12,600 (0.3 per cent) will be *moderately* retarded. The balance of about 110,000 (2.6 per cent) will be *mildly* retarded and, with special training, can acquire limited skills and become relatively independent.[20]

Causes of Mental Retardation

The causes of this major health problem are multiple. Some 70 per cent of the cases are thought to be due to familial or cultural factors. Whether heredity or environment is more important is not known, but environment is probably far more significant than has previously been recognized. Genetic factors including both abnormal genes and chromosomal defects account for some 6 per cent of the cases of mental retardation. Another 4 or 5 per cent are accounted for by prenatal, perinatal, or postnatal infection, trauma, or anoxia. For the remaining 20 per cent, the cause is unknown.[21]

In some cases of mental retardation, no demonstrable, gross brain abnormality may be present, and there may be only mild impairment. In others, minor brain damage too subtle to be demonstrated by present techniques may be a cause. In still others, unfavorable environmental and psychologic influences, such as economic and social deprivation and parental neglect, may contribute to retardation. Early identification and prompt remedial treatment are essential in these cases.

New Approaches to the Problem of Mental Retardation

Many states have already or will soon begin new and vigorous programs in research, prevention, and treatment of the mentally retarded. Largely stimulated by federal funds, efforts to solve the problem of mental retardation include: expanded diagnostic and clinical services, residential care, special education classes, parent counseling, casework, vocational rehabilitation, training of professional personnel, and research in causes and amelioration. Communities are opening local facilities for the mentally retarded where these services can be provided, usually under the direction of a department of mental hygiene. One of the major objectives of such facilities is to help keep as many retarded children as possible out of the large residential institutions. In doing so, a child may be expected to reach a much higher level of development as a consequence of the more personal attention provided by his own family setting. If the family is given help from the local facility, keeping the child at home will not present a major burden.

With the discovery of specific mental retardation preventive procedures, health departments have developed diagnostic and case-finding methods or have encouraged their development by others. The most dramatic of these is in the detection of phenylketonuria, a precursor of mental retardation, which can be reversed by dietary adjustments. The traditional role of the health department in the control of certain childhood diseases has a direct bearing on the prevention of mental retardation. A number of special projects administered by health departments and medical centers are under way for expectant mothers and their infants from the more deprived areas where mental retardation is more prevalent. More crippled children's programs are including the multiple handicapped on their eligibility list and are opening multidisciplinary clinics to better serve their needs.

SUMMARY

Concepts and practices in the field of community mental health include recognizing mental health and illness as community responsibilities; emphasizing prevention, rehabilitation, and treatment of the entire range of mental disorders; and developing various programs and services which will ultimately serve the needs of the entire population.

Concepts of what constitutes mental health and illness have changed over time, and vary from one culture to another. At present, there are several different definitions of good mental health, but criteria for their measurement are difficult to establish. There are also numerous problems in attempting to measure the extent of mental illness in the population, and estimates vary widely depending on the criteria used and the range of severity included. The hospitalized population, although large, accounts for only a portion of all persons who suffer from some form of mental illness. Recently, increasing numbers of persons have been admitted to mental hospitals, but they have been staying for shorter periods of time.

Efforts have been made to develop classification systems for the wide range of mental disorders that exist; a notable example of such a system is that of the American Psychiatric Association. A few mental disorders have been shown to have a physical basis, but for the vast remaining array, exact etiology has not yet been established, although the concept of multiple causation has become generally accepted, and it is believed that various socioeconomic factors, environmental stress, deprivation, and other deleterious characteristics of modern life may play a role. Many research efforts currently are being directed toward investigating the causes of mental disorders, developing criteria for mental health and illness, establishing methods for measuring the extent of mental illness, and gaining an increased understanding of human behavior and characteristics.

Significant developments have occurred in the present century in the provision of community mental health programs and services for the prevention, treatment, and rehabilitation of mental illness. These advances have come only after a long history of neglect and mistreatment of the mentally ill, which extended over many centuries. In the United States, the federal government, the states, and local communities are all participating in the current effort.

In recent years, the United States Congress has enacted legislation designed to combat mental illness on a broad basis; the most recent measure has been the Community Mental Health Centers Act of 1963. This Act supports the establishment of centers offering comprehensive treatment and continuity of care within the community for all who need it. The concept of the community mental health center reflects a marked departure from the traditional practice of treating mentally ill persons in large, often remote, long-term mental hospitals.

Official state mental health agencies are customarily responsible for general planning, coordination, and provision of a variety of services and programs. They have acquired new and important responsibilities in connection with the implementation of the Community Mental Health Centers Act.

On the community level, a growing emphasis on prevention and early treatment of mental illness has led to the development of the concept and practice of *community and social psychiatry*. Several new kinds of community-based mental health facilities have been established over the years, including psychiatric services in general hospitals, outpatient clinics, emergency services, and modified residential services. Impetus to the further development of such facilities is being given by the provisions of the Community Mental Health Centers program.

Future needs associated with the provision of mental health services include solutions to the problems of the cost of care and of personnel shortages and the development of new knowledge in several areas. New knowledge is particularly needed on causes, diagnosis, and cure of mental diseases and mass preventive and treatment methods.

Mental retardation, although varying in severity, affects a large segment of the population. It is due to a number of causes, not all of which are known as yet. Recently, mental retardation programs have been considerably expanded in the areas of prevention, treatment, and research.

REFERENCES

1. MURPHY, JANE M., and LEIGHTON, ALEXANDER H., eds. *Approaches to Cross-Cultural Psychiatry.* Cornell University Press, Ithaca, 1965.
2. OPLER, MARVIN K. *Culture and Mental Health: Cross Cultural Studies.* The Macmillan Company, New York, 1959.
3. BENEDICT, RUTH F. *Patterns of Culture.* Houghton Mifflin Company, Boston, 1934.
4. HALPERT, HAROLD P. Surveys of public opinions and attitudes about mental illness. *Public Health Rep,* **80**:589–97, July 1965.
5. PHILLIPS, D. L. Public identification and acceptance of the mentally ill. *Amer J Public Health,* **56**:755–63, May 1966.
6. LEMKAU, PAUL V. Mental health services. In: Sartwell, P. E., ed. *Maxcy-Rosenau Preventive Medicine and Public Health,* 9th ed. Appleton-Century-Crofts, New York, 1965.
7. SROLE, LEO, LANGNER, THOMAS S., MICHAEL, STANLEY T., OPLER, MARVIN K., and RENNIE, THOMAS A. *Mental Health in the Metropolis: The Midtown Manhattan Study.* McGraw-Hill, New York, 1962.
8. U.S. DEPARTMENT OF HEALTH, EDUCATION, AND WELFARE, Public Health Service. *Patients in Mental Institutions, 1963; Part II, State and County Mental Hospitals.* U.S. Government Printing Office, Washington, D.C., 1964.
9. AMERICAN PSYCHIATRIC ASSOCIATION. *Mental Disorders: Diagnostic and Statistical Manual.* The Association, Washington, D.C., 1957.
10. JACKSON, DON D., ed. *The Etiology of Schizophrenia.* Basic Books, New York, 1960.
11. ZAX, MELVIN, and STRICKER, GEORGE. *The Study of Abnormal Behavior, Selected Readings.* The Macmillan Company, New York, 1964.
12. HOLLINGSHEAD, A. B., and REDLICH, FREDERICK C. *Social Class and Mental Illness.* John Wiley and Sons, New York, 1958.
13. GROUP FOR THE ADVANCEMENT OF PSYCHIATRY. *Urban America and the Planning of Mental Health Services,* Symposium No. 10. The Group, New York, 1964.
14. BERLIN, I. Learning mental health consultation: History and problems. *Ment Hyg,* **48**:257–66, April 1964.
15. CAPLAN, GERALD. *Principles of Preventive Psychiatry.* Basic Books, New York, 1964.
16. JOINT COMMISSION ON MENTAL ILLNESS AND HEALTH. *Action for Mental Health.* Basic Books, New York, 1961.
17. DENBER, HERMAN C. B., ed. *Research Conference on Therapeutic Community.* Charles C Thomas, Springfield, 1960.
18. WORLD HEALTH ORGANIZATION. *Social Psychiatry and Community Attitudes:* 7th Report of the Expert Committee on Mental Health. World Health Organization Technical Report Series No. 177, Geneva, 1959.
19. HARPER, PAUL A. *Preventive Pediatrics: Child Health and Development.* Appleton-Century-Crofts, New York, 1962.

20. U.S. DEPARTMENT OF HEALTH, EDUCATION, AND WELFARE. *The President's Panel on Mental Retardation: A Proposed Program for National Action to Combat Mental Retardation; A Report to the President.* U.S. Government Printing Office, Washington, D.C., 1962.

21. HORMUTH, RUDOLPH P. A proposed program to combat mental retardation. *Children,* **10**:29–34, January–February 1963.

CHAPTER 7

ENVIRONMENTAL HEALTH

The relationship between environment and health

Recent concerns regarding hazards of the environment

Organization of environmental health programs in the United States

The conduct of environmental health programs

Areas of environmental health activity

International environmental health

Summary

The wide range of factors in the environment which affect health either directly or indirectly are described and discussed in this chapter. In the first section of the chapter, a distinction is made between the narrower, traditional concept of environmental health and the present-day, broader concept that recognizes the relationship between man and his total environment. The nature and sources of various recent environmental hazards are described in the second section of the chapter. The third section reviews federal, state, and local organization for the provision of official environmental health services in the United States, and the fourth section describes the various kinds of procedures and methods which are utilized in the conduct of programs. The next section provides an account of the problems encountered and the control measures applied in several different areas of environmental health activity. In the last section, the status and kinds of environmental health programs in developing countries and in European countries are described briefly, and the principal organizations with international environmental health responsibilities are reviewed.

THE RELATIONSHIP BETWEEN ENVIRONMENT AND HEALTH

Long before the development of the modern principles and practices of public health, man recognized certain relationships between his environment and outbreaks of disease. Many of these early assumptions were erroneous and led to various mistaken beliefs. It will be recalled from Chapter 1 that before microorganisms were discovered, the atmosphere was regarded as a probable vehicle of disease. Thus, typhoid and cholera flourished where human waste was allowed to contaminate the environment, and it was assumed by many that the noxious vapors, or miasmas, emanating from such wastes caused the diseases. Similarly, the severe recurring fevers which occurred in lowland areas with much water residue were attributed to the telluric conditions, and the fevers became known as malaria, or "bad air." Only with the advent of scientific knowledge was it established that filth, vapors, and dampness, per se, do not cause disease.

The earliest motivation for public health activity was closely associated with control of serious and widespread epidemics, and public health officials continue to recognize that a primary purpose of environmental health programs is to establish, provide, and maintain conditions necessary for the prevention of disease. This means constant vigilance to see that water supplies are completely safe, milk is pasteurized, food is properly prepared and handled, rodents and insects are kept in check, and wastes are disposed of so as not to pollute the environment or promote breeding of insects and rodents. These are among the traditional "sanitation" activities of public health. However, it has also become recognized that there are many other elements in the environment which affect health, including air free of excessive man-made pollution, control of occupational disease, regulation of exposures to ionizing radiation, suitable housing in a pleasant, quiet environment, and other items having no direct relationship to sanitation as defined traditionally. Thus, the present environmental health objectives of developed countries are to control and modify factors which may more subtly affect man's health and well-being.

In light of the prevailing broadened concept, environmental health may be defined as the science of controlling or modifying those conditions, influences, or forces surrounding man which relate to promoting, establishing, and maintaining his physical and mental well-being. In addition, "optimum" rather than "minimum" control is the objective. The scope and objectives of modern environmental programs are becoming so broad that some favor combining "environmental health" programs with those that may have no direct health implications, thereby developing integrated "environmental control" or "environmental engineering" programs.

The new concept of the impact of the total environment on man is indicated in the following statement by René Dubos: "Man is in general more the product of his environment than his genetic endowment. The health of the people is determined not by their race but by the conditions of their life." [1] Concern is no longer limited to direct and long-range microbiologic, toxic, or carcinogenic effects alone, but in addition, attention also is directed toward all other stresses and forces which affect man. The "population explosion," man's quest for better employment, health, educational and social opportunities, and mechanization of agriculture are producing unprecedented urbanization. Unless properly planned and controlled, urbanization produces serious stresses and problems. Suburbs develop without adequate water supplies, sewerage, solid waste collection and disposal, or building and planning controls. Large families with low incomes crowd into old, poorly maintained, cramped quarters in neighborhoods lacking facilities requisite for good family living. Congestion, traffic, noise, air pollution, refuse accumulations, rodents, and many other problems develop.

The old-fashioned health officer citations and abatement actions do not solve these problems. New, bold, comprehensive approaches must take into account the economic, social, physical, and other factors which contribute to the problems and their solutions. Coordination and collaboration of public health officials with many groups, professions, and agencies are key factors in meeting the public health problems of urbanization. This subject is of such worldwide concern that it was selected as the topic for technical discussion during the 1967 World Health Assembly. More must be learned about the effects of stresses, pollutants, and the many factors which contribute to or mitigate against environmental health. The direct health implications of environmental factors alone create a tremendous opportunity and challenge to a wide variety of specialists in many disciplines and are providing research opportunities and programs of great magnitude.

RECENT CONCERNS REGARDING
HAZARDS OF THE ENVIRONMENT

Some environmental hazards to health may arise unexpectedly from time to time from sources which presumably are well under control. The sporadic appearance of such hazards points up the need for unceasing vigilance and for continued systematic research efforts. Other hazards may be the unanticipated by-products of modern technology or other phenomena of contemporary life. Since hazards of this kind are relatively new, not only may they go undetected for a period of time, but also long and intensive investigation may be required in order to establish their exact source as well as the nature and extent of their harmful effects. The following examples illustrate these different kinds of hazards and the areas of knowledge that still need to be developed before they can be controlled effectively.

For years it was assumed that a water supply was microbiologically safe if it was relatively free of intestinal organisms of the "coliform group." However, in 1965, an outbreak of 18,000 cases of *salmonellosis* in Riverside, California, was traced to a water supply which met current coliform-group-organisms microbiologic standards, and constituted the first-known widespread, waterborne outbreak of a disease formerly considered to be principally foodborne. Previously, in 1955–1956 an epidemic of from 7000 to 29,000 cases of *infectious hepatitis* in Delhi, India, was caused by a public water supply which was treated in a modern rapid sand filtration plant that reportedly met acceptable microbiologic standards.[2] Instances such as these indicate that new laboratory procedures are needed to more adequately evaluate the sanitary quality of water, since it is now known that certain pathogens like the infectious hepatitis virus will survive treatment which removes or destroys the coliform organism.

Air pollution is already a major problem in many metropolitan areas and a growing one almost everywhere. New means of measuring, evaluating, and assessing the type and effects of pollutants and revolutionary changes in sources of energy will be required to meet this challenge. Even today the chemical composition and true health effects of irritants in "Los Angeles smog" have not been fully identified. In general, knowledge on which to base scientific control standards is grossly inadequate.

Chemicals serve man well, and insecticides, weedicides, and agricultural chemicals have come to be accepted as necessary for producing the quantities of food needed for a rapidly growing world population. However, certain chemicals have become suspect, although their deleterious potential is difficult to assess. A vast amount of research and investigation are needed to study possible carcinogenic properties of insecticides, chemical additives to food, substances from containers which "migrate" into foods, air-polluting chemicals, weedicides, and trace amounts of radionuclides. New federal and state programs are oriented toward requiring manufacturers to produce comprehensive proof that new chemicals and substances in foods and drugs are safe before they are placed on the market. To prove a food additive safe may require years of work and hundreds and thousands of dollars for testing by animal feeding. Even then, the question of the validity of results with animals, compared to human beings, is in some doubt. Some groups adamantly demand strict controls and prohibitions, but others are inclined to assess benefits versus risks in making such decisions.

In the field of occupational health, the concentration of deleterious material in the worker's environment which produced no demonstrable injury to workers was, for years, called the "maximum allowable concentration." In recent years, the term was redesignated "threshold limit value"[3] to avoid the assumption that an exposure to such material is acceptable if its harmful effects are not now demonstrable. Periodically, new information is developed to show harmful effects from concentrations which had been considered "safe." In addition, attention is being directed toward reducing concentrations of pollution in the occupational environment which are irritating or seriously unpleasant, even though the physiologic effects are not yet measurable.

Accidents are caused by many different kinds of environmental hazards, and the increasing number of accidents has become of considerable concern in recent years. Automobile safety has been the subject of congressional hearings, and the World Health Organization has taken official notice of the accident problem in the home and elsewhere. This is another field for combined effort of many agencies representing numerous disciplines, and

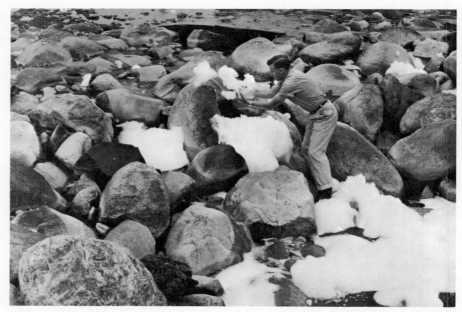

FIGURE 7-1. Detergent foam contaminating a stream. (Courtesy of the Division of Public Health Education, Los Angeles County Health Department.)

one in which public health epidemiologic methods, research, and education are highly appropriate.

In 1964, an Expert Committee of the World Health Organization assessed the various new environmental "threats" to health.[4] The Committee noted the great care with which peaceful use of nuclear energy has been developed and observed that the control which is being exercised over medical radiology and use of radionuclides in medicine and industry results in very little danger to mankind from this source. In connection with the use of chemicals, the Committee noted that the detergents made of stable compounds which produced foam in streams (see Fig. 7-1) and sometimes contaminated drinking water even after modern sewage treatment are being replaced by new compounds which readily yield to normal purification processes. The Committee advocated a similar switch to more unstable, degradable insecticides and chemicals for use in agriculture. With regard to the purity of food, the Committee expressed concern over the possibility of botulism being caused by inadequately sterilized moist foods packaged in the new, transparent plastic airtight wrappers; an instance cited was that of type E botulism organisms which withstood smoke-processing and liberated toxins in fish products packaged in plastic. The Committee noted outbreaks of typhoid in Scotland from beef packed on another continent, and of botulism from tuna canned in California, concluding that contaminated water in which these canned foods were cooled may have entered the cans through fine holes in seams during the vacuum created by cooling.

ORGANIZATION OF ENVIRONMENTAL
HEALTH PROGRAMS IN THE UNITED STATES

In the United States, the national, state, regional, and local environmental health programs cover any element within the broad definition of the field. The scope of each segment of the program and the level of government and the specific agency responsible are determined by the lawmakers. Their actions are influenced by public demand, demonstrated need, and leadership of administrative and technical officials. For instance, air pollution control is given high priority where the problem is acute. To be effective, some programs must be on a national basis, some statewide, and some locally administered. The trend is toward more federal- and state-sponsored programs, although the local level has strong champions who argue that program execution and pioneering in new procedures are most practical at the lowest level of government.

To assure that each program receives appropriate attention at each level of government, careful planning, coordination, and interagency cooperation are required. There is also a need to continue to develop a broad approach to environmental health, rather than one limited to the now outmoded concept that a health program must be justified in terms of disease control. Clean water, decent housing, pure air, and pleasant surroundings are objectives and programs that need not be "sold" on the basis of disease control.

Environmental Health Programs of the Federal Government

Within the U.S. Department of Health, Education, and Welfare the Public Health Service conducts environmental health programs which are largely directed toward research and the development of basic programs, standards, model codes, and techniques for application by state and local agencies. The Service has traditionally avoided becoming involved in large, national law enforcement programs such as the food law enforcement program of the Food and Drug Administration and the meat inspection programs of the U.S. Department of Agriculture. The Public Health Service model codes cover milk, food service establishments, swimming pools, shellfish, and other specialized fields, and are widely adopted by state and local agencies. Water supplies for use on interstate carriers are "certified" on the basis of evaluations by state health agencies for conformance with the well-established Public Health Service Drinking Water Standards.[5] Air pollution control is becoming a large program and research area and is one of the few instances in which the Service is involved in enforcement to abate interstate pollution. A comprehensive radiologic monitoring network resulted from public concern over fallout from nuclear bomb tests, and has become an additional responsibility of the Public Health Service. Another important and valuable function is training of environmental health personnel and the development of educational materials such as pamphlets and visual aids.

The environmental health administrative organization of the Public Health Service includes a Chief Sanitary Engineering Officer in the Office of the Surgeon General. There are also National Centers for Air Pollution Control, Radiological Health, and Urban and Industrial Health within the Bureau of Disease Prevention and Environmental Control, and a Division of Environmental Health Sciences within the National Institutes of Health. These units, together with the environmental health components of many other major organizational units, provide a comprehensive source of skills, research, and assistance for planning, guiding, and staffing programs of all health agencies. Special programs are established as special need arises. For example, research and demonstration grant programs are provided through an Office of Solid Wastes in a new, comprehensive program to develop the best means of disposing of community refuse, agricultural waste products, and even abandoned junked cars which mar the landscape. Studies include means to reduce the volume of the wastes and development of better means for collection, disposal, and processing of materials for reuse.

The Food and Drug Administration is a second agency within the U.S. Department of Health, Education, and Welfare which has environmental health responsibilities. The Administration has seven bureaus, which specialize in scientific research and analysis, medical evaluation, and regulatory and voluntary compliance. To provide nationwide coverage, the United States is divided into 18 district territories, each with headquarters manned by chemists and inspectors and fully equipped with testing laboratories. Within these districts, there are 58 inspection stations located in industrial concentrations. In addition, five field stations span the United States, directing an expanded program for controlling illicit traffic in depressant and stimulant drugs. The Food and Drug Administration has regulatory responsibilities for sanitary conditions, raw materials used, and controls exercised in the production, packaging, and labeling of products destined for interstate shipment. The Administration conducts educational programs to bring about voluntary compliance with legal requirements; undertakes research in the characteristics, safety, efficacy, and toxicity of a wide variety of consumer products; controls the marketing of new drugs; establishes food standards; and monitors the safety and/or efficacy of food additives, pesticides, antibiotics, coloring agents, and household chemicals.

The U.S. Department of Agriculture inspects and identifies meat and poultry approved for interstate shipment. The Department's program includes checking the health of animals, general quality of the product, labeling, and sanitation. It is also involved in the control of brucellosis and tuberculosis in milk cows and in certain aspects of the control of insecticides.

The U.S. Department of the Interior, in 1966, was assigned the national water pollution control program, which is designed to enhance the quality and value of the nation's water resources and to prevent, control, and abate water pollution. The program is administered by a newly created Federal Water Pollution Control Administration. The Department's Fish and Wildlife Service develops voluntary quality standards for fishery products and evaluates rodent control procedures and materials. Its Bureau of Mines has long been concerned with miners' occupational health and has been involved in evaluating personal protection devices such as gas masks and dust-arresting devices.

The U.S. Department of Labor also conducts occupational health and safety programs through its Bureau of Labor Standards, which administers laws related to safety and occupational health. These regulations must be followed by agencies and companies executing federal contracts, and they also apply to all civilian federal workers.

The U.S. Department of Housing and Urban Development, which was created in 1965, has assumed the functions of the former federal housing agencies and is developing programs to cover many other aspects of urban community improvement and development. The Department, by controls tied to federal community improvement grants, is stimulating regional planning. Funds for urban renewal and code enforcement are greatly accelerating local housing and residential improvement programs which will strike at the cause of many urban health problems.

State Environmental Health Programs

Although there is no single pattern for state environmental health programs, every state has a sanitary engineering program which supervises the sanitary quality of community water supplies and conducts other programs of varied scope and magnitude. Some, like New York State, handle the entire water pollution control program under an engineer who is a deputy commissioner of health. Other functions of that unit include air pollution control, general sanitation, certain aspects of housing, residential subdivision control, food and milk, radiologic health, and many other items.

In the California Department of Public Health, the Division of Environmental Sanitation is responsible for food and drug control; for the regulation of public water supplies, swimming pools, and bathing places; for setting air pollution control standards and making studies of its health aspects; for radiologic health; for vector control, including research and advisory services to mosquito abatement districts; and for the provision of consultation, training, and evaluation services for local departments. Other environmental health activities of the California Department of Public Health include occupational health and a regulatory and licensing program for hospitals and nursing homes.

Sometimes important state environmental health programs are under state agencies other than the department of health. For example, in California, water pollution control is largely under State Water Quality Control Boards with the health agencies responsible for only the pathogenic or toxic factors. The State Department of Agriculture is responsible for milk control, meat and poultry inspection, control of pesticide residuals on agricultural products, and labeling of insecticides. The Department of Housing and Community Development regulates housing and mobile home parks. The Department of Industrial Relations is responsible for industrial health and accident law enforcement. The California State Legislature has, however, assigned local responsibilities for some of those programs to local health departments.

The amount of direct services provided by a state to a local unit depends, in part, on how much of the cost is borne by the state. Many states exercise a high level of influence over local programs, principally through subvention or other budgetary allocations to local government.

Local Environmental Health Services

Typical Kinds of Services. Community, county, and other local public health departments usually include an environmental health unit. The unit's staff may range from a single sanitarian or sanitary engineer to several hundred sanitarians and a number of other environmental specialists. The recommended staff is about 1 per 12,000 population, although this may range to less than 1 per 25,000.

The local program usually includes periodic inspections, on a planned basis, of a variety of businesses and activities, including most commercial food preparation, storage, vending, and delivery operations; apartment houses, rooming houses, and mobile home parks; swimming pools and water supply systems; dairies and milk plants; laundries; schools; institutions for the care of children and the aged; industrial plants; users of ionizing radiation; waste treatment and disposal works; and potential sources of air pollution. Other important functions include community rodent, fly, mosquito, and other vector control and nuisance regulation.

Some programs include systems of health permits or licenses to aid in administrative regulation and to help finance activities requiring periodic inspections. For instance, in Los Angeles County, 100,000 businesses are under public health license and pay $2,000,000 a year for this regulatory service.

Differences in Local-State Jurisdictions. In some states there is a trend toward adoption of state regulations which are enforced by local agencies under state supervision. In other states the local programs are more self-sufficient, based on local ordinances and regulations as well as less comprehensive state laws. The amount of local regulatory authority depends, in part, on legally established state-local relationships and on whether local agencies have capabilities in each field. For instance, public water supply and sewage disposal regulation is commonly a state program, but individual water supplies and private, school, and small community sewage disposal systems may be a local responsibility. Milk inspection is another program conducted in a variety of ways. Some responsibilities are usually assigned to the state and some to local health departments. Barbershops and beauty parlors may be under a special state licensing board.

Differences in Local Agency Jurisdictions. From one community to another, there are considerable differences in the allocation of environmental health programs among various local agencies. For example, Philadelphia has a Department of Licensing and Inspection that is responsible for all housing inspection, while the health department has legal responsibility for air pollution control. In Los Angeles County, on the other hand, the air pollution control program is under a special district, while the health department has extensive responsibility for housing code enforcement. Rodent control is usually assigned to the health department. In some programs, the city milk inspection staff checks farms located outside the city, but in certain cities, such as New York, the milk industry is encouraged to do most of the farm milk inspection, while the official agency concentrates on accreditation of the "industry field men" and on health supervision of processing and distribution.

Building departments usually enforce building, plumbing, heating and ventilating, and related codes. They check plans for conformance with their codes and may provide opportunity for the health department to make a separate check for health factors. Some building departments also enforce comprehensive housing codes which require property owners to maintain, repair, and keep all existing housing up to standard. Plumbing inspectors of some jurisdictions enforce codes relating to installation of private sewage disposal, a function which should be closely integrated with the health department's program. In other cases, the principal responsibility for supervision of such installations is assigned to the health department. The plumbing code usually establishes requirements which prevent contamination of the water piping system by cross-connections. Refuse may be collected by a public works department, private haulers, or special sanitation districts. Sewers and sewage disposal may be installed and maintained by the same governmental agency, by a special department, or by a separate sanitation district.

Planning agencies develop master plans and zoning codes and review proposed developments. These agencies are usually receptive to advice on health and sanitation matters which include separation of nuisance-type operations (such as junkyards, certain heavy industries, and sometimes poultry-, animal-, and horse-raising activities) from residential areas. In many communities, separate "community redevelopment" agencies, "housing authorities," and "housing departments" are responsible for urban renewal, slum clearance, and low-rent housing construction, and, in some cases, housing code enforcement.

This summary of the mixed jurisdictional pattern indicates what appears to be a gradual transfer of certain traditional "health" functions to non-health agencies. To assure proper consideration of health factors, the health agency must work closely with other responsible agencies. Ideally, the environmental health unit is represented when building, plumbing, and planning codes are drafted and when plans or programs are being established, revised, or reviewed. The aim of competent local administrators is to minimize duplication and overlapping of inspections. The health agency's goal is to work for the highest health and sanitation standards which are practical, regardless of what agency is responsible for program execution.

THE CONDUCT OF ENVIRONMENTAL HEALTH PROGRAMS

At all levels of government, lawmakers, officials, and the public are taking a new look at traditional health programs. Factors prompting this re-examination include a public demand for more factual data on the long-range effects of environmental stresses on the population; a need for better utilization of scientific data in developing programs and objectives; a desire for a bold, total approach rather than a small, ineffective, piecemeal effort; and a need for utilization of systems analysis and data-processing methods to make long-range assessments of new major programs and to test the effectiveness and efficiency of traditional programs.

A high-priority item in the conduct of environmental health programs is the assignment of the requisite type and number of personnel to various programs. In keeping with the principle of selecting personnel with the appropriate amount of training and education for each task, more attention is being devoted to utilizing technicians and aids for certain routine inspections, sample collection, and monitoring. More highly qualified administrative and technical personnel are thereby freed to plan and guide programs, handle special problems, undertake research, conduct demonstration projects, and perform the more technical inspectional and educational activities.

There was a time when programs were judged by numbers of inspections, citations, court cases, condemnations, and samples collected. While these activities are necessary elements of the program, there has been a shift in emphasis from traditional inspection procedures to the utilization of educational and motivational techniques and the encouragement of business, building, and facility operators, managers, owners, and employees to include environmental health principles in their routine operational procedures.

Development of Codes and Standards

The practice in public health, as in many other regulatory fields, is to include in laws and ordinances only the legal statements of basic objectives and to make provision for a board, commission, or the health officer to develop the more detailed interpretative rules which specify what is required or acceptable. Both the basic laws or ordinances and the rules should be developed in consultation with all concerned groups and interests, thus providing opportunity for the expression of pertinent views. This approach tends to promote understanding of and support for the requirements.

In the development of codes and standards, there is merit in working toward a high degree of uniformity of regulations by adopting model codes provided by the Public Health Service and organizations such as the American Public Health Association. Among the available model codes, standards, and guides are:

Grade "A" Pasteurized Milk Ordinance, recommended by the Public Health Service;

Food Service Establishment Sanitation Manual, recommended by the Public Health Service;

Food and Beverage Vending Ordinance and Code, recommended by the Public Health Service;

Swimming Pool Code, recommended jointly by the American Public Health Association and the Public Health Service;

Housing Code, recommended by the American Public Health Association and developed in collaboration with the Public Health Service;

Model Housing Maintenance and Occupancy Ordinance (Rev. 1967), the American Public Health Association and the Public Health Service;

Manual of Septic Tank Practice of the Public Health Service;

Drinking Water Standards of the Public Health Service;

Recommended State Legislation and Regulations: Urban Water Supply and Sewerage Systems Act and Regulations, Water Well Construction and Pump Installation Act and Regulations, Individual Sewerage Disposal Systems Act and Regulations, the Public Health Service;

Threshold Limit Values of the American Conference of Governmental Industrial Hygienists.

Other sources of data for uniform standards are documents of the World Health Organization, including Expert Committee Reports; the Atomic Energy Commission's national and international committee-recommended standards regarding ionizing radiation exposure; and many other publications and reports covering air pollution control, industrial sanitation, schools, hospitals, and other institutions.

Standards, evaluation criteria, and "seal-of-approval" programs have been developed by several unofficial agencies which have strong support from health agencies. These include the National Sanitation Foundation of Ann Arbor, which has developed standards, criteria, evaluation techniques, and a "seal-of-approval" program covering all commercial food service establishment equipment; plastic pipe for water and drainage systems; swimming-pool equipment; vending machines; and special devices for mobile home waste and "frost-proof" well connectors. The Foundation also has developed procedures for certifying agencies which evaluate x-ray film badges worn by persons such as x-ray technicians.

The Public Health Service, the International Association of Milk, Food and Environmental Sanitarians, and the Dairy Industry Committee, by participating jointly in a Sanitary Standards Committee, have developed many standards and issued seals of approval for milk handling and processing equipment. The Bakery Industry Sanitary Standards Committee is concerned with the sanitary features of commercial baking and bakery ingredient handling or processing equipment, and administers an equipment approval program. The Automatic Merchandising-Health-Industry Committee of the National Automatic Merchandising Association has developed standards for food- and drink-vending machines.

Application of Codes and Standards

The Health Permit and the Grading System. The regulatory *health permit* is a most effective tool for assuring construction, equipment, and materials which meet health agency standards and for correcting serious or repeated violations of standards. The permit should be legally established so it may be withheld or denied until standards are met, and it should be subject to suspension for significant violations of requirements. To comply with good legal and administrative practice, a business owner who believes such action is not justified should be entitled to a formal hearing by the health officer, his authorized representative, or a board.

Some codes provide for "A," "B," or "C" *grading* of food establishments and milk supplies. The concept is that the grade must be prominently posted on the premises or printed on the container. Fear of loss of business when the enterprise or product is graded below "A" encourages management to have a high level of interest in what standards must prevail to maintain the grade. A defect in earlier grading programs was that before reducing a grade, defects were pointed out and time was allowed for correction. Thus, the grade was based on conditions *after* correction and was not a true indication of normal conditions. The newer concept is to base the grade on conditions found at the time of unannounced periodic inspections. Some health officials favor the "permit" system on the theory that all food establishments and milk should meet acceptable standards. Others favor grading on the grounds that they believe enforcement is easier and that the system promotes interest in and support for high standards.

Abatement Provisions. In most large communities, there are usually several kinds of abatement provisions. These include legally requiring vacating of unfit housing, quarantining contaminated foods, providing emergency treatment of water, and abating overflowing sewage. Other provisions may pertain to dealing with contamination by radionuclides, closing grossly substandard swimming pools and beaches, abating heavy rodent or insect infestations, correcting serious occupational health hazards, and other summary abatement procedures.

New Approaches to the Conduct of Environmental Health Programs

The traditional concept of "sanitary inspection" involved noting defects and issuing instructions or a check sheet indicating what improvements were required. Inspections were made periodically, at a frequency based on the size of the inspection staff. Such programs are not as effective as might be expected because, too often, the same or similar unsatisfactory conditions are found repeatedly and are only temporarily corrected. To overcome some of the weaknesses in traditional inspection programs, a more scientific and comprehensive approach is now taken to correct causes and to stimulate continuous maintenance of acceptable conditions rather than to require periodic, temporary compliance. Also, data from past inspections are utilized to indicate which establishments, activities, or programs need more attention and which are almost always in a satisfactory condition. This leads to a frequency of inspection according to need rather than a frequency that is uniformly applicable to all.

Under normal conditions, the steps in the conduct of an environmental health program which produce best results involve a maximum of "preventive sanitation." This begins by the establishment of objectives through studies, applied research, or reference to well-documented, national model codes and standards. Standards are then developed for construction, equipment, and facilities which will aid in accomplishing the objectives. These are written into appropriate codes or rules, and provision is made to check plans, new equipment, construction, and installations for conformance.

Education by on-the-job and "classroom" training of persons with operational responsibilities is a second step. These organized training programs are directed toward groups such as food handlers, milk plant operators, water and sewage treatment plant operators, commercial pest control operators, and swimming-pool operators. Organized classes must be supplemented and in some cases replaced by on-the-job training conducted during inspections. The goal is to educate persons responsible so that they understand what is desired and to stimulate them to want to do what is necessary to follow prescribed procedures. Incentives include certificates to individuals who attend training programs and placards for businesses or plants which carry out the prescribed, continuous sanitary maintenance. Cooperation and participation are stimulated by involving labor union leaders, trade association executives, technical society officials, trade press publishers, and others in program planning and subsequent support and publicity programs.

In the past, there has been a tendency to place too much emphasis on monitoring of, and enforcing codes relating to, physical facilities. Inadequate attention has been devoted to operational activities, which are often of more significance. This is particularly true in programs to reduce food-borne illness. Thus, staphylococcus toxin-type food poisoning is controlled best by keeping toxin-liberating foods appropriately hot or cold. This necessitates careful use of devices for keeping stored hot foods hot and periodic use of food-testing thermometers by responsible food handlers. Similarly, salad and sandwich preparation employees must properly use refrigeration facilities to avoid allowing cold foods to remain too long at room temperature. Salmonella food-borne illness from infected food handlers is best prevented by approved toilet room hygiene and hand-washing practices of persons who handle ready-to-eat moist foods. Care to avoid using utensils, surfaces, or hands which may have become contaminated with raw poultry, for instance, is another element in preventing this type of infection. Another is adequate knowledge of and attention to the cooking temperatures necessary to destroy this organism and other pathogens. Similar examples exist in nearly every branch of environmental health including water purification equipment operation, air pollution control, swimming-pool operation, and maintenance of housing, including mobile home parks. In all of these instances, inspections and code enforcement procedures must be accompanied by programs to train and motivate the responsible employees, managers, and supervisors.

Some programs lend themselves to legally establishing mandatory accreditation of certain persons responsible for health-oriented activities. Included are licensure or certification of water treatment and sewage disposal plant operators, pasteurization equipment operators, swimming-pool operators or service technicians, plumbers who officially test health agency-required check valves that protect the water supply, food-handling employees, milk industry field men who conduct inspections and supervise certain sanitation practices on dairy farms, and others. These programs are usually administered by health departments, which also prepare educational materials or conduct training programs to assist applicants in meeting job qualification requirements.

The evaluation of what is actually being accomplished is another important aspect of the conduct of environmental health programs. Modern data-processing methods are used to assemble and analyze data showing what each employee reports and to indicate the relative condition of the various units subject to inspection. This is an important beginning, but it is recognized that the data simply indicate what was reported. Whether the report accurately represents actual performance and true conditions must be determined by other evaluation techniques. Program evaluation techniques are useful aids in program planning and in supervision. They depend on use of standardized forms and instructions prepared in sufficient detail so that various trained evaluators obtain comparable results. A well-established evaluation method is the Public Health Service compliance ratings for milk control programs in which results are expressed by a numerical score, 100 being perfect. Similar systems have been extensively used for food service establishments and are being developed or are in limited use for various other programs. Some evaluations are conducted by an outside agency, as in the case of a federal rating of a state program or a state evaluation of a local program. Other kinds of evaluations are made routinely by supervisory personnel in connection with the work of their staffs. Some programs build evaluation into each inspection in an attempt to obtain a continuing rating for each unit under routine inspection.

There is a continuing shift in emphasis or priority placed on the various programs in the field of environmental health. Part of the shift is due to the disappearance of certain disease outbreaks which make unnecessary the environmental health programs that had been designed as control measures. This improvement, in turn, is evidence of the effectiveness of the past programs. In general, effectiveness has been achieved not only by requiring good fundamental design and construction of new facilities, but also by encouraging operating agencies and organizations to assume a major share of the health control responsibilities. Examples are the strict operating controls exercised by many agencies which operate water supply, treatment, and distribution systems or sewage treatment facilities. Some maintain and utilize laboratory facilities which are more elaborate than those of many health departments. Similarly, milk companies operate inspection, control, and laboratory programs which include all elements required by health codes plus additional steps considered desirable to improve flavor and quality and to retard spoilage. As such programs become established, the health agency need not duplicate those efforts but may significantly curtail routine inspections and sampling, once satisfied with the methodology applied by the operating agencies. This does not mean that official controls are abandoned, but rather that additional time is available for a more comprehensive over-all program and for evaluation of results. Any time saved by curtailing unessential programs can be well spent in considering and developing controls for new problems.

AREAS OF ENVIRONMENTAL HEALTH ACTIVITY

Water Supply Safety

Urban Water Supplies. As with all effective control programs, community water supply surveillance involves planning, review, and approval of proposed sources, treatment, storage, and distribution systems; periodic inspections; and routine laboratory examination. Water supply sanitation supervision procedures are outlined in the Public Health Service Drinking Water Standards.[5] The first step is the sanitary survey to evaluate the source, treatment processes, storage facilities, and distribution system. The standards suggest the number of samples per month to be collected from various points within the distribution system in order to conduct tests for microorganisms of the coliform group. Standards also are given for color, turbidity, odor and taste, total solids, chlorides, and various chemicals and materials which may be toxic or objectionable.

Community water supplies taken from rivers and lakes are normally filtered. The most common method is by the rapid sand filtration process. A coagulant, usually alum of ferric chloride, is mixed with the water, and slow agitation causes a precipitate to develop, most of which settles out in a few hours and takes with it much of the suspended materials. The water then flows through a layer of sand a few feet thick, at a rate of 2 or 3 gal per minute for each square foot of surface area. Next, the water is chlorinated and flows to a final tank where it remains for about 30 minutes, during which time the chlorine acts on remaining microorganisms. Special treatment is sometimes applied for taste and odor control, usually by use of activated carbon. Some water requires softening or removal of objectionable minerals.

Some water supplies, such as the main supply to Los Angeles, may come from mountain streams and reservoirs which are protected from sewage or industrial wastes. Such supplies are not filtered, but they are chlorinated. Community wells are sometimes used without any treatment if they are built to exclude surface drainage, are located remote from subsurface sewage disposal systems, are over 50 ft from any sewer line, and derive water from sand, sandstone, or a good filtration medium. However, if the water is derived from cavernous or open-jointed limestone, there is hazard of contamination traveling from quite distant sources, and therefore such supplies are usually chlorinated.

Some authorities are advocating that all public water supplies be chlorinated regardless of their origin. Owing to the superior resistance of the infectious hepatitis virus, and possibly other organisms, the trend is toward chlorinating to develop sufficient free chlorine residual to destroy that virus, especially if the supply is derived from a source subject to sewage contamination.

Water supply reservoirs are normally designed to exclude all surface drainage and are screened to exclude birds and animals. When a water supply is stored in an open reservoir which may be contaminated by surface drainage, birds, and other sources, the water flowing out should normally be chlorinated before entering the distribution system. The distribution system must be periodically surveyed to eliminate the hazard of contamination by cross-connections. For example, there may be a direct connection between the public distribution system and an industrial water supply piping system delivering untreated water from a river, canal, or an otherwise unapproved source to be used for processing, cooling, or fire fighting. When the pressure in the unapproved supply exceeds that of the public supply and the interconnecting valve leaks or is opened, serious contamination results. This type of condition has caused several serious outbreaks of waterborne illness. Control is accomplished by prohibiting such direct connections or by special check-valve arrangements which permit the potable water to enter the unapproved water system but prevent flow in the other direction.

Interruptions of pressure in the public water supply may produce vacuums in portions of the water piping systems, which can result in "back-siphonage" from unprotected flushometer valve-operated toilets, from inlets or hoses submerged in contaminated water or chemicals in various tanks and fixtures, etc. Correction is accomplished by installing vacuum breakers which prevent such back-siphonage or by terminating faucets well above the rims of fixtures. Health, water, and plumbing officials, together with plumbers, steam fitters, device manufacturers, and building managers, share in assuring that new installations are safe and that existing hazards are corrected. Special problems with hospital equipment necessitate avoiding direct connections between sewers and autoclaves, instrument sterilizers, and water sterilizers by using a funnel-type drain arrangement to avoid backup of waste water or sewage into these devices.

One of the most common water treatment processes is softening by zeolite. This is sometimes done for an entire public supply such as in the treatment plant of the Metropolitan Water District of Southern California. It is also the method used in most household and commercial softeners. Hardness is caused by the presence of bicarbonates and sulfates of calcium and magnesium in the water. When these chemicals pass through a mass of zeolite crystals, they exchange their calcium or magnesium for sodium from the zeolites, thus producing sodium bicarbonate and sulfate, which do not cause hardness effects. The increase in sodium is not a health factor except for a person with a strict limitation on sodium intake.

An optimal amount of fluoride ion in the water supply has been shown to reduce dental caries by over 60 per cent in persons consuming such water since childhood. While the fluoridation of water is a subject of public controversy in some communities, optimum amounts of fluoride ion produce no ill effects and there is no technical difficulty in adding the appropriate amount to a public water supply. In the Public Health Service Drinking Water Standards, the optimum amount is given according to the mean annual daily maximum temperature and ranges from slightly under to slightly over 1 milligram per liter or part per million (ppm).

Rural Water Supplies. Since it is normally uneconomical to extend public water supply systems to rural homes and buildings, these are normally served by private supplies. However, most health officials strongly advocate developing a community water supply system in preference to developing individual, private supplies for suburban subdivision developments. Household water treatment systems cannot economically provide safeguards normally expected from public supplies. Operation is likely to be neglected or not correctly carried out. For these reasons most rural household supplies are obtained from wells and springs.

Wells may be drilled, driven, bored, or dug. Except where driven wells are practical, most modern wells are drilled. They are located 100 to 150 ft or more from subsurface sewage disposal systems and lesser distances from sewers. Usually every effort is made to locate the well on higher ground than nearby septic tank systems. The casing, platform, and pump are built and arranged to effectively exclude surface drainage or leakage. The casing should normally not terminate in a subsurface pit or basement because of the danger that flooding will cause contamination to enter the well.

After wells are drilled, pumps installed, and piping connected, the well and system should be heavily chlorinated, allowed to stand full of chlorinated water, pumped out to remove the chlorine residual, and subjected to the coliform test. The water also should be checked for chemical content, except where the content of the region's well water is known. Any well pump which must be primed, or wells and springs from which water may be dipped, are too subject to contamination to be considered safe (see Fig. 7-2). Water from wells, particularly those in limestone or similar formations, should be periodically checked to be sure it is free of contamination.

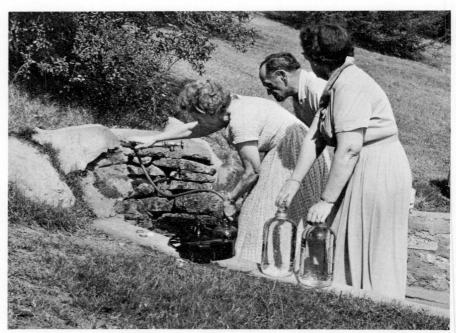

FIGURE 7-2.   Unsafe spring water. (Courtesy of the Division of Public Health Education, Los Angeles County Health Department.)

Milk Sanitation

The control of diseases of cattle that are transmittable to man is largely a function of state departments of agriculture and involves tests for tuberculosis and brucellosis and the slaughter of reactors. Currently, much effort is devoted to the control of mastitis in cows, even though no direct human disease problem is normally involved. It is also important to prevent transmission of human pathogens from milk handlers to milk. The main factor in control of milkborne disease is pasteurization followed by processing and packaging in a manner to prevent recontamination.

Pasteurization is heat processing which destroys all organisms that may be pathogenic when ingested. It does not destroy spores or heat-resistant organisms, but these are not pathogenic when ingested. Pasteurization of fluid milk is accomplished under a wide variety of time-temperature conditions. Currently, the most common method is the high temperature–short time method, 161°F for 15 seconds, in a unit which employs heat exchange principles to utilize the hot pasteurized milk to warm the cold incoming milk and vice versa. Controls and recorders, checked periodically by the health official, assure conformance with time-temperature requirements. Other temperature-time combinations include 145°F for 30 minutes, and 194°F for 1 second.

Pasteurization is checked by the phosphatase test, which is based on the fact that the enzyme phosphatase, naturally present in raw milk, is inactivated by pasteurization. Standards limit coliform organisms to ten per milliliter on the presumption that the presence of this organism is evidence of improper pasteurization or of contamination subsequent to pasteurization; the coliform organism is destroyed by pasteurization. The rickettsial organism which causes Q fever is also destroyed by pasteurization; this disease is thought to be transmitted by air as well as by contaminated milk.

The Public Health Service code provides detailed explanations of all important features of dairy farm and milk-processing sanitation. The most common test is the standard plate count, which indicates, principally, improper cleaning of equipment and inadequate refrigeration. Tests which health departments perform on milk samples include: tests to discover watering of milk; butterfat tests; nonfat solids tests; bioassay tests for vitamins; tests for radionuclides (most significant when nuclear bombs were being tested); microbiologic growth-inhibiting tests for presence of antibiotics used to treat cows; and insecticide residue tests to determine that milk meets the "zero tolerance" requirement for chlorinated hydrocarbons. Tests of milk-processing procedures include: timing tests to be sure milk is held at pasteurization temperature for required time; control-valve tests to see that milk cannot leave the pasteurizer except at required temperature; pressure tests to be sure pasteurized milk in heat exchanger units is always at higher pressure than raw milk, so that the latter cannot leak into pasteurized milk; and total plate counts of milk cartons to check for compliance with microbiologic standards.

Although most municipalities in the United States require milk to be pasteurized, some allow raw milk if it is "certified," which means it is produced under the additional supervision of a Medical Milk Commission and is subject to additional tests. In the production of certified raw milk, cows and milk-handling employees are subject to special health examinations and total plate counts must be low (5,000 to 10,000 per milliliter compared to over 100,000 permitted for raw milk which is to be pasteurized). Most health officials believe modern pasteurization does not destroy or adversely affect any significant component of milk and that pasteurization is the best process to assure milk which is free of pathogens. The Public Health Service code no longer makes provision for raw milk.

Pasteurization of dairy products, other than milk, is also important. This applies to ice cream, butter, cottage cheese, many other cheeses, etc. Dry milk, to meet Public Health Service standards, must be made from "grade A" pasteurized milk. Unfortunately, some dry milk products are made from raw, manufacturing-grade milk and may not be properly pasteurized if dried under a vacuum which permits "boiling" at relatively low temperatures.

High standards for fluid milk are enforced, in part, by regulations which permit "degrading" of the milk for significant violations. In some systems this means that the label on the cartons must then be changed from "A" to "B." In other jurisdictions, it means that, when degraded, the milk can be used only for manufacturing such products as butter, cheese, and certain other items.

Dairy inspection, especially for those close to urban developments, includes control of manure handling to minimize fly breeding and nuisances and proper drainage for mosquito control. Modern dairy operation involves milking machines, sometimes directly connected to pipelines which deliver milk to a refrigeration unit and an insulated storage vat from which it is pumped directly into a tank truck.

Plant inspection includes checking recording devices which indicate pasteurization temperatures and setting and sealing pasteurizer pumps to assure milk is processed slowly enough to provide the required holding time. Proper cleaning and bactericidal rinsing of most pipelines and equipment, both in the modern dairy and at the plant, is by clean-in-place methods which surge rinse water, detergent, and sanitizing solutions through all equipment. This does a satisfactory job, avoids contamination by hands, and saves labor. Much of the milk industry's effort is directed toward quality control. This includes control of off-flavors from the cow's feed, oxidation, overpasteurization, etc., and reduction of psychrophiles (cold-thriving organisms) in order to prolong the "shelf life" of milk. The Public Health Service provides a program of certification of interstate shippers of milk. Participating state milk control officials are qualified to check and rate local inspection services, including their laboratories and their level of conformance with the code. Milk from qualifying areas and plants then is accepted in other states which participate in the program.

Food Sanitation

One category of food sanitation programs involves those wholesale food-processing, packaging, and distribution operations which are interstate in nature and are largely under the control of the Food and Drug Administration and the U.S. Department of Agriculture. These programs are primarily concerned with labeling, adulteration, misbranding, control of botulism, regulation of meat and poultry slaughter and wholesale processing, long-range effects of toxic or carcinogenic ingredients, and control of sanitation and insect or rodent contamination of such foods.

The second category of food sanitation programs applies to operations which are normally subject only to state and local control. The state and local programs are more directly concerned with administration of laws and ordinances governing food service, preparation, processing, sale, and distribution on a local level. The objectives of the programs are to minimize food poisoning and infection; to provide clean, sanitary, and vermin-free establishments; to provide foods that are sanitary, safe, and wholesome; to provide sanitary utensils; and even to regulate, to a degree, the esthetic conditions of food establishments as they broadly relate to health and sanitation. The most commonly reported foodborne illnesses are from a toxin liberated in certain ready-to-eat foods which were contaminated with staphylococcus organisms and allowed to remain at room temperature for hours. Fewer salmonella than staphylococcus toxin cases are reported but more probably occur due to salmonella from intestinal discharges from human beings, poultry, animals, and rats. Other causative organisms of foodborne illnesses include enterococci and *Clostridium perfringens*.

Local food sanitation programs cover restaurants, markets, bakeries, bakery distributors, vending machines, caterers, food demonstrators, itinerant restaurants, food service operations at carnivals and festivals, bars, soda fountains, and a wide variety of other types of businesses and establishments.

As mentioned earlier, a food sanitation program is most effective if a license or permit, or a grading placard, must be obtained and displayed before operations begin. This is issued only after it is determined that the establishment is designed and equipped to facilitate proper maintenance. A food establishment should have design features to exclude rodents; screens or self-closing doors to exclude flies; lighting to facilitate sanitary operation; surfaces and materials which can readily be kept clean; and equipment to protect foods from contamination by leakage or by customers, including protective devices for unpackaged food displays. Special provision should be made for hand-washing facilities convenient for the employees, preferably in food preparation areas. There should be equipment such as drainboards, garbage disposers, and preflushing devices, and sinks or dish-washing machines for utensil and equipment washing. The provision of facilities to permit orderly storage of foods at safe temperatures is par-ticularly important. Facilities should be provided to properly prepare foods, including washing of fruits and vegetables to be eaten raw; cutting boards and slicing machines capable of being kept clean; and arrangements to keep utensils, containers, and surfaces used for raw foods such as meat, fish, and poultry separate from those used for ready-to-eat products. In-structions and training should be provided to assure capability to operate in compliance with health standards.

The customary measurement of the effectiveness of a sanitizing process is the "rim count" test (standard plate count) indicating a recovery of less than 100 microorganisms from each utensil "swabbed" in a prescribed manner. To meet this requirement it is usually necessary to expose utensils to hot water at about 180°F in a sink or spray-type machine or to immerse them in a 100-ppm chlorine solution or in an equivalent iodine or quater-nary ammonium compound solution.

Special precautions are necessary in order to ensure safe preparation of poultry and meats in markets. In such establishments, facilities may be inadequate; raw products may contaminate finished foods; inadequate temperatures may permit salmonella to survive the cooking process; and food "warmers" may be so designed, loaded, or used that foods are held at temperatures which favor multiplication of microorganisms.

Other food service operations which present special problems include central commissaries which distribute food to several establishments or schools. The main concern in such cases is maintaining temperature control during the distribution process. Similarly, catering of foods to special pri-vate parties may be hazardous unless properly regulated. Modern lunch trucks which serve industrial plants and carry full meals of both hot and cold foods also have temperature control problems unless proper equipment is provided. A special danger may exist if leftover perishables are kept overnight on a truck that is not equipped with electrically or gas-operated refrigerators and hot-holding units.

"Food poisoning" investigation is an important program, especially when results of such studies are used in developing preventive programs through education of the health department staff and the food industry. One study found that over 80 per cent of foodborne illness from meals in the United States was due to meat or meat products. A second most common cause was found to be custard made of egg and dairy products. Prevention of staphylococcus "food poisoning" is principally accomplished by tempera-ture control since staphylococcus organisms practically stop multiplying at below 45°F and above 118°F. Codes usually require perishable foods to be kept at below 45°F or above 140°F, except during processing. Hand washing is another high priority item, especially after using the toilet, in order to prevent spread of salmonella from food handler to foods. Salmonella infection is commonly traced to food handlers, unpasteurized egg products, and inadequately cooked poultry. Since symptoms do not occur until 12 to 24 hours after eating, this illness is very inadequately reported, with probably less than 1 per cent of the cases being made a matter of official record.

Waste Disposal Control

Liquid Waste Disposal. Primary objectives in liquid waste control are to prevent contamination of surface or underground sources of water supply, to preserve the sanitary quality of waters used for swimming and recreational purposes, to avoid nuisances and health hazards from overflowing septic tank systems and cesspools, and to prevent contamination of water supply sources with chemicals, insecticides, weedicides, or other materials which may be toxic.

One approach to regulating liquid waste disposal is by requiring approval by the official regulatory agency of plans and specifications for the treatment facilities. The other approach is through "performance standards" whereby conditions required to be maintained in the waste-receiving waters are specified by a regulatory board and the means employed to comply are left to the ingenuity of the designers.

The degree of treatment provided for community sewage and liquid industrial waste depends on the use of the receiving water and the quantity of waste in relation to the quantity of water available for dilution. For example, the degree of removal of potentially pathogenic microorganisms needs to be much higher when the effluent is discharged into a stream or lake used as a source of a public water supply than when it is discharged into the ocean at a point remote from recreational areas or shellfish beds.

In Los Angeles, sewage is discharged into the ocean through multiple outlets a few hundred feet deep and miles from shore. This procedure meets requirements after only "primary" treatment to remove suspended and floating solids. The removed material (sludge) is digested in a closed, heated tank to break down grease and organic solids, producing a large quantity of gas used for power generation. The digested sludge is then discharged to the ocean from the treatment plants.

For more complete treatment to discharge into fresh water or ocean water near beaches or shellfish beds, large cities and many towns use the activated sludge process to produce a much more highly purified effluent. This process includes introducing air bubbles into sewage held in tanks for 6 to 12 hours or longer, thereby promoting the growth and multiplication of aerobic organisms which feed upon sewage constituents and convert nitrogenous material into stable nitrites and nitrates. These organisms then clump together, or flocculate, to produce a brownish "activated sludge," which settles out in a final settling tank. Part of this sludge is returned to the aeration tank to maintain that desired concentration of microorganisms needed to accomplish good treatment, the balance being disposed of, usually by drying after digestion. The effluent may be further "purified" by chlorination or chlorination plus filtration and may be used for irrigation, recreational lakes, recharge of underground water supply "basins," industrial processing, and other beneficial purposes.

Simple and efficient sewage treatment also is accomplished by a process applicable to small communities and some industrial wastes. The sewage is simply discharged into one or a series of "stabilization ponds" about 3 ft deep in algae, which in the presence of sunlight liberates oxygen that, in turn, is used by microorganisms to stabilize and purify the waste. About an acre of water surface is required for each 200 to 1000 population. While originally used only in warmer climates such as California and Texas, the process now operates even in cold northern states. It is especially suitable for developing countries.

Health agency participation in community or regional planning and in real estate subdivision approval programs lends support to a practice of extending public sewerage systems or of requiring properly designed treatment systems for community sewage. Such systems are desirable alternatives to the unsatisfactory practice of allowing suburban developments with a septic tank system for each home. Septic tank systems eventually overflow or stop functioning and cause waste to back up in plumbing fixtures. When public sewers and community disposal systems are not practical, the subdivider should be required to provide lots which are large enough and laid out to provide ample area for sewage disposal systems, and other controls should be established to assure that private sewage systems are not allowed except where conditions are favorable to their successful operation.

There are other sources of concern and problems yet to be solved in connection with liquid waste disposal. Industrial wastes discharged to streams and lakes may deplete the dissolved oxygen, causing fish to die and odors to develop. Reclamation of waste water by proper treatment is a desirable objective. Another problem arises from the presence of phosphates and other nutrients in the effluent from sewage and waste water treatment processes which are satisfactory in all other respects. These nutrients promote the growth of algae which are undesirable in recreational and other lakes since they cause cloudy and sometimes odorous water and produce undesirable bottom deposits, as has happened in Lake Erie. This phenomenon is causing international concern and is leading to interstate action as at Lake Tahoe on the California-Nevada boundary.

Solid Municipal Waste Disposal. Community collection and disposal of solid waste, and public cooperation in its proper storage, are necessary to minimize rodent problems, fly breeding, and nuisances from improper storage and disposal (see Fig. 7-3), as well as to abate smoke from burning in improperly designed and operated incinerators. Improperly regulated public dumps for solid wastes produce flies, rats, and smoke.

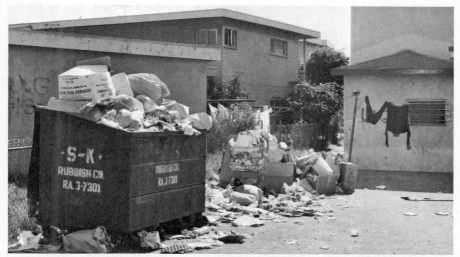

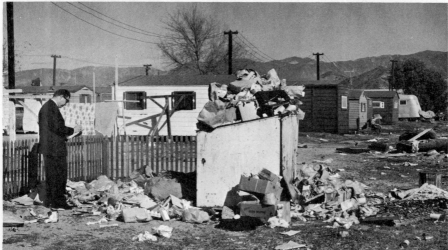

FIGURE 7-3. Improper disposal of waste. (Courtesy of the Division of Public Health Education, Los Angeles County Health Department.)

Health agencies usually have major responsibility for promoting or requiring sanitary storage of waste materials at living quarters, markets, and elsewhere and for preventing rat, fly, and nuisance conditions at the refuse disposal site. Public works officials are responsible for collection and disposal. They usually want to economize by collecting refuse and garbage only once a week, while some health officials favor twice-a-week collection. Health agency studies in California show that cans or other receptacles containing garbage produce thousands of flies per week when collection is only once a week, and that the number of flies is greatly reduced by a twice-a-week collection. However, it has been shown that even when twice-a-week collection is provided, 50 per cent of the cans are set out for collection only once a week. No ordinary garbage can is "flytight" since adult flies crawl under a "tight lid" to lay eggs, and larvae crawl out under the lid to pupate in nearby ground. Devices for discharging garbage to the sewer are a big factor in reducing this problem.

Sanitary landfills provide a reasonably satisfactory method for disposal of community refuse. The material is deposited in marshes, canyons, abandoned gravel pits, etc., compacted by bulldozers, and promptly covered with earth before fly breeding or rat feeding can occur. The land reclaimed by the filling operations provides much-needed parks and "open space." Care is taken to locate sites where they will not pollute underground water supplies, and to locate and operate to minimize neighborhood nuisances from blowing papers, dust, and odors.

Incineration of refuse and garbage in well-designed and operated community units is practical, but costs about five times as much as disposal by sanitary landfills. The incinerator must be designed to predry very moist material, to introduce a controlled amount of air to support combustion, and to provide a combustion chamber of such size and design that it will allow enough time and air mixing (turbulence) to promote complete combustion at a temperature above 1200°F. Devices to collect "fly ash" from the stack gases are installed and operated to prevent neighborhood nuisances from dust and charred paper.

Agricultural Wastes.   Unless properly regulated, agricultural wastes produced by commercial chicken and poultry raising, dairies, and horse raising, particularly in suburban fringe areas, cause serious fly problems. The most important step in preventing fly breeding and nuisances from animal manure is to arrange, operate, and maintain the animal-raising premises to facilitate prompt drying of the manure. Fly larvae feed and develop when manure is moist, but not when it is reasonably dry. This objective involves covering chicken-raising pens and coops to exclude rain, design to facilitate ventilation, and regular removal of manure or raking to mix with already dried manure. Manure from cows raised in feeding corrals causes little problem in dry, warm weather but serious problems when the manure remains moist and warm. The magnitude of the problem is indicated by the fact that each cow produces 9 tons of manure a year, so that at large dairies with up to 1000 cows or more there may be 25 or more tons of manure produced per day.

Manure and certain other solid wastes, if provided with the right amount of moisture and air, will heat themselves to destroy any form of insect life (and weed seeds) and become a valuable soil conditioner and fertilizer. Composting of animal waste is usually economically practical, but composting of mixed municipal refuse in the United States has not been as economically successful.

Solutions to agricultural waste problems are being developed by collaboration between health officials and agricultural interests such as farm advisors, Farm Bureau Federation officials, and university specialists. Large numbers of research and demonstration projects on all aspects of solid waste management and disposal are being supported by Public Health Service grants. One important point already agreed to is that the problem must be approached on a regional basis.

Housing, Urban Renewal, and Building Inspection

When housing is considered in the context of a broad definition of public health, there is no doubt about a direct relationship to health. The American Public Health Association has long been active in promoting and developing standards for healthful housing. The Association's "Basic Principles of Healthful Housing" has served as a guide and goal for designing new housing and for developing codes and evaluation procedures for existing housing; the appraisal procedures are characterized in terms of "facilities," "maintenance," "occupancy," and "environment."

New Housing. As was stated by Lawrence Veiller, an authority of the early 1900's, housing programs should begin by assuring that future housing is properly designed, built, located, and equipped. The health agency's role in this phase is largely advisory and consultative and includes supporting and participating in the development of master plans and zoning regulations which will ensure good residential environmental conditions. Such conditions include space for light and ventilation; freedom from avoidable traffic hazards, noise, and air pollution; separation of housing from undesirable industrial and commercial activities; and provision of requisite community services and facilities such as water, sewers, drainage, play and recreational facilities, green belts, refuse collection services, and other elements of a good neighborhood.

Building codes should be reviewed to be sure that new housing, built according to the code, will satisfy the "Basic Principles of Healthful Housing." Health official participation in developing building codes should provide expert advice regarding space (including separation of functional parts of the living quarters), light, ventilation, plumbing, accident prevention, heating, insect and rodent control, and all other items with health implications. Special consideration should be given to standards for legal conversion of large, old homes to multiple occupancy for apartments, "light-housekeeping" units, rooming houses, or boarding homes; occupancies intended for the aged; mobile home parks; condominiums; and multistoried buildings, especially those intended for large numbers of families with children.

Maintenance and Occupancy. Health departments traditionally have had some responsibility relating to sanitation and vermin control in housing. In some states, such as California, they have had authority to enforce state laws regulating sanitation, maintenance, ventilation, and occupancy of all housing, including a single family home occupied by its owner. Enforcement of such regulations by periodic, planned inspections of all multiple occupancies which operate under a "health permit" and of all housing in older neighborhoods has prevented development of those grossly insanitary and delapidated conditions which characterize slums. Authority to require vacating of grossly unfit housing is a valuable administrative tool when suitable substitute housing is made available through cooperative programs among health officials and public housing authorities, welfare officials, relocation specialists of community redevelopment agencies, and other agencies or groups with resources for relocating displaced families.

Unfortunately, code enforcement, alone, does not completely correct unsatisfactory housing conditions, and citations and fines are not effective in producing lasting results. In some cases, occupants must be educated and motivated to properly use and maintain housing. In addition to the traditional evils of unsympathetic absentee landlords, it is impossible to provide and maintain housing satisfactory for modern living at rents which poor, large families can afford to pay. It is also impossible to enforce a law requiring individuals or couples who live, sleep, cook, and eat in a one-room unit to move to a unit with a private toilet and bath, separate kitchen, and separate living and sleeping areas when they are living on limited pensions. Such persons cannot afford more than a single light-housekeeping room with shared toilet and bath facilities. Health officials must take a realistic approach to these problems and work for the best housing attainable within the economic limitations of the occupants.

Public Housing and Urban Renewal. Federal financial assistance has helped many communities to provide new public housing for low-income families at rents they can afford to pay. Proper utilization of such programs provides acceptable housing for that segment of the population which cannot otherwise afford suitable quarters. In some communities this program is well accepted and supported, while in others, groups have objected to such an extent that no public housing is being built.

There are a wide variety of federal financial assistance programs available for improving housing and the environment. Some must be administered by a special housing agency authorized by state law and organized by local government. To qualify for such programs, the community must first adopt a "workable program" with several requisite elements, including adequate codes and ordinances; acceptable administrative procedures and financing; assistance for displaced families to find "decent, safe, and sanitary housing at rents they can afford to pay"; citizen participation through communitywide and neighborhood housing committees; a program to evaluate and appraise existing housing; and a master plan to guide future development and redevelopment.

When its program is approved, a community is eligible to receive federal financial aid in various forms. For instance, two federal dollars are available for each local dollar to finance an approved *community renewal project*, which is a comprehensive study of physical, social, and economic factors to plan and program future community improvement programs. Health departments can be, and in some cases are, active participants, and contribute much to the success of these programs.

Community redevelopment programs provide federal financial assistance for the acquisition of areas so unfit or poorly planned that they should be cleared, replanned, and rebuilt. The cleared land is sold to private developers who build according to the local agency's plans. *Assisted rehabilitation* is a program in which federal funds are available for staff to administer and operate area improvement programs and to help property owners plan improvements. Qualifying property owners may obtain government-insured financing to make improvements, and completely unfit units may be purchased and demolished to make room for play areas, parks, or automobile parking. *Code enforcement* assistance is available to pay for extra inspection staff and to finance surface improvements such as paving and street lights.

Financial aid and loans are available to help qualified, needy property owners make necessary repairs and improvements. These programs, as in Birmingham, may be administered by a health department. "Demonstration cities," rent subsidies, and other programs give promise of further stimulating a more massive approach to housing and community improvement.

In the conduct of these programs, the health agency should be an expert advisor on health, sanitation, and environmental subjects and should be a participant in appraisal and code enforcement. Economic and social factors must be considered, in addition to the old, traditional concept of housing code enforcement by "criminal prosecution."

Rodent and Insect Control

The control of insects and rodents is commonly called vector control because of their disease transmission potential. The rodent is the host for the flea, which is the vector, or carrier, of plague and endemic typhus. Anopheles mosquitoes transmit malaria, which, until this decade, caused up to 300 million cases and 6 million deaths a year. Even without their disease transmission features, the control of rats, mosquitoes, and flies is justified. Control is normally most effectively achieved by modifying and regulating the environment to reduce or prevent their propagation. This is particularly applicable in cities and developed areas.

Rodent Control. As in nearly all health programs, rodent control involves cooperative work of many groups, organizations, and the public. Buildings should be constructed to prevent rodents from entering and from nesting inside. Food wastes should be stored and disposed of so that they are inaccessible to rats. When necessary, extermination measures through poisons, trapping, and gassing should be undertaken.

Trapping is relatively slow and difficult. Suitable poisons, mixed with the rodent's favorite food or water supply and placed along runways, are most effective. This is done by commercial pest control operators and some public agencies, including health departments. Some poisons are deadly to man, and their placement must be carefully controlled. Some, such as anti-coagulants mixed with cereals, are quite effective and, since feedings are required over several days, are less hazardous to children than the more fast-acting poisons. A reasonably effective material, when properly used, is red squill, which kills rodents because they cannot regurgitate, but acts as an emetic to human beings, poultry, and animals other than rodents. To be effective, rodent control programs require constant community education and periodic inspection visits and consultations.

Mosquito Control.   Since mosquito eggs hatch and the larvae and pupae develop only in quiet water and under certain conditions, mosquito control is most effectively accomplished by eliminating or modifying these waters. Each species has a special preference for the type of water accumulation in which it develops. Anopheles mosquitoes prefer clean, shallow water. *Aedes aegypti*, which transmit yellow fever and dengue, prefer small quantities of water near concentrations of people, including rainwater accumulations in discarded containers. *Culex tarsalis*, the vector of encephalitis, breeds in a variety of nonsalty waters including surplus irrigation water. A vicious daytime-biting aedes species lays its eggs on dry salt marsh flats where it remains until submerged in salt water. *Culex fatigans*, which causes urban filariasis, prefers water heavily contaminated with human wastes.

Control programs include draining and filling marshes and low areas; planting a species of fish (*Gambusia affinis*) which eats the larvae; fluctuating water levels to cause larvae and pupae to be exposed to waves and currents; applying larva-killing sprays; improving irrigation practices; designing better gutters and drainage systems for new subdivisions; and conducting public education programs on control procedures.

Some health departments have active mosquito control programs. However, in New Jersey, California, and some other states, mosquito control is the responsibility of well-organized, -staffed, -equipped, and -financed mosquito abatement districts which operate heavy grading and ditching equipment, airplanes for spraying, and special vehicles to spray the water in gutters and catch basins. Ponds are also maintained to stock Gambusia fish for planting where needed and for distribution to persons who maintain garden pools in which mosquitoes may breed.

Fly Control.   The public expects the modern urban environment to be reasonably free of flies. As with mosquito and rodent control, fly control is most effective when its breeding habits are understood and the program is directed toward eliminating conditions favorable to fly development. With but few exceptions, the fly's eggs must be deposited in moist organic material on which the emerging larvae can feed. After about three or more days of feeding, the larvae leave the very moist material, burrow into the ground or reasonably dry material, where they develop shells to become pupae, and then, a few days later, emerge as adults. The housefly, *Musca domestica*, prefers animal manure; the lesser housefly commonly develops in chicken manure; and the shiny "blowflies" prefer garbage and decomposing meat.

Fly control involves keeping flies from their preferred larvae-developing materials; disposing of such materials before the larvae are fully developed; arranging and operating poultry and animal-raising facilities to dry the manure before the larvae are fully developed; and substituting units to dispose of garbage in the sewer instead of in garbage containers. Adult flies are excluded by screens and self-closing doors. The use of fans to exclude flies from markets and restaurants has been promoted, but studies in Los Angeles failed to demonstrate any statistical correlation between presence or absence of fans and the number of flies. Further studies showed fans must produce an air velocity of over 1700 ft per minute to exclude flies, and this was objectionable to customers and employees so that fans of adequate capacity were not routinely turned on.

Extermination of adult flies requires continuous attention. As new insecticides are developed, the fly develops resistance, so that new products must constantly be developed. Strict control to prevent contamination of milk and certain foods with DDT-like compounds has reduced the use of these chemicals on dairy farms and in food establishments. Lindane vaporizers are not favored because they may cause contamination of foods and are a suspected cause of a few cases of aplastic anemia. Pyrethrum sprays have been used for many years, are effective if the mist strikes the fly, and are relatively nontoxic.

Air Pollution Control

The effects of air pollution range from localized nuisances of smoke, soot, dust, and odors to huge areawide fumigations which cause serious physical discomfort, possible injury to health, and sometimes deaths.

Causes and Control of Air Pollution. St. Louis and Pittsburgh, long noted as smoky cities, found their sources to be principally smoke from coal burned in furnaces, boilers, and industrial operations. By requiring the coal to be relatively free of sulfur and by enforcing codes requiring "smokeless coal" or efficient automatic stoking devices, those cities made miraculous progress in air pollution control. Smoke control is accomplished by efficient combustion in properly designed and operated equipment.

Large power and heat-generating plants in which coal is burned may produce large quantities of fine ash which is discharged through the chimney. This is especially true when coal dust is burned in a boiler equipped with fans which produce a heavy draft. Dusts are also produced in certain steel-making processes and in many other industrial operations. These dusts may be collected in any of several types of dust collectors. Relatively coarse dust is collected by centrifugal force in a device called a cyclone. Some dusts are trapped in devices which function like a vacuum cleaner bag. Fine dusts are collected in an electrical precipitator in which a high voltage between wires and metal plates causes the dust to be precipitated on the plates from which it is periodically removed.

Odors are controlled by various processes. Some are soluble in water and disappear when the odorous air is passed through a suitable water spray. Some odorous vapors, such as those from rendering (pressure-cooking) meat scraps and dead animals, are condensed and drained to the sewer. Various other controls include beds of activated charcoal, chlorine, odor-neutralizing or -masking compounds, and incineration of odorous gases.

Smog. The greatest public interest and concern are expressed about concentrations of atmospheric pollutants which have caused deaths, as in Donora, Pennsylvania; have covered a whole community or area such as New York City and much of the East; and have produced the well-known Los Angeles "smog" and somewhat comparable air pollution situations in various parts of the world (see Figs. 7-4 and 7-5). Heavy, areawide concentrations of air pollution are usually associated with meteorologic conditions which do not permit normal dispersion and dissipation of pollutants from an area. The most common condition is known as a temperature inversion. This refers to the fact that the air temperature normally decreases about 5°F for each 1000 ft rise in elevation. On some days, for various reasons, a cooler layer of air remains near the earth's surface while the sun warms the air above that layer. The elevation above which the air temperature drops, with a rise in elevation, is known as the base of the inversion. Its height varies from a few hundred to a thousand or more feet. The lower the elevation, the more intense the "smog" because all pollutants accumulate beneath and cannot escape beyond that elevation until the sun warms the lower air mass and breaks the inversion condition. The inversion is accompanied by calm air with very little horizontal or vertical motion.

The other factor in some "smog" formations is a photosynthetic reaction which promotes chemical reactions that transform nonirritating substances to irritating or lacrimatory chemicals and change transparent gases to cloudy materials. In Los Angeles studies, it has been shown that unsaturated hydrocarbons from unburned gasoline or automotive exhaust combine with nitrogen dioxide, ozone, or other "oxidants" to produce complex chemicals which induce irritation. Control involves attempts to eliminate discharge of unsaturated hydrocarbons by blocking their escape from the engine's crankcase and by developing devices or methods to more completely oxidize or burn the fuel. Oxides of nitrogen are produced by a chemical union of oxygen and nitrogen of the air when exposed to high temperatures in

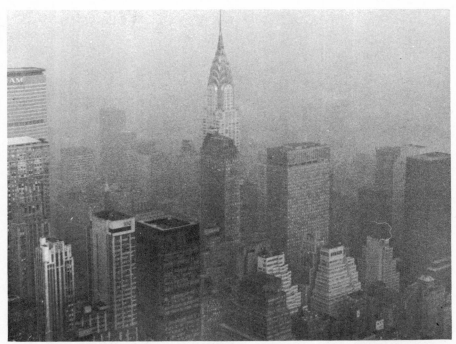

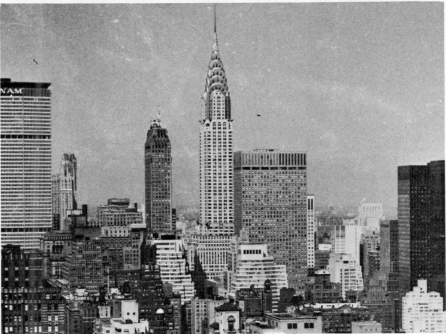

FIGURE 7-4. Midtown Manhattan (New York) blanketed by smog; same view on a clear day. (Courtesy of United Press International.)

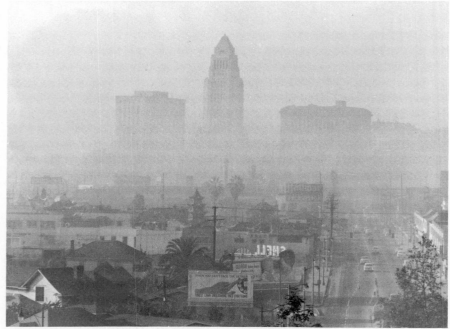

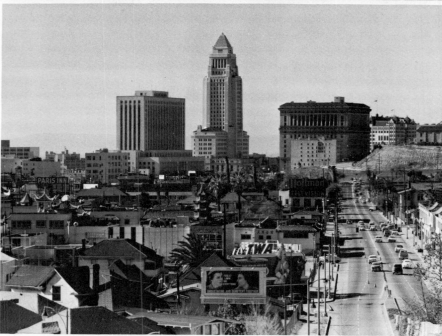

FIGURE 7-5. Downtown Los Angeles blanketed by smog; same view on a clear day. (Courtesy of the Division of Public Information and Education, Los Angeles County Air Pollution Control District.)

boilers of power plants and to combinations of temperature and pressure in the internal combustion engine. Oxides of nitrogen produce a reddish-brown tinge to the atmosphere and some become involved in photosynthetic reactions. In above-normal concentrations they are toxic and irritating.

In some areas, the automotive vehicle is the principal source of air pollution. Control of this source is a serious problem in an area of frequent, marked temperature inversions and heavy automotive traffic. The solution will include more use of electric rapid transit and ultimately, possibly, substitution of other sources of power such as new, more efficient batteries to power vehicles and controlled atomic energy for major power-generating stations.

Radiologic Contamination Control

Public interest and concern over radioactive contamination reached a peak during the period when nuclear bomb test explosions were releasing huge quantities of man-made radioactive pollution. Radioactivity was easily detected by simple geiger counters in the visible dust accumulations which occurred, and contamination was found in water, food, and milk. The cessation of tests has greatly reduced this problem. Much of the concern was based on calculations which purported to show that genetic damage would affect millions of people in posterity. Another concern was for strontium 90, which accumulates in the bones, including the backbone, and emits ionizing radiation to bombard blood-forming body substances. A further concern was for iodine [131], which was found in milk, water, and food shortly after nuclear blasts. It may accumulate in the thyroid and thereby increase the risk of cancer of the thyroid or other conditions. Fortunately, iodine [131] loses half its strength every eight days. The Public Health Service and state departments of health continue monitoring the environment for these substances in food, milk, and water.

The conclusion drawn from assessments of hazards from radiologic contamination is that man is likely to receive much more ionizing radiation from medical application than from fallout. This lends support, for example, to comprehensive control programs aimed at eliminating, as far as possible, unintentional exposure to x-rays. Health physicists and radiation control technicians of health departments encourage and require, or actually install, devices to limit the size of the x-ray beam so it exposes only the area required for the desired film or treatment. Lead-containing aprons shield the gonadal region. "Filtration" of the beam through aluminum removes soft, useless, but somewhat undesirable rays. Fast film, more sensitive fluoroscope screens, better fluoroscopic techniques, and more efficient units all aid in that objective. Shoe-fitting fluoroscopes (see Fig. 7-6) and units of some practitioners of the healing arts which produced long exposure for relatively useless purposes are outlawed in most places.

Atomic Energy Commission licensing of users of man-made radionuclides

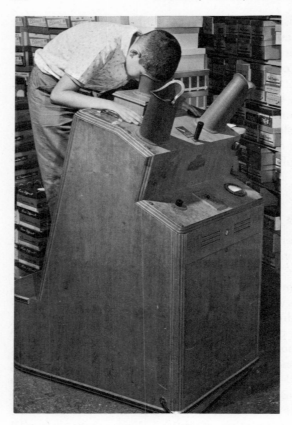

FIGURE 7-6. Child using a potentially dangerous fluoroscope in a shoe store. (Courtesy of the Division of Public Health Education, Los Angeles County Health Department.)

and persons who may dispose of radioactive wastes provides a high degree of protection. Fifteen state health departments now assume these functions in their states. A few redelegate the function to qualified local health agencies. A good, comprehensive program carefully regulates all users of man-made radionuclides in medical, industrial, research, and teaching activities. The Atomic Energy Commission reserves to itself control over reactors and similar masses of the material.

Occupational Health

Health programs particularly directed toward workers and their families are in the category of occupational health. This term is preferred to "industrial health" because it is broad and includes agricultural and all other kinds of occupations in addition to those found in industry. Industrial hygiene is primarily concerned with industrial sanitation and control of those specific materials which are known to produce particular occupational disease. Occupational health usually means a more broad program which covers the total public health field as it relates to employees and sometimes their families.

The earliest industrial hygiene programs resulted from the discovery that workers who were exposed to certain substances, usually over an extended period of time ranging from hours to years, developed specific symptoms which came to be associated with such exposures. Breathing lead fumes or ingesting lead produced peculiar conditions such as the "blue line of the gums" and "wrist drop" recognized as symptoms of lead poisoning. Years of exposure to silica dust as in "hard-rock" mining and sandblasting reduced the oxygenation capacity of the lungs and accelerated the ill effects of tuberculosis and other lung diseases. Mercury compounds used in preserving rabbit furs for felt hats produced a nervous irritability which led to the saying "mad as a hatter." Workers not adjusted to exposure to zinc oxide developed a nighttime chill known as brass founder's ague. Scientific study was made of cause and effect by teams including the industrial physician, industrial hygienists, and industrial health chemists. Long-term correlation of symptoms with types and levels of exposures led to adoption of the "threshold limit values."

Control of the Working Environment. A good occupational health program includes checking plans for new plants and new proposed processing operations in order to identify potential hazards and to "build in" appropriate controls. New chemicals are checked and tested for deleterious effects before workers are exposed to them. This kind of industrial hygiene should be carried out in conjunction with all other interested environmental control program administrators. For instance, processes are checked to assure that discharges from workroom ventilation systems meet air pollution control requirements. The source of water supply is checked to be sure that it is safe, and water-piping plans are checked to assure no cross-connections will contaminate the supply. Industrial liquid and solid waste-handling proposals are reviewed. Proposed installations of x-ray units or facilities for use of radionuclides are reviewed. Plans for lighting, ventilation, air conditioning, noise control, first aid, drinking fountains, toilet rooms, dressing rooms, special safety eye showers, and all other items related to health are checked.

A well-rounded program establishes a planned, periodic inspection program for most places of employment. This should cover the entire working environment, including water supplies and cross-connections, stream and air pollution potentials, sanitation, and housekeeping as it relates to safety.

Control of Hazards to the Worker. Control to limit worker exposure to injurious materials is effected by a combination of procedures. Thus, harmless substances are substituted for those which have a deleterious effect, as in the case of the substitution of a nontoxic glue for liver-damaging benzol as a rubber adhesive. Particular kinds of processes are isolated, such as the handling of all lead oxide for batteries in a closed, vacant, glass-sided room until mixed and made into the dust-free battery plate. Local exhaust ventilation is provided in order to draw contaminants away from workers, such as in paint spray booths. Various personal protection devices are used such as aprons and gloves to protect against acids and air-line respirators for sandblasters who cannot be otherwise protected.

In the decade from 1953 to 1963, the number of hearing-loss claims filed by workers against their employers rose dramatically. This started with a New York court case in which, for the first time, substantial compensation was awarded for partial hearing loss, a condition for which such awards previously had been limited to medical costs and lost wages. Awards of over $20,000 have since been made in certain cases. Control of industrial noise exposure includes reduction of noise at its source, isolation of noise-producing operations in sound-proofed areas or rooms, and use of suitable noise-reducing earplugs or muffs. Regular hearing tests are advocated for all employees subject to sound levels which approach 85 decibels for a considerable part of the working day. This level of noise is much below that which produces the sensation of pain and is approached on the busy street corner of a large city.

Since workmen's compensation laws make occupational diseases compensable (as explained in Chap. 5), physicians report suspected cases. Investigations and tests are made to determine whether a cause-and-effect relationship is demonstrated, and suitable corrective measures are recommended as required.

Prevention of Occupational Diseases. Pre-employment and periodic examinations are part of a good occupational health program and include special tests to enable measurement of incipient, adverse health effects from the working environment. Such examinations include special blood and urine tests, x-rays, hearing tests, and whatever else may be necessary to learn whether exposure to dusts, fumes, chemicals, noise, and special stresses (such as excessive temperatures, vibration, strains, and other adverse working conditions) are producing measurable deleterious effects. Beyond this, the program may tie in with a total preventive and case-finding health program for the worker and his family. Some exemplary programs bring together the entire applicable resources of the employer, the unions, and the official health agency.

Occupational health physicians and nurses observe for dermatitis and its causes, this being the most common occupational disease. Special effort is made to reduce exposure to excessive temperatures or repeated motion which causes strain. Facilities are provided to make the employees' environment as healthful and pleasant as practical. For outdoor workmen such as telephone linemen, advice is offered on controlling exposure to, and effects of contact with, poison ivy or poison oak. Agricultural workers are given information on methods of protection from toxic sprays, and mechanics are advised on skin-damaging effects of various solvents, cutting oils, and chemicals.

Industrial medical, nursing, and consultation services may be operated in conjunction with other official health agency, private agency, or labor organization programs. Programs of this kind may include case-finding for tuberculosis or more broad medical provisions similar to those now existing under certain private and government sponsorship. There must be close collaboration with the workmen's compensation and safety officials of labor departments and with industrial safety experts so that all understand and agree on systems of referrals and avoid conflict and overlapping. While officials of public health agencies are interested in accident prevention, that program is largely the responsibility of labor or industrial welfare agencies, with whom health officials collaborate. Many industrial plant organizations include good combined occupational health, radiologic health, and safety programs, and such a combination would be desirable within health agency programs.

The Role of Official Health Agencies in Occupational Health. The staff of the occupational health units of those state and local health agencies which have a formal program usually include one or more physicians, engineers, nurses, chemists, industrial nurse consultants, and a number of industrial hygienists and field inspection personnel. Some occupational health inspection and survey programs are operated only on a consultant basis, responding to requests of other governmental agencies, industry, and labor. Good support has been given, however, to those agencies which make routine visits to all places of employment, comprehensively survey the total working environment, and require necessary corrections. Local health departments sometimes combine this type of program with sanitation inspections of food service, general sanitation, and cross-connection control in places of employment. They then refer observed suspected occupational hazards to industrial hygienists, engineers, nurses, or physician for follow-up or consultation. In California, local occupational health programs are mandatory activities for the more populous counties. In several states, local health departments are empowered to enforce state labor law provisions related to occupational health, as well as to enforce all health and sanitation codes. This makes it possible to develop a comprehensive program.

State programs vary according to what department is assigned primary responsibility for occupational health. In some states, rather full legal authority is assigned to health departments. In most, the primary legal authority is assigned to another agency with the health agency serving in a consulting role. However, there is need for an occupational health unit in every state health department in order to provide advice, at least, on health problems of industrial, agricultural, transportation, mining, and construction programs.

Current Status of Occupational Health Programs. Occupational health programs are strengthened by federal laws which require health controls in industries and by activities which are federally financed or under federal contracts. Educational systems such as colleges and universities have established strong occupational health programs for their employees, research workers, and students by combining occupational and radiologic health, sanitation, and safety in an integrated program. Some large industries have well-organized and -staffed, full-time occupational health programs covering medical, nursing, engineering, environmental, radiologic, physiologic, and psychologic problems of workers. The main unmet need for industry-operated programs is to find ways to provide more complete programs for small industries, especially those with fewer than 500 employees.

Accident Prevention

The number of deaths from accidents in the United States has been mounting steadily over the past decade. On the other hand, the death rate per 100,000 population has been declining somewhat. These facts are illustrated in Table 7-1, which shows an increase in accidental deaths from

TABLE 7-1   Deaths and Death Rates from Accidents, United States, Selected Years

	Number of Deaths	Rate per 100,000 Population
1950	91,249	60.6
1955	93,443	56.9
1960	93,806	52.3
1963	100,669	53.4

Source: Adapted from U.S. Bureau of the Census. *Statistical Abstract of the United States, 1965,* p. 62.

about 91,000 in 1950 to over 100,000 in 1963, but a decline in the death rate from 60.6 per 100,000 population in 1950 to 53.4 in 1963.

Table 7-2 shows that considerably more accidental injuries occurred at home than at places of employment. Thus, in 1964, there were 12.6 injuries

TABLE 7-2   Rates of Persons Injured, by Class of Accident and Sex, United States, 1964 *

	Rate per 100 Population		
	Male	Female	Both Sexes
While at work	7.8	1.6	4.6
Home	12.5	12.7	12.6
Other (incl. motor vehicle)	14.7	8.3	11.4
Total	35.0	22.6	28.6

Source: Adapted from U.S. Bureau of the Census. *Statistical Abstract of the United States, 1965,* p. 84.
* Data refer to the civilian noninstitutionalized population, including Alaska and Hawaii. Includes only persons with injuries involving one or more days of restricted activity or medical attention.

per 100 population incurred at home and only 4.6 while at work. Compared to females, males have an over-all higher rate of accidental injuries, the difference being accounted for by a higher injury rate while at work and from other sources, including motor vehicles; the rate of home accidents is similar for both sexes.

Health departments have in some places stimulated development of good accident-reporting and analysis programs in what is known as the epidemiology of accidents. This provides factual data for use in educational and control programs. Such programs may include measures to reduce poisonings of children by various causes, the most common cause being improper storage of drugs and chemicals. Health officials in Baltimore and Philadelphia have long recognized that children who chew on the old, blistered paint from poorly maintained housing develop lead poisoning. This led to educational and enforcement programs, including efforts to obtain substitution of paint which is free of lead.

Industrial accidents are receiving much attention, and programs of safety groups and state accident commissions have produced a dramatic reduction in injuries and deaths from this cause. Institutions and housing for the aged and handicapped persons provide a good opportunity to study causes of accidents and to develop corrective programs involving construction, maintenance, wiring, and various types of handholds. In fact, accident prevention is an integral part of any comprehensive housing inspection, enforcement, and educational program.

Food establishment inspection programs and accident prevention are closely related. The apparent conflict between requiring "smooth, readily cleanable floors" and the need for floors rough enough to prevent slipping when wet or coated with grease is being evaluated with a view toward relinquishing some degree of cleanliness for greater safety. Burns, cuts, lost fingers from grinders, falls due to use of improvised stands for reaching high shelves or because of poor lighting, and slippery and littered floors and stairs are examples of conditions of special safety interest in food establishments. Grease fires in broilers and from grease-laden filters or parts of kitchen exhaust systems are common and may be minimized by proper design, operation, and maintenance.

Motor vehicle accidents have become an increasing concern in recent years. There are now about 50,000 *deaths* a year from such accidents. With respect to *injuries* due to moving motor vehicle accidents, Table 7-3 shows that the age group of 15 to 24 years has the highest injury rate. Thus, in the period 1959 to 1961, there were 30 injuries per 1000 population in this younger age group compared to about 18 injuries per 1000 population among those aged 25 to 64. Driver-training courses in schools, other kinds of educational programs such as those conducted by the National Safety Council, and the accident prevention programs of official health agencies are all directed toward reducing motor vehicle accidents. There is also a growing national participation by health professionals in programs to im-

TABLE 7-3   Rates of Persons Injured, by Type of Accident and Age, United States, 1959–1961 *

| | Rate per 1000 Population | | |
	Moving Motor Vehicle Accidents	Other Accidents	Total
Under 15 years	9.3	294.5	303.8
15 to 24	30.0	261.6	291.6
25 to 44	17.2	210.6	227.8
45 to 64	18.8	199.5	218.3
65 and over	13.7	175.8	189.5
Total	16.4	238.8	255.2

Source: Adapted from U.S. Bureau of the Census. *Statistical Abstract of the United States, 1965,* p. 84.
* Annual average for July 1959–June 1961. Data based on household interviews conducted by the National Health Survey and covering a sample of the civilian noninstitutionalized population, including Alaska and Hawaii. Includes only persons with injuries involving one or more days of restricted activity or medical attention.

prove automotive safety. This includes such diverse activities as conducting studies to aid in developing safe traffic arrangements in new residential areas, participating with others in learning the causes of automotive accidents and injuries, and developing corrective measures. Health authorities are conducting research to learn what automobile design factors will minimize injury from collision and what human reactions are related to the causes of accidents.

INTERNATIONAL ENVIRONMENTAL HEALTH

Environmental Health in Developing Countries

For developing countries, the disease control aspect of environmental health is still paramount. In many such countries waterborne diseases remain a leading cause of illness and death. A study of water supply conditions of 75 developing countries [6] showed that 40 per cent of the urban populations and at least 70 per cent of the total populations had no access to piped water within reasonable distances of dwellings. In many cases the water supplies were unsafe or the pressures so intermittent that contamination of the distribution system resulted, even though the source was satisfactory.

Where piped water is not available at each dwelling, water often is stored in vessels which provide breeding places for *Aedes aegypti* mosquitoes, the cause of extensive outbreaks of dengue fever. Inadequate sources of safe water and the presence of unsafe piped-water outlets in residential areas are a major reason why cholera persists in Calcutta. When water is piped into communities in which there are no sewers and where the soil is impervious, waste water accumulations develop and provide excellent breeding conditions for the mosquito *Culex fatigans,* which transmits "urban filariasis." An attack rate of 20 per cent was reported for Georgetown, in what was British Guiana. Similar conditions developed in Rangoon, Burma, and elsewhere.

Malaria eradication is still a big, future job in many countries, especially with resistances developing to insecticides and antimalaria drugs. New dams and irrigation projects are increasing the already high rate of schistosomiasis (called bilharziasis in many countries), an infection from contact with water contaminated by small, free-swimming cercaria which develop in snails. The infection is through skin contact with the water, as well as possibly through ingestion. A challenge to health educators is to persuade people to avoid contact with such water and to research specialists to develop more effective snail-killing chemicals (molluscicides).

The vast majority of the inhabitants of many developing countries live in villages and rural areas. Under these circumstances, environmental health services may range from simple health education on sanitary excreta disposal to well-organized programs to provide convenient, safe water supplies for villages and rural dwellers. Rustic and improvised housing is commonly made of the most convenient, locally available materials, such as straw and palm leaves in some regions and mixtures of mud, straw, and bamboo elsewhere. Water may be taken from somewhat distant streams, from dug wells subject to contamination, or from ponds or improvised catchment areas to collect rainwater.

The current mass movement to cities is creating huge, uncontrolled, unplanned, and grossly insanitary areas surrounding many cities of developing countries. People with no money and no skills erect makeshift shacks, haul their water from distant faucets, have no sanitary facilities for excreta or waste disposal and no organized health or sanitation services. Within the many modern cities of developing countries the environmental problems are quite similar to elsewhere and include congestion, air and water pollution, occupational health problems, and many other conditions which necessitate collaboration of health, planning, construction, and operating agencies in order to minimize the possible ill effects of urbanization.

National planning which integrates health programs with economic, social, and physical planning on a broad scale is an effective means of promoting rural environmental health in developing countries. An example is the Venezuelan program of improving living conditions in villages in order to arrest the mass movement to "ranchos" of squatter families ringing cities such as Caracas. The program is linked to a national agrarian reform movement and is successful partly because it is carried out under a combined welfare and health agency. By combining into one unit the disciplines and authorities necessary for a comprehensive program, and in collaboration with the agricultural department, a remarkable program emerged. Planners and economists on the health staff, working with agricultural specialists, plan and build villages surrounded by farm plots for each family.

The health department's sanitary engineers build the village water systems and streets. Natives with special aptitude are encouraged to become small private contractors who, under health department supervision, build the homes. These are provided with running water to a kitchen sink, a laundry tub, toilet, and shower. Homes are surrounded by flowers and small garden plots. Social workers select families most likely to be stable and successful and assist them in adjusting from life as seasonal cane sugar fieldworkers living in crude shacks to a new life in a self-governed community. Families, in their spare time, have built elementary schools, clinics, village halls, and churches. The income from farm produce provides a good living for most families. The high level of sanitation plus other health services provided by periodic medical-nursing team visits to the clinics produces dramatic improvements in health.

Environmental Health Administration and Programs in European Countries

European health administrations have never adopted the American practice of including a strong sanitary engineering unit in their organization. Environmental health programs are largely administered by medical administrators, assisted by various kinds of inspectors. Engineering programs related to public health are principally conducted through national public works or other agencies. Housing programs are centered in housing and building departments. At the national level and to a lesser extent at the local level, the assignment to health administrations of responsibility for large medical care programs and the recognition of the desirability of combining environmental health with other environmental improvement and control programs are leading to the assignment of all environmental responsibilities to agencies other than health departments. For instance, most national environmental health programs in England have been moved to the Department of Housing and Local Affairs. At the local level, most traditional health agency environmental programs of Britain are under the Chief Public Health Inspector, and some of the programs are operated as a separate department directly under the local governing council.

In the U.S.S.R., the health ministry has major environmental health responsibilities and does a large amount of research on this subject, working with and through research institutes. The studies cover a wide variety of subjects with emphasis on learning the adverse effect on human beings of long-range exposure to small concentrations of deleterious substances and to various types of noise. Experimental tests also are conducted on the effects of modified features of housing and community design and arrangement. Health-regulatory programs in the U.S.S.R. are conducted by "sanitary physicians" aided by college-trained assistants called "feldshers."

The level of health standards varies from country to country, but in many there is less emphasis on elements which are stressed in the United States.

The consumption of wine and beer in place of water may be due to the fact that there has not been adequate emphasis on water supply sanitation to enable people to drink water without concern for their health. Similarly, much raw milk is being sold, some dipped into the customer's container by the milkman. However, the Scandinavian countries and certain others have effective programs to assure the highest quality of milk products as well as other exemplary sanitary controls. Raw meat and even processed meat, which are potential sources of foodborne illness, are commonly displayed or hung in markets and restaurants without refrigeration. Glasses and dishes are washed in a single basin sink with only a cold-water faucet, and no facilities are provided for bactericidal treatment, even at many of the newest and most modern bars and restaurants. Self-service smorgasbords are common, but very few are equipped with typical American protective glass shields.

Community collection and disposal of solid wastes in Europe is generally by modern packer-loader trucks, or in some countries, by collecting whole cans and leaving cleaned, empty containers. Special effort is made to provide clamped-on lids, rubber covers, etc., in recognition of the fact that ordinary lids do not exclude flies and confine odors. This may, in part, account for the lack of fly problems at sidewalk cafes and elsewhere. Composting and incineration are most common since land is generally too scarce for use as sanitary-landfill sites.

Stream pollution control is well advanced in many countries, with some exemplary international programs such as the cleanup of the Rhine River, which was subject to heavy municipal and industrial pollution. An international conference on water pollution control research in Munich in 1966 indicated a large amount of work in this field. The new concern about algae growth in lakes owing to nutrients in liquid wastes is receiving attention. For instance, all communities around Lake Zurich are building new sewage treatment plants, or are modifying existing ones, to utilize ferric chloride to remove most phosphates. Temperature inversion effects on air pollution were recognized when an oil-burning steam plant to generate electric power was built in the Rhone Valley with its smokestack located high on the mountainside, well above the level where temperature inversions would cause concentration of this potential source of air pollution.

Much study is directed toward establishing housing and environmental conditions to provide optimum satisfaction of "human requirements." Extensive studies are conducted under the Housing, Building, and Planning unit of the Economic Commission for Europe. An example is a comprehensive inquiry made by that unit to learn what objectives have been established for all housing and environmental factors such as space, air, water, esthetics, light and sunlight, noise, and many other factors. Planning and housing conferences consider such topics as the allocation of land for housing, the construction of new towns, and how to rebuild old cities to accommodate the increasing numbers of automobiles.

England is concentrating considerable resources on a new town movement directed toward establishing self-sufficient, modern communities. The aim is to avoid further growth and congestion of cities such as London. Similarly, the U.S.S.R. is activating a policy to "decongest" its largest cities by locating most new industries at planned communities of 30,000 to 300,-000 inhabitants. The planned communities are designed to provide clusters of neighborhoods, or "microrayons," with shops, services, schools, child-care centers, central heating, laundries, and related facilities located in each. The microrayons are separated from each other by green belts and are designed to minimize traffic within the area and to minimize travel to the place of employment by locating the factories in nearby, especially designated zones, which are termed "compulsory observance of health-protection zones."

The British and U.S.S.R. new towns are providing examples of how planning aids in providing optimum environmental health. Similar examples are being developed in Sweden, Denmark, the Netherlands, and elsewhere. Under socialistic and similar governments, physical planning is closely linked with national economic and social planning, and the resulting policies determine what part of the country's economy will be devoted to housing and the environment.

International Environmental Health Organizations

Several organizations and agencies conduct programs and deal with problems in environmental health on an international scale. Many countries participate in the organizations, and the programs are conducted for the benefit of all nations, but particular attention is paid to coping with the environmental health problems of rural and urban areas of developing countries. The principal objective of such international environmental health programs is to develop and control those environmental factors which are most essential to the control of disease.

The World Health Organization includes environmental health and malaria eradication among its major programs. A significant function of the Organization is to develop reports, papers, and other publications which provide the latest, most authoritative data, advice, and opinion on specific topics in various fields involving the environment. This is accomplished by collaborating with other international organizations, by utilizing the assistance of expert environmental health advisors and consultants, and by periodically convening "expert committees" representing many geographic areas. Notable projects include use of special funds to engage consulting engineering firms to make surveys, financing of studies, and recommendations as the basis for planning comprehensive environmental health programs for metropolitan regions or even entire countries.

Two other units of the United Nations also have responsibilities for certain environmental health programs. The International Labor Organization in Geneva is the principal international agency concerned with the protection of the health of industrial, agricultural, and other workers. The program includes industrial hygiene and the broader considerations of the health of workers and their families. The Food and Agricultural Organization, with headquarters in Rome, works in collaboration with the World Health Organization on the environmental health aspects of milk, meat, and other foods.

The Pan-American Sanitary Bureau, as the executive organ of the Pan-American Health Organization, conducts environmental health programs in the Western hemisphere. In Latin America, the Bureau develops training facilities in sanitary engineering and conducts short courses on selected subjects for practicing engineers. A major activity is developing plans and building or supervising the construction of community water supply systems. Other activities include the establishment, in 1964, of the Institute of Occupational Health and Air Pollution Research, sponsored by the Chilean government, the United Nations Special Fund, and the World Health Organization. Malaria eradication has a high priority. A new program was started in 1964 in parts of the United States, Puerto Rico, and the Virgin Islands to eradicate the *Aedes aegypti* mosquito and eliminate dengue fever as well as yellow fever. In connection with the Central American Common Market, food sanitation studies have been made in Central America by Bureau consultants to assist in setting minimum sanitation standards.[7]

The Agency for International Development includes environmental health among the several fields for which it provides funds and technical assistance to other countries. It conducts programs and helps to train persons in participating countries to take over technical and administrative responsibilities in environmental health. It also stimulates the use of local resources and funds for programs such as the construction of self-supporting water supply and sewerage systems. In order to aid such programs, the Agency publishes various technical manuals in several languages.

SUMMARY

Environmental health programs in the United States traditionally have been concerned with water supply, milk processing, food preparation and handling, waste disposal, and rodent and insect propagation. Extensive control measures in these various areas are directed toward the prevention of specific diseases, and have long constituted the basic sanitation activities of public health. The success of the control programs is indicated by the marked reductions that have occurred in various diseases which are waterborne, foodborne, or attributable to any one of the other sources. However, the traditional areas of concern continue to require attention not only in order to maintain the reduced disease rates that have been achieved, but also because of the development of new, unanticipated hazards from time to time.

A broadened concept of environmental health which recognizes the influence of the *total* environmental on man, combined with the emergence of hazards arising from modern urbanization and industrialization, has generated additional areas of concern and has led to the development of new kinds of environmental health programs. These programs include air pollution control, radiologic contamination control, occupational health, housing in its many aspects, and accident prevention.

Several agencies of the federal government have environmental health responsibilities which, in the aggregate, cover a broad range, including the conduct of programs to improve the quality of various specific aspects of the environment; the development of standards and model codes; the enforcement of legal requirements with respect to various interstate environmental health matters; the conduct of research, testing, and analysis; and the support of training programs. On the state level, the official health agency usually has responsibility for several specific environmental health programs, but in certain states, responsibility for some of the programs may rest with other agencies; furthermore, the allocation among agencies may differ from state to state. Similar mixed jurisdictional patterns occur with respect to official state-local programs, and also in connection with the allocation of responsibilities among local official agencies.

Although the development and application of codes and standards continue to be important aspects of the conduct of environmental health programs, they are guided by several new concepts, including the use of model codes and standards in an effort to achieve some degree of uniformity; the involvement of relevant groups and interests in the code development process in order to promote understanding and support; the conduct of sanitation inspections according to need rather than on a fixed-frequency basis; and the use of a variety of educational and motivational techniques to gain compliance as a preferable alternative to citations and court actions. Other aspects of the conduct of environmental health programs include attention to the quality of operational activities as well as physical facilities; accreditation, certification, and licensure procedures; and provisions for evaluating the effectiveness of programs.

On the international level, environmental health in *developing countries* presents a marked contrast to the United States with respect both to needs and the status of control measures. Waterborne and vectorborne diseases remain principal causes of illness and death in many developing countries, and thus, the provision of safe water supplies and vector control constitute major objectives. In *European countries*, although the level of health standards varies from one country to another, there are numerous instances of significant advances in the several specific areas of environmental health concern. There are a number of organizations and agencies which promote environmental health on an international scale and thus aid countries throughout the world, particularly the developing nations.

REFERENCES

1. Dubos, René. *Man and His Environment.* Pan American Health Organization Scientific Publication No. 131, Washington, D.C., 1966.
2. Senn, C. L., Berger, B. B., Jensen, E. C., Ludwig, H., and Shapiro, M. A. Coliform organisms as an index of water safety. *J Sanitary Engineering Division, Amer Soc Civil Engineers,* 87, No. SA6, November 1961.

3. AMERICAN CONFERENCE OF GOVERNMENTAL INDUSTRIAL HYGIENISTS. *Threshold Limit Values of Industrial Atmospheric Contaminants.* The Conference, published annually.

4. WORLD HEALTH ORGANIZATION. *Environmental Change and Resulting Impacts on Health.* World Health Organization Technical Report Series No. 292, Geneva, 1964.

5. U.S. DEPARTMENT OF HEALTH, EDUCATION, AND WELFARE, Public Health Service. *Public Health Service Drinking Water Standards, 1962.* Public Health Service Publication No. 956, U.S. Government Printing Office, Washington, D.C.

6. DIETERICH, B. H. and HENDERSON, J. M. *Urban Water Supply Conditions and Needs in Seventy-five Developing Countries.* World Health Organization, Geneva, 1963.

7. HORWITZ, ABRAHAM. *Health and Progress in the Americas.* Pan American Health Organization Miscellaneous Publication No. 80, Washington, D.C., 1966.

ADDITIONAL READING

AMERICAN PUBLIC HEALTH ASSOCIATION. *Accident Control in Environmental Health Programs—A Guide for Public Health Personnel.* The Association, New York, 1966.

AMERICAN PUBLIC HEALTH ASSOCIATION, Subcommittee on Radiologic Health. *Ionizing Radiation.* The Association, New York, 1966.

ANDRZEJEWSKI, A., BERJUŠOV, K. G., GANEWATTE, P., HILBERT, M. S., KARUNARATNE, W. A., MOLNER, J. G., PEROCKAJA, A. S., and SENN, C. L. *Housing Programs: The Role of Public Health Agencies.* World Health Organization Public Health Papers No. 25, Geneva, 1964.

BACKETT, E. MAURICE. *Domestic Accidents.* World Health Organization Public Health Papers No. 26, Geneva, 1965.

BELL, ALAN. *Noise—An Occupational Hazard and Public Nuisance.* World Health Organization Public Health Papers No. 30, Geneva, 1965.

EHLERS, V. M., and STEEL, E. W. *Municipal and Rural Sanitation,* 6th ed. McGraw-Hill, New York, 1965.

PAN AMERICAN HEALTH ORGANIZATION. *Environmental Determinants of Community Well-Being.* The Organization, Washington, D.C., 1965.

SALUATO, JOSEPH A., JR. *Environmental Sanitation.* John Wiley and Sons, New York, 1958.

U.S. DEPARTMENT OF HEALTH, EDUCATION, AND WELFARE, Public Health Service. *Grade "A" Pasteurized Milk Ordinance—1965 Recommendations of the United States Public Health Service.* Public Health Service Publication No. 229, U.S. Government Printing Office, Washington, D.C.

WORLD HEALTH ORGANIZATION. *Environmental Health Aspects of Metropolitan Planning and Development.* World Health Organization Technical Report Series No. 297, Geneva, 1965.

WORLD HEALTH ORGANIZATION. *Epidemiology of Air Pollution.* World Health Organization Public Health Papers No. 15, Geneva, 1962.

CHAPTER 8

ACUTE COMMUNICABLE DISEASES

Historic aspects of communicable disease and international implications

The communicable disease process

Public health roles in acute communicable diseases

Principal prevention and control measures

Community aspects of prevention and control

Some common communicable diseases

Summary

This chapter discusses some of the basic principles and problems of the communicable diseases. The historical significance of these diseases and the measures which have developed for their control are reviewed in the first section of the chapter. The next section describes the basic components characterizing infectious diseases and outlines the procedures in identifying suspected disease. Public health objectives in communicable disease programs and responsibilities for control, surveillance, and research are discussed in the third section. Principal methods and various community aspects of prevention and control are reviewed in the next two sections. In the last section of the chapter, the characteristics of several selected communicable diseases are described.

HISTORIC ASPECTS OF COMMUNICABLE DISEASE AND INTERNATIONAL IMPLICATIONS

Communicable diseases have always afflicted mankind and influenced important turns in human history, as has been described in Chapter 1. Leprosy resulted in the phenomenon of "social outcast" and the social obligation of verbal warning by the diseased person that he was "unclean." Epidemics over the centuries have killed more soldiers than weapons of war and turned significant victories into defeat. The Black Death of the Middle Ages carried off intellectual and artistic communities that might have contributed to the earlier enlightenment of the Western world. Pandemics hastened decay of the older civilizations. Tropical fevers such as malaria inhibited development of Asia, and yellow fever had a vivid connotation in "the white man's grave" of West Africa.

The control of these diseases was largely empirical for many centuries. Thousands of years before proof of the germ theory of disease transmission, the enforced requirement for lepers to separate themselves from normal social intercourse was an early form of quarantine. The establishment of Adriatic quarantine stations by the Venetian maritime powers in the sixteenth century was the direct forerunner of the present international quarantine covering six pestilential diseases: smallpox, cholera, plague, louseborne typhus, louseborne relapsing fever, and yellow fever.

Jenner's observation of the protective power of cowpox inoculation in 1798 led to the practice of vaccination decades before the basic principles of microbiology and immunology were even contemplated. Louis Pasteur, less than a century ago, applied the new objective scientific methods of observation and controlled experiment to establish the modern science of microbiology. As a result, he successfully dealt with rabies, a problem that today still challenges the most sophisticated virologic and immunologic techniques and public health practice. Sir Patrick Manson, Sir Ronald Ross, and Walter Reed established the principles of arthropod transmission of filariasis, malaria, and yellow fever.

Provision of pure water supply, sewage disposal, and drainage was the basis for the successful opening of Asia and Africa in the past century. The European introduction of these controls for infectious diseases has been responsible for the emergence of many of the newly developing nations of the world today.

Modern means of communicable disease control have contributed so significantly to the current human population explosion that some of the frightened beholders of the results have even suggested withholding means of disease prevention from those most in need. However, history has shown that the intelligence of man has adapted new boons to his own social betterment and that serious trouble results when people selectively judge who will survive. In fact, the greatest problem preventing self-development of *newly emerging nations* is the creation of a healthy and productive people by conquering the communicable diseases (see Fig. 8-1) which have vitiated their capability to learn and work competitively with those who have largely achieved such control. Communicable diseases are still the number-one health problem of the vast majority of human residents of the earth. Economic self-sufficiency and world peace will not be within reach until communicable disease control and prevention effectively reach all people wherever they may be.

In these days of highly sophisticated developments in surgery, chemotherapy, and massive chronic and mental disease control programs, it is seldom recognized that the knowledgeable worker in infectious diseases

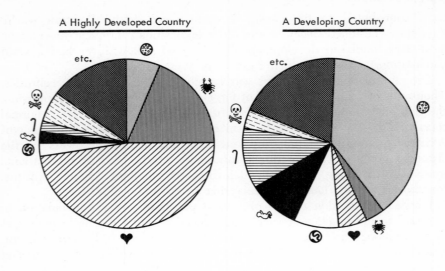

A Highly Developed Country   A Developing Country

⊛   Infectious and parasitic diseases

🦀   Cancer

♥   Diseases of the heart and blood vessels

🕤   Ulcer, appendicitis, intestinal obstruction, gastritis, etc.

👶   Birth injuries, infections of newborn, other infancy diseases

⊐   Old age

☠   Violent death, including accidents, murder, suicide

etc.   All other causes

FIGURE 8-1. Patterns of causes of death: a highly developed country and a developing country. (Source: World Health Organization, Geneva, 1967.)

possesses the resources, opportunity, and obligation to alleviate more suffering and save more useful lives than in any other field of medical science or public health practice.

Various other public health problems such as air and water pollution that have arisen as a result of the affluent society have obscured the needs associated with communicable diseases, which, sometimes through neglect, have been relegated to international health authorities. These authorities are the World Health Organization and Pan-American Health Organization, which are given financial and technologic contributions for the conduct of programs that are merely token compared to the need. Actually, long-term self-interest should stimulate special attention and adequate support in dealing with communicable disease problems abroad.

Although such international organizations have attacked certain communicable disease problems such as malaria and smallpox through specific technical assistance programs, effective application of knowledge to many problems such as yellow fever and schistosomiasis has not been possible because of limited resources. Their most effective performance so far has been in the realm of communication of information and the provision of consultation. The communication is formalized in frequent epidemiologic reports of quarantinable and other diseases, general information in periodic chronicles, and outlets for scientific advances and research through technical publications. In addition, comprehensive presentation of specific areas of knowledge is provided through special technical reports and monographs; orientation and general education are provided through widely distributed publication of interesting and readable elementary information in brochures and periodicals. Localized or epidemic problems are dealt with by provision of expert consultation or participation in investigation and control efforts. Resources and mechanisms for long-term research and investigation of specific prevalent or potential communicable disease problems have, unfortunately, not yet been attained.

THE COMMUNICABLE DISEASE PROCESS

Most organisms have parasitic relationships to other living forms, i.e., one organism lives in or upon, and at the expense of, another. Man as an organism is constantly parasitized by myriad microbial forms. The processes and manifestations of such parasitism are medically characterized as the infectious diseases. Because public health efforts for detection, control, and prevention are focused more toward mechanism of transmission than the process of infection (invasiveness), infectious diseases in the context of preventive medicine and public health are more commonly referred to as communicable diseases.

Terms Relevant to Infectious or Communicable Disease

Etiology is the specific microbial cause of an infection. An *etiologic agent* is the causative infectious agent, such as virus, bacterium, or protozoan parasite. *Susceptibility* is the condition for establishment of an infection by invasion of the etiologic agent. *Resistance* is the condition of lessened susceptibility that may result from immunization, changed nutritional status, and influences of age, sex, race, and heredity. *Diagnosis* is the factual or deduced conceptual terminology for the disease, which usually conveys a specific etiology. *Infection* is the process by which a microbial organism invades and establishes a parasitic relationship to the host. *Pathogenesis* is the course of multiplication, further invasion, dissemination, and destruction of tissue by the etiologic agent following infection. The entire process of infection, pathogenesis, and immune response is often encompassed by the term *infection*. *Incubation period* is the elapse of time from initial infection through evolution of pathogenesis to first appearance of symptoms and signs of disease. It characteristically reflects biologic features of the infectious agent and may be precisely limited in time for certain diseases such as measles, for which the incubation period is ten days. Other diseases have variable incubation periods which may reflect initial mass of infectious material introduced into the host, longer if in small amount, shorter if from a large infectious dose. *Tropism* is the tissue selectivity of the parasite. *Viscerotropic* means that the organism has a proclivity for invasion of the abdominal organs, as in amebic hepatitis. *Neurotropic* is the affinity for the central nervous system, as with the viruses of rabies or poliomyelitis.

Clinical course is that stage of the disease pathogenesis from the time symptoms are first observed to point of recovery: cessation of fever, absence of infectivity, and beginning of convalescence. *Communicability* and *infectivity* are terms that apply to the period that the host is infectious, either by extraction (as with blood-sucking arthropods), secretion (as with sputum), excretion (as with urine and feces) or shedding (as with dermal scales and pustules in smallpox). Infectivity may precede onset of the clinical course of disease. *Immune response* is the capacity of the host to develop specific antibodies to an antigenic stimulus involving either invasion and multiplication of microorganisms during an infection or as a result of active immunization. *Immunity* is the physiologic status that prevents or limits invasion and parasitism by specific etiologic agents or effect of specific endo- and exotoxins. *Sequelae* are deleterious effects such as physical defects and paralyses that result from an infectious disease. A *contact* is a potentially susceptible individual who has been in the proximity of a case, possibly during the period of communicability. *Inapparent infection* is an invasion and limited pathogenesis of an infectious agent without causation of recognizable disease but with stimulation of an immune response. A *zoonosis* is an infectious disease that has its origin in a cycle involving a nonhuman vertebrate reservoir. A *reservoir* is an animal or situation in which etiologic agents are maintained and from which vectors are infected. A *vector* is a carrier or transmitter of an etiologic agent from reservoir to susceptible host. Some vectors, such as ticks, may serve as effective reservoirs.

Communicable diseases may be sporadic, endemic, epidemic, or pandemic. *Sporadic* disease is a separately occurring case by locality or time. An *endemic* disease is one which is always present in terms of locality or time. *Epidemic* refers to disease occurrence beyond that usually expected, either as a new entity or an increase above expected numbers of an endemic disease. A *pandemic* is a sweeping epidemic in terms either of a large number of a specified population being afflicted or of a rapid extension geographically, usually beyond the national borders where it was originally recognized as an endemic or epidemic disease.

Basic Components Characterizing
Infectious Disease

There are three basic components that must be defined in characterizing an infectious disease: (1) pathogen or etiologic agent, (2) host, and (3) mechanism of transmission. Functional health of man is the absence of disease. Continued health depends on host resistance to an upset in the equilibrium which allows excessive influence on the host of the other two components. Survival of the parasite as a threat to human health through causation of infectious disease is dependent on maintenance of equilibrium in the interdependent parasitic cycle.

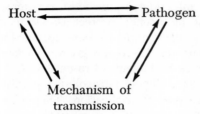

Infectious diseases can therefore be defined and the potential threat understood in terms of these three basic elements.

Host. The term "host" can apply to nonhuman vertebrates and lower animals that harbor pathogens in an unobtrusive or inapparent maintenance cycle, the factors which influence the human host also being applicable to these other forms. Among these are: (1) exposure, (2) susceptibility (age, sex, race, heredity), (3) pathogenesis, (4) resistance, (5) immune response, (6) alteration of susceptibility through immunization and treatment, (7) mechanism of pathogenesis, (8) sporadic or epidemic nature of appearance, (9) occupation and social behavior, (10) social impact, (11) symptoms and signs, (12) indirect detection of infection by laboratory means, and (13) control and prevention of invasion and pathogenesis.

The host component required for occurrence of an infectious disease not only applies to the susceptible individual, but also encompasses the community as a collective host. While measles may produce a sporadic case in a susceptible individual child, epidemic manifestation may occur in a school community of children, the community having in context the same attributes as the individual child.

Pathogen. Infectious diseases can be and are classified in a number of ways. One is by geographic distribution of occurrence. Another is by mechanism of infection. Another is by clinical manifestations such as the exanthemic diseases, diarrheal diseases, and central nervous system diseases. However, the most basic, versatile, and universally applicable classification is based on the character of the pathogen. Generally recognized categories are viruses, rickettsia, bacteria, fungi, protozoa, metazoal parasites, and ectoparasites. In dealing with a wide spectrum of infectious diseases, this kind of classification is the most rational framework in which to comprehend the variety of events that progress to the parasitic causation of ill health, i.e., disease.

Viruses are the smallest pathogens and in one respect the most successful form of parasite. They consist of a template chemical that borrows from the living cell the enzymatic and nutritional elements necessary to reproduce. In doing so they deleteriously deplete or destroy the cells, which ultimately leads to organic dysfunction. As obligate intracellular parasites they can only replicate (reproduce) inside a living cell, a phenomenon which characterizes virus infections as the most insidious. The cells, tissues, and organs of the host in essence protect the virus from chemotherapeutic attack, which is the conventional means for dealing with the other categories of etiologic agents. There is a greater variety of viruses than of any other category of microbial agents of disease.

Rickettsia are also obligate intracellular parasites but are susceptible to antibiotic suppression of replication. They also differ from viruses in being visible under a conventional microscope by special staining techniques.

Bacteria can readily multiply outside of living cells. This makes them amenable to cultivation on artificial media. They are also readily visualized by appropriate staining techniques. The detection and identification of a bacterial cause of disease is therefore much simpler relative to the special facilities and techniques necessary to detect, isolate, and identify viruses and rickettsia.

Fungi are the lowest form of infectious agent that bridge the gap between free-living and host-dependent parasites. Being of uni- or multicellular form, they are rather easily characterized visually under the microscope and can be grown on selective artificial media.

Protozoa, as the term implies, are single-celled organisms. They are large enough to fix and stain for definitive microscopic identification according to nuclear and cytoplasmic structure. Although as living cells their nutritional and physiologic requirements are complex, some can be readily cultivated, which aids in their detection and identification. Forms vary from intracellular (malaria) to hematogenous (trypanosomes).

Metazoal parasites, because they are multicellular, occur in widely varied form that reflects the special adaptation characteristic of their parasitic cycles, which are reflected by the categorical terms trematodes, nematodes, and filaria.

Ectoparasites range from those which superficially affect the host, like lice and scabies mites, to those which invade the integument, such as larvae of dipterous flies.

Mechanism of Transmission. A parasitic species must gain exit from its supportive host to continue its existence. It must then survive until it finds and successfully invades another susceptible host. There it reproduces to initiate a further cycle which perpetuates the species. Means for exit of a pathogen is not only of significance in survival of the parasite; it characterizes the infectivity of the host to others and determines the hazard of the infected host to the environment it occupies. This is of significance relative to the chance of contaminating a vehicle such as air, water, or food, directly inducing further infection of susceptible hosts by contact or infecting an intermediate host which may serve as a reservoir or vector of the pathogen.

The period during which the pathogen can escape from the infected host is the period of infectivity or communicability. It is the time during which means for isolation and control against further transmission can be applied. The pathogen exists as constituents of tissues and body fluids: nasopharyngeal secretions, saliva, sputum, urine, feces, and blood. These can induce infection of a susceptible host directly by *contact* through inhalation of aerosols such as those produced by coughing or laboratory procedures, transfer by intimate contact with mucous membranes as in kissing or venereal exposure, ingestion as with contaminated finger to mouth, or injection with a contaminated instrument (hypodermic needle) or penetrating animal bites (rabies).

Environmental substances such as air, dust, water, food, and sewage may be contaminated by the pathogen. Such substances are called *vehicles.* Pathogens may survive for substantial periods of time in such vehicles, which may also carry pathogens for long distances to produce infection by inhalation and ingestion. They can also infect by contamination of mucous membranes or traumatized tissues such as skin (tetanus and gas gangrene).

Vectors extract blood or other tissues containing pathogens of the infected host. By mechanical transfer or following multiplication in tissues of the vector (extrinsic incubation period), the pathogen is introduced into a susceptible host during a subsequent penetration of the skin by probing or bite for another blood meal.

The features which support passage of the pathogen from infected to susceptible host constitute the mechanism of transmission. Perpetuation of the infectious process obviously depends on successful completion of this chain of events.

Procedures in Identifying
Infectious Disease

The interdependency of the basic components of an infectious disease and their influencing factors emerge as an inseparable complex that must be fully comprehended before definition of the problem and means for dealing with it can be rationally accomplished. Epidemiology is the methodology for systematic characterization of the complex situation. By application of statistical, laboratory, descriptive, and interpretative techniques, based on scientifically accepted criteria and previous experience, various aspects of the infectious disease process in a community can be shaped into visual images most commonly presented as statistical tables and graphs.

The response of the epidemiologist to a reported disease is to determine in time, numbers, and geographic range the extent of the communicable disease process. The basic approach is *case finding*. Starting with inquiry of the person who detected the earliest or first suspected case, called the index case, other suspected cases are located by telephone, house calls, hospital visits, and a variety of other means encompassed by the term "shoe leather epidemiology." On the basis of clinical suspicion and epidemiologic clues as to the etiology, appropriate specimens—blood, urine, feces, sputum, throat washings, skin scrapings, or purulent substances—are collected from cases and contacts. These are submitted to the public health laboratory for isolation, characterization, and identification of the causative agent or for serologic determination of the etiology.

As case finding locates additional suspect patients, information is obtained that focuses on the time and location of exposure, possible source of infection, incubation period, pathogenesis, clinical course, status of outcome (recovery, sequelae, or death), and pattern of dissemination. On receipt of laboratory characterization of the etiology, the fundamental basis for confirmation of suspect cases is established. Definition of the disease as to origin, time, evolution, and dissemination can be accurately assessed on the basis of epidemiologic data. Intelligent means for control and possibly prevention of other infections can then be applied.

Epidemiologic definition of a communicable disease in a human population is dependent on quantitative determination of incidence and prevalence of either infection or disease. Incidence is the occurrence at a point or within a unit of time. Prevalence may be considered the amount within a particular population. The more acute the process, the closer incidence approximates prevalence, as with measles. The more insidious, the greater variance between the two. For example, the incidence of active tuberculosis at any time in a community is distinctly less than the prevalence of persons showing past infection by x-ray or tuberculin test. Another example is the relationship of the annual incidence of overt cases of St. Louis encephalitis as compared to the prevalence of accumulated immunes owing to previous, usually inapparent infections as manifest by presence of specific antibody in serum detected by serologic tests.

Statistically, incidence is represented as number of detectable cases (numerator) among number of persons present or observed (denominator) at a point or in a unit of time; $I = \dfrac{C}{O}$, where I is incidence, C is cases, and O is total observed. Prevalence is the number of cases accumulated (numerator) from the persons observed (denominator) over a course of time; $P = I \times D$, where P is prevalence, I is incidence, and D is duration of observation.

PUBLIC HEALTH ROLES IN ACUTE COMMUNICABLE DISEASES

Communicable disease saps the well-being and productivity of individuals, communities, nations, and societies of human beings. A primary goal of public health is to prevent occurrence of recognized communicable diseases and to avoid potential diseases that threaten to intrude from elsewhere. Therefore, the priority objective in any acute communicable disease program is prevention. This involves application of the most up-to-date means of sanitation, immunization, and quarantine.

Although present-day healthy communities, which are largely free of pestilential diseases of the past, exemplify extensive success of such measures, the relentless threat of parasitism requires continued awareness. In the United States even in relatively recent years, communicable diseases have shown a variety of patterns in frequency of occurrence. Several specific diseases have declined, but others have increased, or remained fairly constant, or fluctuated. Table 8-1 illustrates a few of these patterns, showing

TABLE 8-1   Selected Reportable Diseases—Cases Reported, United States, Selected Years

	1945	1950	1955	1960	1963
Pertussis (whooping cough)	133,792	120,718	62,786	14,809	17,135
Malaria	62,763	2,184	522	72	99
Diphtheria	18,675	5,796	1,984	918	314
Brucellosis (undulant fever)	5,049	3,510	1,444	751	407
Typhoid fever	4,211	2,484	1,704	816	566
Poliomyelitis, acute	13,624	33,300	28,985	3,190	449
Psittacosis	27	26	334	113	76
Salmonellosis	649	1,233	5,447	6,929	15,390
Measles	146,013	319,124	555,156	441,703	385,156
Streptococcal sore throat and scarlet fever	185,570	64,494	147,502	315,173	342,161

Source: Adapted from U.S. Bureau of the Census. *Statistical Abstract of the United States, 1965,* p. 82.

the *number of cases* of several reportable communicable diseases during selected years from 1945 to 1963. Thus, whooping cough, malaria, diphtheria, brucellosis, and typhoid fever have declined markedly since 1945. Acute poliomyelitis and psittacosis increased in the early 1950's, but declined subsequently. Salmonellosis is particularly notable because it increased steadily and strikingly from 1945 to 1963 (Table 8-1). Measles and streptococcal sore throat, including scarlet fever, have shown variable patterning and had among the highest number of cases of all the reportable diseases in 1963 (being exceeded only by the venereal diseases).

Objectives of Acute
Communicable Diseases Programs

The principal objectives of communicable disease programs are: (1) detection of disease occurrence, (2) adequate facilities for expeditious confirmation of etiology, (3) means for determining incidence and prevalence, (4) technical capability for elucidation of transmission, (5) adequate resources—material and technical—for application of control, (6) facilities for improving prevention, (7) capacity to utilize experience for research, and (8) long-term capability for elimination of a disease which exists.

Responsibilities for Control Programs

An effective agency-designated responsibility for dealing with acute communicable disease problems must have authority, properly equipped physical facilities, adequately trained personnel, and a continuous systematic program for keeping current by research and training.

Like other spheres of public health concern in the United States, communicable disease control is the responsibility of each sovereign state. The state health officer customarily delegates this full-time activity to a division of communicable diseases. A staff of physicians, public health nurses, and veterinarians works closely with the public health laboratory and state epidemiologist in detection, diagnosis, assessment, and control of communicable diseases. Because of their separate magnitude, tuberculosis and venereal diseases are often handled by associated divisions, specially designated for those diseases.

On the recommendation of the infectious disease experts, legislation is promulgated requiring every physician, practitioner, veterinarian, dentist, coroner, and responsible director of dispensaries, clinics, and hospitals to notify local health authorities (city or county) of the occurrence of cases of specified reportable diseases. This information is relayed to the state health department, where it is statistically tabulated. The information may be of such type or extent to require further investigation or outside support and augmentation of local measures for control.

Such further investigation can be requested by the local authority or suggested by the state experts. An epidemiologist or other qualified person may be sent to investigate the reports and circumstances to determine whether it is a sporadic case or a component of an impending or current epidemic. Field and laboratory methodology and resources are utilized expeditiously to obtain a clear assessment of the situation. Where these are limited, the state health officer may request assistance from the National Communicable Disease Center of the Bureau of Disease Prevention and Environmental

Control, Public Health Service (the Center is located in Atlanta, Georgia). The Center's epidemiology and laboratory programs can provide skilled investigators and laboratory techniques of a type and quantity that may not otherwise be obtainable within state resources.

In an affluent nation such as the United States, tax-supported public investment in community pure-water supply and sewage disposal facilities, associated with well-regulated privately owned home and industrial sanitary systems, has virtually eliminated a number of diseases that were prevalent two generations ago. Typhoid fever and bacillary dysentery are but two examples of diseases that were once common but now appear only occasionally, when there is a breakdown in the sanitary systems, i.e., failure of private individuals to comply with generally accepted standards and regulations for food handling and sewage disposal.

On the other hand, this same affluent society has fostered a much greater mobility of its citizens and an accelerating shift from rural to urban and suburban ecologic conditions that in themselves generate an environment for new communicable disease problems. It is obvious that local concern, through local health authorities, in regard to communicable diseases of importance to regional units such as states has effectively contributed to the improvement and maintenance of health and a decline in the threat of many communicable diseases.

The Elusive Goal of Eradication. The eradication of communicable disease is frequently assumed to be the ultimate goal of communicable disease control programs. It is unfortunate that so much "promotion" has been disseminated regarding projected attempts to eradicate one or another infectious disease or vector of transmission. Uncritical use of the word *eradication*, which really means to extirpate, has led to misconceptions of biologic feasibility. Naive expectations of various lay groups will ultimately see as a failure the continued existence of a "semantically eradicated" disease entity when, in fact, its incidence will have been reduced to a level below the serious status which brought upon it the aim to eradicate.

If eradication is interpreted to mean extirpation, the ultimate objective must necessarily be the elimination of the last viable representative of a specific pathogen from the earth. The enormity of such an accomplishment challenges imagination and does not seem practical. Other "eradicators" simply mean removal of a pathogen from a geographic region or population group. Still others envisage eradication to mean suppression of an infection or disease below an apparent or detectable level in a community or other definable situation. It is obvious that pursuit of any one of these goals of eradication can bring about effective disease control and actually accomplish widespread prevention of disease.

Potential and actual deleterious effects of eradication campaigns are important considerations. Pressures on survival of biologic forms force manifestation of biologic means for survival. Genetic mutation, as has been observed in the development of antibiotic-resistant bacteria and insecticide-resistant mosquito vectors, has produced more perplexing communicable disease problems than existed before means were applied to eliminate these species.

Removal of the immunizing prevalence of endemic infections such as malaria or poliomyelitis may result in intrusion of other parasitic forms that have, until now, not reached the human population. Unsuccessful attempts universally to immunize a juvenile population by active immunization for a disease like measles may delay infection in sufficient numbers of persons who will then suffer more severe and more frequently fatal complications of the adult disease. The objective of disease eradication is a constructive public health concept provided there is a clear understanding of what is really meant.

Surveillance

The increased rapidity and frequency of human movement have brought increasing dependence for recognition of communicable diseases beyond the confines of the sovereign state. This has evolved into a collective communication of state information to the Public Health Service, which tabulates and assesses the data on a national scale. The resulting information is produced as the *Morbidity and Mortality Weekly Report* of the National Communicable Disease Center.[1] The reports list the communicable diseases which are reportable in most states. Often, only on a national scale can current or evolving problems requiring urgent attention be visualized. An example of this is the cumulative reporting of hundreds of malaria cases in American service men returning in 1966–1967 from Southeast Asia to a nation where malaria as an indigenous problem was eliminated 25 years ago. Person-to-person-transmitted virus diseases such as influenza and poliomyelitis emerge from the national picture as a completely different order of importance for the attention of local and state public health personnel than if the status of these diseases was available only at the state level. Therefore, the national reporting has not supplanted the basic state provision of information for its own localities. It has given an additional and very useful perspective which is at the disposal of those who must detect and combat communicable diseases.

It must be reiterated, however, that without the local observers such as the private practitioner and other individual health personnel, who see or suspect a patient with an infectious disease, the higher echelons of information gathering, collation, and action would be impossible. The corollary is that without the individual professionals in various medical and health pursuits, measures of prevention and control derived from the regional and national assessments would be impossible. The local practitioners and health institutions are therefore the beginning and the end, initiator and recipient, of the essential chain of events which leads to control and prevention of communicable disease.

Research

It seems apparent that amassing of knowledge for defining and controlling infectious disease has far outrun its application. There are those who suggest that research for further knowledge about infectious disease and its prevention not be stressed relative to the need for similar knowledge in other fields (i.e., cancer, heart disease, mental disease). However, being biologic phenomena, infectious diseases are continually shifting in nature to adapt to the changing patterns and circumstances of human behavior. It is therefore important to recognize the basic value of a vigorous, well-oriented research program in any continuing campaign to lessen the impact of infectious disease on individual and community health. Only through such continued study can appropriate means be applied for disease control. Such research ranges from basic laboratory studies to field investigations leading to detection, diagnosis, epidemiology, surveillance, and application of control.

Too often the relative importance of such a wide variety of problems as that encompassed by the area of communicable disease is overlooked. There are legitimate differences of opinion about whether to apply limited resources to the application of existing knowledge rather than devoting a substantial portion to acquisition of new knowledge by research. Sometimes, eradication of one disease is promoted to the exclusion of effective control of several others which may collectively have a more significant impact on the health of the community, be it local or international.

Just as the infectious disease process is a complex manifestation, research on the cause and control of such diseases cannot be clearly divided into singular approaches or limited areas of delegated responsibility. Often the key to recognition of the problem is a local physician, health officer, laboratorian, epidemiologist, or county or state professional.

Different from most other types of human disease, communicable disease occurrence is nature's fortuitous experiment that can be scientifically exploited to yield fundamental information that no specially designed experiments could ever produce. Therefore, knowledgeable professionals, scientifically trained and provided with adequate facilities and appropriate equipment, are continually applying these resources to detection and definition of natural occurrence of infectious diseases in sporadic and epidemic form, systematically deriving data that can be formulated into new knowledge, interpretable in terms of new concepts and as a basis for application of new methods of disease control.

While the definition of a communicable disease situation is often attempted by observational and statistical epidemiology, the use of the public health laboratory as an investigative and etiologically confirmatory instrument is inseparable. In fact, for the most expeditious elucidation of most communicable disease problems, the public health laboratory is essential as the spearhead of the epidemiologic investigation.

The federally supported facilities and programs for dealing with infectious disease problems cannot be definitively characterized as to area of function or specific mode of approach. The National Institute for Allergy and Infectious Diseases within the National Institutes of Health is related only organizationally to the other institutes where research efforts are being made, for example, to elucidate the infectious nature of the cause of cancer or of neurologic disease and blindness. Yet the Institute pursues in depth problems ranging from the common cold to exotic hemorrhagic fevers. Its primary mission, function, and goals are toward research.

On the other hand, the National Communicable Disease Center cannot carry out its responsibility of detection, definition, evaluation, characterization, surveillance, control, prevention, and dissemination of information about infectious diseases without a substantial research capability and performance. Research is the root, foundation, and spearhead along a broad front of communicable disease control. So the difference between these two monumental efforts of the Public Health Service is one of emphasis rather than means and capability for research.

The National Communicable Disease Center has an intimate, very often human and personal as well as intuitive, relationship with state health authorities, which, as the primary point of responsibility, influences the success or failure of collaborative research efforts in decisive ways. Many significant advances in knowledge of infectious disease definition and control could only have been achieved through such collaborative exploitation of nature's experiments in one or another geographic situation encompassed by a sovereign state. So it must be remembered that successful solution of infectious disease problems is not solely dependent on research facilities and organizational goals; also involved are human attitudes, organizational flexibility, and administrative intelligence that in its most useful operation reflects the epitome of the democratic system on which communicable disease control ultimately depends.

As public health practice and publicly supported means for communicable disease control and prevention have matured and expanded, the relative importance of the pioneering research and control efforts of such privately supported agencies as the Rockefeller Foundation has diminished. However, recognition and understanding of the research, administrative, and intellectual evolution of currently accepted and widely practiced techniques (viz., for hookworm, malaria, yellow fever) are important for any insight into the national and global capability for communicable disease control. In perspective it is also important to recognize that no substitute for the privately supported, special-group, investigative field and laboratory attack on infectious disease problems has yet been evolved. This may be cause for reinstituting in greater measure this approach by those who have inherited this tradition and capability from the past.

PRINCIPAL PREVENTION AND CONTROL MEASURES

Quarantine

Quarantine is the process of detecting infectious agents, infected persons, or other implicated hosts and vectors and preventing their introduction into a susceptible locality or population. Quarantine can be applied at the geographic source, which in the world at present is possible only under sanctions of the World Health Organization. It is usually applied at points of entry into a susceptible locality which is free of the agent in question. Thus, quarantine is one of the most effective measures for prevention of communicable disease occurrence in various parts of the world, particularly in the United States. Quarantine measures have prevented outbreaks of smallpox and possibly the introduction of yellow fever. They have slowed and sometimes stopped the movement of cholera and often work in concert with other preventive measures, such as immunization, to prevent geographic expansion of a variety of infectious diseases.

Immunization

Immunization is a process by which susceptible hosts are artificially prepared to resist infection by a specific disease agent. Immunization of a community to a calculable extent is a means for preventing establishment of a communicable disease. There are two types of immunization: active and passive.

Active immunization is the introduction of a specific antigenic substance to produce a specific immune reaction in the form of antibodies. The antibodies formed will oppose or combine with a specific infectious agent preventing its invasion and multiplication in the tissues of the host or prevent effect of a toxin. Antigens may be living, attenuated forms of the virulent agent, as in 17 D yellow fever vaccination, or they may be substances in which the infectivity is inactivated without destroying the antigenicity that stimulates the specific immune response. Examples of the latter are typhoid and cholera vaccines in which the virulent organisms have been chemically killed. It is apparent that if a person is actively immunized against the agent for which quarantine is performed prior to entry into a susceptible area, it is unlikely that the specific infectious agent can escape to infect another susceptible host.

Passive immunization is accomplished by the introduction of specific immune substances which act directly against exposure to an infectious agent within a reasonable period of time. For example, infectious hepatitis is sufficiently endemic and widespread in the human population to have produced specific antibodies in a large number of human beings. Immune globulin, extracted from blood plasma pooled from many people, contains in concentrated form specific antibodies against the virus of infectious hepatitis. Therefore, a sufficiently large dose of pooled human immune globulin inoculated into a person likely to be exposed to infectious hepatitis virus infection while traveling or living abroad (as with Peace Corps volunteers and troops fighting in Southeast Asia) will provide protection for up to six months, by which time the antibodies in the immune globulin will no longer persist in sufficient strength. Prolonged exposure requires periodic reinoculation with passively immune substances such as gamma globulin.

The Vaccination Assistance Act of 1963 has put at the disposal of state and local health authorities the means for immunizing large sections of the population against such diseases as smallpox, diphtheria, pertussis, and measles. The combination of quarantine to keep exotic infectious agents such as smallpox out of a locality and community immunization to raise the collective resistance of society against communicability of specific disease agents is preventive medicine in its most objective form.

Environmental Control Measures

Preventive measures of a more permanent nature evolve from environmental control. Accomplishments of sanitary engineering such as pure water supply and proper disposal of sewage and other potentially infectious material has been legislated into building codes, city planning, state laws, and federal regulations to the point where they are almost an automatic, routine procedure in the physical development of the environment occupied by the growing population of the United States.

Associated with this, however, are biologic phenomena that so far have frustrated engineering design for exclusion. These are the zoonotic sources of infectious agents, i.e., vertebrate reservoirs and arthropod vectors. It is therefore necessary to maintain surveillance for the implicated vectors and reservoir animals. For instance, *Culex tarsalis* and *Culex pipiens quinquefasciatus* mosquitoes are vectors of arbovirus encephalitis. It has not been possible to engineer them out of existence, so continuous monitoring of their breeding and activity in previously affected or potentially susceptible localities is necessary. In the same way, dairy cattle reservoirs for Q fever and domestic canine and wild vertebrate hosts for rabies must be continually watched for the appearance of infected animals that could become a source of transmission of disease to man.

It is obvious that resources must also be developed, maintained, and continually changed in order to provide effective vector and vertebrate reservoir control. Every health authority responsible for a population in a mosquito-infested environment should have not only pest mosquito control but also means for dealing specifically with mosquito vectors of disease. The important role of the public health veterinarian pertains not only to the surveillance, but also to the control, of zoonotic sources of infectious agents.

In the realm of environmental control is the capability of disinfecting potentially infectious materials and premises, procedures which may well be within the capacity of a sanitary organization that effectively deals with vectors and animal reservoirs. Such a capacity would range from the rodenticidal control of rats to the fumigation and decontamination of rooms bacterially contaminated with such agents as staphylococcus or anthrax.

Control of Human Carriers

Human carriers of such diseases as typhoid, amebiasis, and infectious hepatitis as vertebrate reservoirs must be kept under surveillance, detected, and controlled in a manner similar to other vector-reservoir species. It is often necessary physically to control human carriers by varying degrees of isolation. These may range from enforcement of rules segregating infected food handlers from eating establishments, to hospitalization of actual or suspected carriers for surgery or chemoprophylaxis. Examples are the extirpation of the *Salmonella typhii*-infected gallbladder, the chemotherapy of staphylococcus-infected nasopharynx or other lesions, and the suppression of *Neisseria meningococcus* by sulfa drugs. These means, which are often used on an individual basis, may on occasion be extended to a population such as the military personnel of a unit in which meningococcic meningitis exposure or epidemic has occurred, recognizing that one result may be the development of resistant strains, as has occurred in hospital infections with staphylococcus.

COMMUNITY ASPECTS OF PREVENTION AND CONTROL

As means for control of communicable diseases have become more effective and widely applied, there has been a shift in emphasis from control to prevention. Laws and regulations enforcing reporting, investigation, rectification of sanitary and environmental deficiencies, isolation of cases, and disinfection are now infrequently applied and only under exceptional circumstances, because the conditions they were written to improve have now become part of a way of life.

On the other hand, as preventive and curative medical services have become more universally available through prenatal, well-baby, school, and outpatient clinics, new types and more effective vaccines have been given to a much larger segment of the population. The widespread use of Sabin oral polio vaccine is an example. Regulations for commercially distributed foods in regard to absence of bacterial contamination are becoming more rigid. Animal inspections and meat product-processing standards are being used to prevent disease by enforcing sanitary practices consistently. This is far more effective than using such methods merely for the detection and prosecution of offenders after a disease outbreak has occurred.

Increasing educational level, lay dissemination of public health information about communicable diseases, and enormous growth of the public health establishment under aegis of the American Public Health Association have given visibility to the absence of disease resulting from preventive measures.

The previously mentioned affluence of society has provided an increased standard of living that routinely provides sanitary housing that was beyond reach of a majority of citizens a generation ago. The increased tax base supports additional public health programs. Increased income allows preventive visits to clinics and physicians that were unthinkable a few years ago when vaccination for one serious disease was a major expense.

However, there is another aspect which must be contemplated in the awareness that communicable disease control has never been more effective than at the present time. As good control isolates the human host from infectious disease agents, a nonimmune segment of the population is being developed which, in the future, may be exposed with more serious consequences following some catastrophe or change in occupational pursuit, or as biologic shift in pathogens, environment, or mechanism of transmission occurs. Abroad are human reservoirs of these diseases that will threaten with increasing frequency as intercontinental travel expands.

The widely held misconception of a decade or so ago that infectious diseases were passé because of antibiotics, chemotherapy, new vaccines, and sanitation is no longer assumed by knowledgeable leaders in medicine. However, not enough medically oriented young people are selecting infectious diseases as a career as will be necessary to maintain vigilance in the United States and effectively deal with the exotic diseases abroad in terms of what has been achieved in acute communicable disease control at the present time. Education of qualified professionals in the clinical, laboratory, epidemiologic, and preventive aspects of communicable diseases is one of the most important objectives to be pursued by those engaged in medical science. As a challenge, these diseases persist. They will continue to lurk, sporadically threatening—with some new ones developing—as far as can be seen into the medical future of mankind.

SOME COMMON COMMUNICABLE DISEASES

The remainder of this chapter provides accounts of selected communicable diseases in order to illustrate the varieties of etiologic agents, incubation periods, hosts affected, and mechanisms of transmission. The examples also illustrate means for control and prevention, including methods for passive and active immunization. Two other kinds of communicable diseases, namely, the venereal diseases and tuberculosis, are discussed in Chapter 9 and Chapter 10, respectively. Descriptions of the etiologic, epidemiologic, and clinical manifestations of some 148 communicable diseases appear in a publication of the American Public Health Association entitled *Control of Communicable Diseases in Man.*[2] Information is also available in numerous textbooks of infectious disease, medicine, and preventive medicine.[3-7]

In the following descriptions, if a nonhuman host vector is *not* mentioned, the disease is dependent on a human host and is transmitted person to person by nasopharyngeal secretions, dermal contact, or anal-oral contamination.

Rubella (German Measles)

Rubella is a virus infection which is highly infectious by person-to-person contact with nasopharyngeal secretions. It may be aerosol-transmitted after a 14-to-21-day (average 18 days) incubation period; fever, catarrhal symptoms, and maculopapular rash with cervical lymphadenopathy and leukopenia develop. It is an epidemic disease usually seen in spring and summer. Infectivity lasts up to four days following onset. While it is a disease of childhood, it has often occurred in young adults, military recruits, and pregnant women. If it occurs in the first trimester of pregnancy, it causes congenital defects in the fetus frequently enough that termination of pregnancy is considered. The epidemic of 1964–1965 produced congenital defects in thousands in the United States. The erythematous-to-maculopapular rash often causes diagnostic confusion of single or sporadic cases with other erythematous and exanthemic diseases such as measles, erythema infectiosum, exanthem subitum, Boston exanthum (ECHO virus infection), and Coxsackie A virus infection.

Treatment is symptomatic. An effective attenuated virus vaccine is currently under evaluation which promises to give lifelong protection and will be most useful prior to marriage. Since it is a mild disease, voluntary exposure of female children to epidemic cases has often been practiced as means for early infection and immunization.

Infectious Hepatitis (Epidemic or Catarrhal Jaundice)

Infectious hepatitis is an acute febrile infection with a heat-resistant gastrointestinal virus transmitted by finger to mouth, person-to-person contact, food handler-contaminated food, or fecal- or sewage-contaminated water. Incubation period is weeks to two months resulting in onset of fever, marked anorexia, nausea, malaise, gastrointestinal discomfort, and often jaundice. Leukopenia is frequent. Anicteric cases of mild nature are frequent. Fatalities due to liver damage are rare but occur more frequently in adults, pregnant women in particular.

Infectivity occurs prior to onset and continues for at least a week. Carriers may be infectious for many months. Sporadic cases may occur, but the disease is often seen in epidemics. While it is thought to be caused by a single virus type, providing lifelong immunity, there is a possibility that there are several types.

Best protection is by personal hygiene and good sanitation with emphasis on feces disposal and pure or treated water supply, and by pre-employment examination, history, and surveillance of food handlers with isolation of suspects or cases from contact with food. Patients should be isolated during the first week of jaundice.

Effective prophylaxis for persons exposed or at high risk (e.g., personnel assigned to overseas occupations, Peace Corps workers, missionaries, or military personnel) in poorly sanitated areas is by pooled human gamma globulin (5 ml) every six months. The virus has not been isolated in other-than-human volunteers; so no active immunization is yet available.

Serum Hepatitis (Homologous Serum Jaundice)

Serum hepatitis is an acute infection by heat-resistant virus causing a disease indistinguishable from infectious hepatitis. It has a distinctly longer incubation period of two to six months, usually 60 to 120 days. Transmission has long been considered possible only by inoculation, as in vaccination with contaminated needles or by blood and plasma transfusion. Recent evidence suggests occasional transmission by the oral route. There is no cross-protection with infectious hepatitis virus; so repeated attacks of clinical jaundice are possible.

Prophylaxis is also by pooled human gamma globulin, although it is not so certain. Prevention is by use of disposable single-use needles and transfusion equipment. Where necessary, disinfection by heat-penetrating steam (autoclave or pressure cooker) and nacent halogen disinfectants (Clorox) is the only reliable means. Even *prolonged boiling* cannot be relied on to inactivate heat-resistant serum hepatitis virus. No vaccine is available.

Arbovirus Encephalitis

Western equine encephalitis (WEE), eastern equine encephalitis (EEE), St. Louis encephalitis (SLE), and California encephalitis (CE) are North American diseases that are caused by some of the smallest viruses. These are antigenically related to others which cause similar diseases in other areas of the world. They are maintained and disseminated in a mosquito-vertebrate-mosquito cycle in nature and are therefore zoonotic viruses which only tangentially infect man, an accidental host, thus resulting in a dead-end infection. The vectors and vertebrate hosts differ according to the region, ecologic situation, and type of virus.

Culex tarsalis mosquitoes are widespread, breeding in rural flood and irrigation water west of the Mississippi, and they transmit WEE and SLE viruses during the summer months. The viruses are picked up from viremic wild birds in the late spring and summer dissemination of virus. If enough mosquitoes are infected, the viruses, after an extrinsic incubation period of

10 to 14 days in mosquitoes, are transmitted to man, resulting in sporadic or epidemic infections.

Originally in St. Louis, and recently associated with urbanization of human populations in the United States, epidemics of SLE have resulted from transmission by *Culex pipiens quinquefasciatus* mosquitoes, which breed in poorly drained or sewage-contaminated waters in suburban and urban localities. They are commonly infected by feeding on birds that customarily inhabit backyards.

Culiseta melanura is a bird-feeding mosquito that maintains and transmits EEE virus in swamp-associated reservoir cycles in southeastern United States and east of the Appalachian Mountains, as far north as Massachusetts, where severe epidemics have been reported. Because *C. Melanura* only occasionally bites man, Aedes mosquitoes such as *Aedes sollicitans* are implicated in the transmission of EEE to man.

California encephalitis has recently emerged as an important epidemic central nervous system disease in the Ohio Valley and Middle West, where it has been called "farm encephalitis" because of the recognized association with rural exposure on farms or while hunting, fishing, picnicking, and camping. The wild cycle is scattered because of wood-breeding Aedes vector species that get CE virus from wild mammals.

WEE commonly afflicts very young children in rural towns and farms. Epidemic EEE also affects children predominantly, although cases have been observed in all age groups. SLE is a disease of the elderly, almost all fatalities being reported of persons over 55 years of age. California encephalitis is another children's disease, more than 90 per cent of patients being under 16 years of age, and apparently it results in a significant incidence of severe and long-lasting sequelae such as behavioral problems and loss of ability to learn in school. Infection with any one of these arboviruses induces lifelong immunity. Overt disease occurs in only a small percentage of those infected.

It is obvious that avoidance of mosquito bites breaks the chain of transmission. Any measures, such as repellants, screens, and mosquito control with insecticides, that accomplish this induce control of epidemics and are the basis for prevention of human infection. There are no chemotherapeutic or immunizing substances available to prevent infection or that will alter the course of disease once infection occurs.

Rabies

Rabies is a neurotropic virus invasion of the central nervous system resulting in acute encephalitis, hydrophobia (aversion to water), muscle spasms, paralysis, convulsions, and death. The virus is maintained and transmitted in a zoonotic cycle in dogs and cats and wild vertebrates such as foxes and skunks. Bats also serve as a reservoir, vampire bats possibly sustaining latent infection over long periods without becoming rabid. Airborne transmission in closed spaces such as caves may occur.

The virus infects and multiplies in salivary glands. Human infection follows the saliva-contaminated bite of a rabid animal. The incubation period is usually four to six weeks, but possibly many months. If the wound is on the head and neck, or close to a profuse nerve supply, a short incubation occurs. The stage of infectivity in animals may precede rabid signs and continues until death.

Rabies is one of the few virus infections amenable to prophylaxis following exposure. This is accomplished by thoroughly washing and flushing the bite wound with soap and water, detergent and water, or water alone as soon as possible after exposure. There follows a medical cleansing with 20 per cent green soap or 1 per cent solution of quaternary ammonium compound. Hyperimmune antirabies serum is topically applied and flushed through the wound, which is left open. Additional antirabies serum is infiltrated by injection around the wound site.

To determine whether rabies will develop, dogs and cats are incarcerated for at least ten days' observation following infliction of a bite. Other animals are observed for 14 days. If disease develops, a section of brain is examined by special staining for Negri bodies and specific staining by a fluorescent conjugate. Brain material may be inoculated intracerebrally into mice, which, if infected, will show signs in 10 to 14 days.

If no break in skin or abrasion is apparent, and the attacking animal does not become rabid in ten days, no systemic treatment is recommended. However, if clinical signs of rabies develop in the animal, vaccination is started immediately. If a bite is evident and there are suggestive signs that the attacking animal has rabies, hyperimmune rabies serum is administered immediately, followed by a full course of vaccination. If bites are multiple and severe, serum should be given without delay. No vaccine is indicated until the animal shows signs of rabies. If the animal escapes or is not available for observation, a full course of vaccine should be given.

The slight risk of postvaccinal encephalitis indicates conservative judgment in the case of mild exposure to an animal that does not develop rabies. In persons anticipating hazard of exposure, such as veterinarians, active immunization can significantly lessen the chance of infection.

Community prevention is dependent on a well-administered vaccination program for household pets and a stray-dog collection and disposal facility.

Q Fever

Q fever is caused by a rickettsia, *Coxiella burnetii*, type of intracellular parasite that in other rickettsial disease entities is transmitted by acarine (ticks and mites) vectors, infected from viremic mammals. While *Coxiella burnetii* may be harbored by ticks in a reservoir state, it is transmitted by contact with or aerosol exposure to unpasteurized milk and infected placentas of livestock.

Control and prevention are by pasteurization of milk and adequate disposal of placentas and sanitary livestock handling. Q fever is susceptible to treatment by broad-spectrum antibiotics, and effective vaccines have been developed experimentally that protect persons at high risk of infection.

Ornithosis (Psittacosis)

Ornithosis is infection with intracellular agents that infect and replicate like a virus. However, because of their large size and susceptibility to antibiotics, they are considered to belong to a distinguishable group of infectious agents called Bedsoniae which evolved from bacteria. Originally recognized as a natural infection of psitticine birds (parrots), it is now recognized to be common in many avian species, the most important being pigeons, burrowing seabirds, turkeys, and other gallinaceous birds. Zoonotic transmission is by contact and airborne infectious particles, hence the infection of persons in close contact with infected birds or feathers, droppings, or nests.

After an incubation period of 4 to 15 days, there is acute onset of fever and headaches with pneumonic involvement and development of unproductive cough which subsequently produces mucopurulent sputum. Anorexia and constipation are sometimes severe, and human cases can be infectious until the causative pulmonary agents are eliminated from the respiratory tract, usually by tetracycline therapy.

Control is by elimination of the unusually hardy infectious agents by feeding antibiotics to infected birds before allowing close contact with human beings. Organized public health surveillance includes such means as marking birds to detect origin and follow-up of laboratory-proved cases to isolate or destroy an infected bird or flock. There is no immunizing substance.

Staphylococcal Infections

Staphylococcal infections include a variety of disease manifestations resulting from infection, growth, and contamination by a group of selectively cultivable, antigenically closely related bacteria, morphologically identifiable as staphylococcus.

Impetigo (Impetigo Contagiosa). Impetigo is a dermal infection and purulation that produces dermatitis with vesicular and crusted seropurulent lesions that are highly infectious by person-to-person contact. Control is by maintenance of cleanliness, isolation of lesions and affected persons, and treatment of the infection.

Focalized and Systemic Staphylococcal Disease. Impetigo and systemic infections, including those of the eye (conjunctivitis) and nasopharynx, may be a source of more serious staphylococcus infections. These are furuncles and carbuncles seen most often in the young; deep-seated tissue infections such as tonsillitis and pneumonia; and suppuration as in emphysema and osteomyelitis, leading to organic abscesses and septicemia in the debilitated and elderly. These more serious complications may result in death, particularly with antibiotic-resistant strains.

The widespread use of antibiotics, which were initially almost universally effective in the control of staphylococcal infections, has resulted in the evolution of antibiotic-resistant strains of these bacteria. They are particularly hardy, often escape even diligent attempts at disinfection, and cause widespread postsurgical and contact infections that are not amenable to antibiotic therapy. Because clinical facilities, particularly hospitals, focalize diseased people, the problem of hospital, antibiotic-resistant staphylococcal infections has become a major communicable disease problem. It results in serious complications of intractible postsurgery infections and epidemics among newborn babies.

Only through careful disinfection, application of sanitary and isolation measures, and selective use and testing of antibiotics can safety and intelligent control be accomplished.

Staphylococcal Food Poisoning. Certain strains of staphylococcus grow well in artificial media as provided by prepared foods, such as those made with milk, eggs, and chopped meats. Unrefrigerated, at room temperature, the bacteria grow rapidly and produce an enterotoxin which results in severe gastrointestinal reactions. These reactions include abrupt and often violent nausea, vomiting, diarrhea, and prostration which, although serious, are rarely fatal because of expulsion of the toxic material. Staphylococcal food poisoning occurs soon (one-half to four hours) after consumption of prepared foods which have been held unrefrigerated for a substantial period of time, often being initially contaminated by a food handler shedding staphylococcus from a dermal or nasopharyngeal infection.

Staphylococcal food poisoning is most frequently manifest as a common food source epidemic of short incubation period. It follows consumption of a food contaminated by enterotoxin-producing bacteria, usually easily identifiable by case history and by culture.

Prevention is by surveillance of food handlers for infection or lesions and sanitary preparation and refrigeration of food. Treatment is symptomatic. Cases are not directly infectious to others.

Meningococcic Meningitis

Meningococcic meningitis is an inflammation of the coverings of the brain and spinal cord caused by morphologically distinct diplococcal bacteria.

They grow and are secreted in the nasopharyngeal tissues; so transmission is by contact or aerosol from infected cases and asymptomatic carriers. Early dramatic success with treatment by sulfa drugs and antibiotics has been followed by development of drug-resistant strains that are refractory to any known chemotherapeutic regime.

Meningococcic meningitis has returned to its status of damaging disease, with significant mortality. Its recent occurrence as a sporadic and epidemic disease in the military forces has led to closure of training camps in order to eliminate foci of exposure to civilian communities. The patients should be isolated, a search for asymptomatic carriers initiated, and surveillance established to detect the earliest case so as to prevent exposure of others in a concentrated human population such as exists in military barracks and dining halls. Administration of oral sulfa drugs to an exposed population group for prophylaxis has been practiced, but may have contributed to development and dissemination of drug-resistant strains.

Typhoid Fever (Enteric Fever)

Typhoid fever is a bacterial infection by *Salmonella typhosa* which multiplies in the enteric tract to produce a systemic disease that affects many organs including the lymphatic tissues and spleen. Untreated, it is characterized by prolonged fever, often with daily cyclic fluctuation, reaching a high peak after several days. There may be a mortality rate of 10 per cent unless the disease is treated by broad-spectrum antibiotics. It is person-to-person transmitted by exposure to fecal contamination, sewage-polluted or untreated water, food handled by an unclean carrier, or contact with an infectious case. Infectivity of a case or carrier continues as long as bacteria are excreted.

The incubation period is one to three weeks, averaging about two. Clusters of cases occur, such as family outbreaks in rural situations. Some convalescents become chronic carriers by permanent infection of the biliary tract, intermittently or continuously excreting bacteria into the intestine. These may resist elimination by antibiotics and require cholecystectomy. In a society with high-level sanitation, chronic carriers are the main source of sporadic cases. Continuous vigilance, surveillance of food handlers, and enforcement of rules of cleanliness by public health authorities are therefore extremely important.

Although the protective value of active immunization for all vaccinated persons is not absolute, immunization of those likely to be exposed during foreign travel or who are anticipating residence in an endemic or poorly sanitated area is of significant protection. Massive exposure can break through such immunity. The best protection is proper sewage disposal, consumption of treated water, and personal cleanliness.

Tetanus (Lockjaw)

Clostridium tetani is an anaerobic (grows in absence of oxygen) bacterial species of characteristic "clubstick" morphology. The organisms multiply and produce an exotoxin in deep wounds, burns, and tissue sites that have been contaminated by dirt or other fecally soiled substance that carries spores of this desiccation-resistant organism. The exotoxin produces a neuromuscular disease sometimes manifest by lockjaw, but also involving muscle spasm near the site of injury, such as tetanic spasms of neck and dorsal muscles (opisthonos). Painful spasm of any muscles can be precipitated by slight stimuli.

Found in the intestinal tract of man and many other animals, it has a ubiquitous distribution and is particularly common in areas which for a long time have been under cultivation with association of grazing animals. Its resistance makes unreliable disinfection by ordinary heating, boiling, or the usual chemical antiseptics used in hospitals and medical practice. The only reliable means is by autoclave. Extensive débridement of contaminated wounds, opened to the air, lessens the chance of anaerobic bacterial growth.

Specific active immunization with tetanus toxoid in infancy, followed by booster injections at the time of subsequent injury, or at least every five years, provides protection. In exposures of those not so immunized, passive protection can be accomplished by injection of substantial quantities of specific antitoxin, more being required the longer the time lapse following infection. Tetanus is a disease that can be prevented by appropriate immunization.

Brucellosis (Undulant Fever)

Brucellosis is caused by *Brucella abortus, B. suis,* or *B. melitensis* bacterial infection. It is a chronic febrile systemic disease which fluctuates in severity. It is characterized by intermittent bouts of fever, malaise, headache, chills and sweating, arthralgia, and generalized aching. Brucellosis is a zoonosis, the bacteria being ingested in milk from infected cows, swine, and goats or by exposure to other excretions of infected animals.

Although the etiologic agent may be excreted, person-to-person transmission is rare. The incubation period is variable from a few days to many months. Treatment with broad-spectrum antibiotics will control and eliminate the infection. Because the relapse rate is high, effective treatment is prolonged for at least three weeks. Long-term immunity is not evident; so reinfection can occur.

Prevention is by detection and disposal of infected animals and pasteurization of milk, as well as by enforcement of environmental sanitation in and around premises where potentially infected domestic animals dwell. No regimen for immunization has been devised.

Histoplasmosis

A free-living mold, *Histoplasma capsulatum*, as a yeast parasitizes the human respiratory tract producing an acute, benign respiratory disease characterized by malaise, weakness, fever, chest pains, and productive or dry cough. Rarely the infection may disseminate to other organs, producing splenomegaly, septic fever, prostration, and death if not properly treated. Histoplasmosis is susceptible to the antibiotic amphotericin B.

The incubation period is commonly ten days following inhalation of spores that are highly concentrated in soil composed largely of bird droppings in and around chickenhouses and wild-bird and bat roosts.

Protection by masks is indicated during occupational exposure to such foci. Prevention is by avoidance of inhalation and contact with such environments. As a common, inapparent infection, resistance develops which is protective except to massive exposure. No artificial means for induction of immunity have been devised.

Malaria

Malaria is caused by a protozoal parasite which invades, multiplies in, and destroys red blood cells in a cyclic rhythm varying from 48 to 72 hours. The sporozoites of any of four species of *Plasmodium* (*vivax, falciparum, malariae*, and *ovale*) which develop by sexual reproduction in the definitive Anopheles mosquito host are injected into the intermediate human host during the process of taking blood. After invasion of the parenchymal cells of the liver, mesozoites form, which are released into the blood to invade red cells to form schizonts. It is the schizogony that produces cell destruction resulting in febrile paroxysms.

The incubation period may be as short as 11 or 12 days, but may take months or even years. The sudden onset of fever and shaking chills is characteristic but of limited duration, is called a paroxysm, and occurs intermittently. During the interim, the patient is usually afebrile, apparently normal, but may feel weak.

Control of malaria has been by protection from bite by anopheline vectors and by destruction of vectors through use of residual insecticides such as DDT, dieldrin, and malathion. While this is directed at breaking the transmission chain, elimination of the parasite from the blood and liver is attempted by chemotherapy with drugs such as chloroquine, daroprim, primaquine, and quinocrine. Development of drug-resistant strains of plasmodia has led to use of natural quinine for treatment, intravenously in the case of cerebral malaria. The drugs are also used prophylactically for prevention of malaria attacks.

Toxoplasmosis

A protozoan parasite, *Toxoplasma gondii*, produces widespread infection in man, only occasionally resulting in overt disease. Prenatal infection of a fetus can cause death in utero, residual manifestations apparent at birth, or subsequent postnatal development of chorioretinitis, cerebral calcification, hydrocephalus, microcephalus, psychomotor retardation, and convulsions. Signs of acute infection in the newborn, resulting from transplacental or postnatal infection, are fever, jaundice, maculopapular rash, hepatomegaly, splenomegaly, xanthochromic spinal fluid, convulsions, lymphadenopathy, and lymphocytosis.

The parasite is found in a wide variety of domestic animals, including dogs and cats, with which man has close association. The incubation period is weeks to months following exposure. Other than intrauterine infection of the fetus, the person-to-person transmission mechanism is unknown, because infection of man from what is considered to be a zoonotic reservoir has not been demonstrated. Therefore, aside from personal hygiene, a system for protection against Toxoplasma infection has not been devised.

Amebiasis (Amebic Dysentery)

In amebiasis initial infection of the intestinal tract is by ingestion of hardy cysts of a morphologically identifiable protozoal parasite, *Endamoeba histolytica*. Multiplication in the intestine may result in dysenteric signs of abdominal discomfort, constipation, and diarrhea. While it is primarily an intestinal disease, amebae may be spread in the blood stream to lodge in other organs, particularly the liver. Amebic hepatitis and amebic abscesses are serious complications because they are difficult to treat and may result in death before control can be achieved.

Endamoeba histolytica is an obligate parasite of man and is transmitted by fecal contamination. It is a common contaminant of wet foods such as leafy vegetables in environments where sanitary disposal of feces is not practiced. Untreated cases become carriers and often transmit in eating establishments through handling food.

The only protection is personal hygiene, sanitary sewage disposal, pure water supply, and avoidance of consumption of raw foods that may have come from a contaminated source.

Trichinosis

Trichinella spiralis is a metazoal parasite that encysts and survives for long periods as male and female forms in muscles of mammalian hosts such as bears, marine mammals, wild canines, swine, and man. Infection occurs by ingestion of viable encysted worms in inadequately cooked pork. Trichinosis is therefore classified as a zoonosis. The incubation period is about nine days, but may be shorter or up to three times as long.

In the gastrointestinal tract, the worms emerge from the cysts. The female Trichinella produces larvae, which penetrate the intestinal wall into the blood; the blood carries the organisms to various muscles and organs where they encyst. An acute febrile disease occurs, often marked by edema of the upper eyelids, followed by various hemorrhages in the eye. Muscle soreness, remittent fever, pains, gastrointestinal symptoms, weakness, prostration, and eosinophilia ensue, the severity and recovery depending on whether vital organs such as the brain and heart are invaded. Critical signs of such complications appear three to eight weeks after infection. Under civilized circumstances, person-to-person transmission is not possible.

Prevention is by avoidance of inadequately cooked pork products or of those domestically produced and therefore not required to be frozen below −16°C for 36 hours. Imposition of statutes requiring cooking of garbage has significantly diminished swine infection in areas where such regulations are enforced. No means for immunization exist. Reinfection occurs with subsequent exposure.

Filariasis

Filariasis is a general term for a variety of diseases caused by growth in various tissues of filarial worms injected by arthropod vectors during probing for a blood meal. In contrast to onchocerciasis, which is Simulium-transmitted, filariasis usually refers to mosquito-transmitted *Wuchereria bancrofti* or *Brugia malayi*. Larval sexual forms are introduced by vector mosquitoes of many genera and species (*Aedes polynesiensis* in the Pacific, *Culex quinquefasciatus* in Southeast Asia). On maturation and mating in the lymph glands, these forms produce asexual microfilaria which circulate cyclically in the blood.

Filarial fever and elephantiasis result from the lodging of and reaction to these worms in the lymphatic system with subsequent blockage of lymph drainage. Treatment by diethylcarbamazine kills the filaria and microfilaria. This destruction of the microfilaria prevents reinfection of mosquitoes and breaks the parasite transmission chain.

Sanitation and insecticide application control breeding and exposure to vector mosquitoes and are the most effective control and method of prevention of transmission by infected arthropod vectors.

Hookworm Disease (Ancylostomiasis)

As the name implies, the infection is by one of two worms, *Ancylostoma duodenale* or *Necator americanus*, the larvae of which penetrate human skin and are carried by the blood to the intestine, where they develop into adult male and female worms that hook onto the lining of the gut. There they suck and ingest blood. Heavy infestation results in a hypochromic microcytic anemia, which causes varying degrees of disability. About six weeks after infection, eggs are produced by the females which pass out with the feces. In favorably warm, moist environments, the eggs hatch to produce the larvae, which seek penetration of human skin to start the invasive cycle over again. There is no immune mechanism which prevents infection; so people can be infected repeatedly. Control is by sanitary disposal of feces, elimination of the worms, and protection of skin by wearing shoes in fecally contaminated areas where larvae may be lurking.

SUMMARY

History has been influenced by the scourge of communicable disease, which for centuries took a heavy toll in sickness and death. Whereas early methods of communicable disease control were largely empirical, modern methods are based on the principles of several branches of science, including microbiology, immunology, and virology. These scientific advances and the application of environmental sanitation practices have reduced the threat of communicable diseases in some countries, such as the United States. However, for the vast majority of the world's population, these diseases still constitute the principal health problem, and as yet adequate resources are not available to cope with such hazards.

The basic components which characterize an infectious disease are the pathogen or etiologic agent, the host, and the mechanism of transmission of disease. These components are interdependent and form an inseparable complex in the communicable disease process. Epidemiology is the methodology for systematically evaluating various features which constitute a specific disease process.

Communicable disease control is the responsibility of the individual states and is based on legal requirements regarding the reporting of cases of specified diseases. Surveillance of the communicable diseases is made possible by the assembly of information on disease occurrence on a local, state, and national basis. Continued, vigorous research programs on the infectious diseases are required because the nature of these diseases is continually changing.

Although several diseases that were prevalent in the United States some years ago have been virtually eliminated, mobility of the population gives rise to the possibility of new communicable disease problems. Another potential problem stems from the development of a segment of the population which lacks immunity to certain infectious disease agents.

Principal methods of preventing communicable diseases are quarantine, immunization, environmental control measures, and control of human carriers. In the United States, there has been a shift in emphasis from control to prevention of communicable diseases, as the means for control have become more effective and widely applied.

REFERENCES

1. PUBLIC HEALTH SERVICE, National Communicable Disease Center. *The Morbidity and Mortality Weekly Report*. The Center, Atlanta, 1967.

2. GORDON, JOHN E., ed. *Control of Communicable Diseases in Man,* 10th ed. American Public Health Association, New York, 1965.

3. SARTWELL, PHILIP E., ed. *Maxcy-Rosenau Preventive Medicine and Public Health,* 9th ed. Appleton-Century-Crofts, New York, 1965.

4. ANDERSON, G. W., ARNSTEIN, M. G., and LESTER, M. R. *Communicable Disease Control,* 4th ed. The Macmillan Company, New York, 1962.

5. TOP, FRANKLIN H. *Communicable and Infectious Diseases: Diagnosis, Prevention, Treatment,* 5th ed. The C. V. Mosby Company, St. Louis, 1964.

6. HUNTER, G. W., III, FRYE, W. W., and SWARTZWELDER, J. C. *A Manual of Tropical Medicine,* 4th ed. W. B. Saunders Company, Philadelphia, 1966.

7. BEESON, P. B., and McDERMOTT, W., eds. *Cecil-Loeb Textbook of Medicine,* 12th ed. W. B. Saunders Company, Philadelphia, 1967.

CHAPTER 9

VENEREAL DISEASES

Significance of venereal diseases

Incidence of syphilis and gonorrhea

Types of venereal diseases

Pattern of spread of venereal diseases

Problems of prevention and control

Social control measures

Future needs in venereal disease
control

Summary

The venereal diseases are singled out from the other communicable diseases for special attention in this chapter because of their particular characteristics and because their recent history is of considerable import to public health. After a brief review in the first section of the chapter of the reasons these diseases are particularly significant, the second section discusses the trends in the incidence of the major venereal diseases in the general population and points out the segments of the population which are at special risk of infection. The third section describes the causative organism, incubation period, developmental characteristics, diagnosis, and treatment of each of the principal types of venereal disease. Elements in the pattern of spread of these diseases are discussed in the fourth section, followed by an account of some of the major problems in prevention and control. The last two sections of the chapter describe the current status of several different kinds of venereal disease control measures and the provisions which must be made in the future in order to minimize the threat of these diseases.

SIGNIFICANCE OF VENEREAL DISEASES

The venereal diseases are communicable and thus are related to the diseases discussed in Chapter 8. However, unlike most of the other communicable diseases, only human beings serve as reservoirs and vectors, and the mode of transmission is almost exclusively sexual intercourse. If untreated, the venereal diseases become chronic requiring more comprehensive treatment and management for rehabilitation or restoration and, therefore, are related to the kinds of conditions which are discussed in the next chapter.

The stigma of having such diseases, the tendency to chronicity if untreated, the remote sequelae of some of them, the length and cost of treatment, and the resulting personal inconvenience complicate the problem both for the individual and for public control. The individual who contracts a venereal disease comes into conflict with society's mores, and, in addition, public law requires that his case be reported to the health department. He may, therefore, be reluctant to seek diagnosis and treatment for fear that public identification of himself and his contacts may result in social ostracism and legal harassment. The confidentiality of official venereal disease records and epidemiologic follow-up is well protected by law and practice, but this fact is not fully recognized by the public or the medical profession.

The significance of the venereal diseases from the public health standpoint is that they are communicable, they are preventable, they affect relatively large numbers of people, they may appear as epidemics and remain endemic in many population groups, they are influenced by the prevailing social philosophy and mores of segments of society, and they require organized social action and individual responsibility for control. Most communities require by law that health departments and the medical profession take some positive, sustained action in the prevention and control of venereal diseases.

The public attaches little significance to early signs and symptoms of venereal disease and sometimes is opposed to public education on the subject, yet the risk of chronic physical and mental disease is great and costly. Complications of untreated or inadequately treated *syphilis* may lead to heart disease, blindness, paralysis, infected newborns, psychoses, and pathologic changes in many tissues and organs of the human body. It is known that over $55 million is spent annually in the United States for the care of patients with central nervous system disorders due to syphilis. Although the cost of care of syphilitic heart disease patients is not known, this condition is even more common than disorders of the central nervous system. *Gonorrhea* is still considered by many persons as nothing worse than a common cold, but there are, in fact, serious potential complications of sterility and urinary obstruction, especially for females.

INCIDENCE OF SYPHILIS AND GONORRHEA

The two most common venereal diseases are gonorrhea and syphilis. Statistics pertaining to syphilis usually distinguish between two major categories which reflect the stage of development of the disease. The first category is subdivided into *primary* syphilis, which indicates the initial point of contact and infection (usually the genitalia), and *secondary* syphilis, which indicates the early systemic involvement (usually skin lesions are present and are indicators of bodywide infection of all other organs). The second category consists of *latent* and *late* syphilis, which are the chronic stages of the disease and include the involvement and destruction of selected tissues and organs remote from the usual sexual point of initial contact and infection. Manifestations of this stage of development of the disease may be delayed for months or even years.

It is generally agreed that incidence figures (the number of new cases per year) and prevalence figures (the total number of cases in various stages of diagnosis, treatment, and rehabilitation at any given time) underestimate the magnitude of both syphilis and gonorrhea. The figures are influenced by the stage of the disease, the number of persons who seek diagnosis, and the number who are treated in public clinics versus by private physicians. Thus, the venereal disease problem reveals itself like an iceberg showing only a small part of its total mass; the bulk of the problem hides unreported in the community.[1] It has been estimated, for example, that California has more than 200,000 new cases annually rather than the 45,000 cases reported.[2] Many of the individuals with undetected venereal disease may be unaware that they are infected because they have only minor symptoms or none at all. Although all cases treated in public clinics are reported, it has been estimated that only about 25 per cent of the cases of syphilis and gonorrhea which are diagnosed by private physicians are reported to health authorities.[3] However, in spite of the problems resulting from the various kinds of gaps in reporting, available data probably do indicate at least the general direction of actual trends and differences, even if not the precise amount.[4]

Trends in Syphilis and Gonorrhea Incidence

Trends in the incidence of syphilis and gonorrhea have differed from one another and have undergone notable changes during the present century. In 1919, the incidence of gonorrhea somewhat exceeded that of syphilis (total, all stages), but shortly thereafter the gonorrhea rate declined slightly and leveled off, whereas the incidence of syphilis began increasing, particularly after 1935, until it reached a peak of 447 cases per 100,000 population in 1943. With the discovery of penicillin in 1943 as effective therapy for both major venereal diseases, the rate for syphilis dropped sharply. The incidence of gonorrhea, on the other hand, began increasing in the early 1940's and reached a peak of 284 cases per 100,000 in 1947 after which it, too, declined, but from then on, it remained consistently higher than the rates for syphilis.[4]

Table 9-1, which shows incidence for the period 1950–1966, reveals that the downward trend in the rate of gonorrhea continued until 1959; at that time it again began to increase, reaching about 174 cases per 100,000 in 1966. In contrast, the downward trend in syphilis rates (total, all stages),

TABLE 9-1 Cases of Syphilis and Gonorrhea and Rates for 100,000 Population Reported by State Health Departments, Fiscal Years, 1950–1966

Fiscal Year	Primary and Secondary Syphilis		Early Latent Syphilis		Late and Late Latent Syphilis		Total Syphilis *		Gonorrhea		Total Infectious VD (P&S Syphilis & Gonorrhea)		Total VD (Syphilis † All Stages & Gonorrhea)	
	Cases	Rate	Cases	Rate	Cases	Rate	Cases	Rate	Cases	Rate	Cases	Rate	Cases	Rate
1950	32,148	21.6	64,786	43.5	112,424	75.5	229,723	154.2	303,922	204.0	336,070	225.6	533,645	358.2
1951	18,211	12.1	52,309	34.7	107,133	71.1	198,640	131.8	270,459	179.5	288,670	191.6	469,099	311.3
1952	11,991	7.9	38,365	25.2	101,920	66.9	168,734	110.8	245,633	161.3	257,624	169.2	414,367	272.1
1953	9,551	6.2	32,287	20.8	100,195	64.7	156,099	100.8	243,857	157.4	253,408	163.6	399,956	258.2
1954	7,688	4.9	24,999	15.9	93,601	59.4	137,876	87.5	239,661	152.0	247,349	156.9	377,537	239.5
1955	6,516	4.1	21,553	13.4	84,741	52.7	122,075	76.0	239,787	149.2	246,303	153.3	361,862	225.2
1956	6,757	4.1	20,014	12.2	89,851	54.8	126,219	77.1	233,333	142.4	240,090	146.5	359,552	219.5
1957	6,251	3.8	19,046	11.4	96,856	58.1	130,552	78.3	216,476	129.8	222,727	133.6	347,028	208.1
1958	6,661	3.9	16,698	9.8	85,974	50.5	116,630	68.5	220,191	129.3	226,852	133.2	336,821	197.8
1959	8,178	4.7	17,592	10.2	86,776	50.1	119,981	69.3	237,318	137.0	245,496	141.7	357,299	206.3
1960	12,471	7.1	16,829	9.5	84,195	47.6	120,249	68.0	246,697	139.6	259,168	146.7	366,946	207.6
1961	18,781	10.4	19,146	10.7	80,942	45.0	125,262	69.7	265,685	147.8	284,466	158.5	390,947	217.5
1962	20,084	11.0	19,924	10.9	78,264	42.9	124,188	68.1	260,468	142.8	280,552	153.8	384,656	210.9
1963	22,045	11.9	18,683	10.1	81,736	44.1	128,450	69.3	270,076	145.7	292,121	157.6	398,526	215.0
1964	22,733	12.1	18,104	9.6	72,184	38.4	118,247	62.9	290,603	154.5	313,336	166.6	408,850	217.4
1965	23,250	12.3	17,315	9.1	67,633	35.7	113,018	59.7	310,155	163.8	333,405	176.1	423,173	223.5
1966	22,473	11.6	16,974	8.8	66,149	34.3	110,128	57.1	334,949	173.6	357,422	185.2	445,077	230.7

Source: The Association of State and Territorial Health Officers, The American Public Health Association, The American Venereal Disease Association, and The American Social Health Association: A Joint Statement. Today's VD Control Problem. American Social Health Association, New York, 1967.

* Includes congenital and other syphilis.

† Excludes chancroid, granuloma inguinale, and lymphogranuloma venereum.

which began after 1943, has continued fairly consistently, although a plateau occurred during the period 1958–1963. However, Table 9-1 also shows that, if the rates for primary and secondary syphilis, only, are considered, the trend is similar to that for gonorrhea: the downward trend lasted until 1959, when it began to rise and reached 11 or 12 cases per 100,000 in the period 1962–1966; both the syphilis rates and the numbers of cases, however, have remained markedly lower than those for gonorrhea.

It is evident, then, that the advent of penicillin, combined probably with the intensive venereal disease educational and control programs which were conducted during World War II, served to reduce the rates of gonorrhea and syphilis by the mid- or late 1940's. As a result of the success with penicillin, the point of view developed that treatment alone would eliminate these diseases. Organized community venereal disease control programs were de-emphasized, and many physicians gave these diseases a low priority in differential diagnosis and treatment management. The identification of new cases and of their contacts and sources of exposure were no longer considered a major public health problem. As a consequence, federal, state, and local support waned. However, the reversal of the downward trend and the resulting increase in the rates of gonorrhea and of primary and secondary syphilis which began in 1959 emphasize the fact that continuing surveillance, vigilance, and community programs must be maintained in order to minimize the risk of these diseases.

Population Groups at Risk

The increase of venereal disease in recent years is found in the younger age group, with 56.2 per cent of the total reported infectious cases occurring in persons under 25 years of age in 1964.[5] The greatest increase of infections has occurred among boys and girls between 10 and 14 years of age and among teen-agers 15 to 19 years of age. In fact, the teen-age case rate for infectious syphilis in the calendar year 1964 was 22.7 cases per 100,000 population, or nearly double the national average of 12.1 for all ages during the same year.

Gonorrhea, as well as syphilis to a somewhat lesser extent, is more likely to be reported among males than females, and both diseases are more likely to be reported among nonwhite than white groups. Both diseases are also reported at far higher rates in the Southern and Southwestern states than in the rest of the nation. However, all these differences may be overstated owing to wide variations in completeness of reporting.[4] Thus, venereal disease reporting for males is probably more complete than for females because of the greater visibility of symptoms among males and because males may be less reluctant to seek treatment. Nonwhite persons are more likely to be diagnosed and treated in public clinics and hence become cases reported, whereas whites are more likely to be treated by private physicians. The state or city with the highest venereal disease rate may merely reflect more cases identified, and not necessarily that there is more community infection than in another state with a reported lower rate of infections. Furthermore, a local, relatively isolated outbreak can cause the rate for a state to rise sharply.

Public health authorities are nevertheless concerned about these differences in venereal disease rates among population groups and about the reasons which may account for the differential reporting. Certain other groups have also become of special concern in recent years because of suspected high rates, or because they present particularly difficult control problems. These groups include homosexuals, migrant workers, military personnel, and American Indians on reservations.[4] There is also reason to believe that higher socioeconomic groups are involved with increasing frequency.

TYPES OF VENEREAL DISEASES

There are five separate and distinctly different venereal diseases: as mentioned earlier, syphilis and gonorrhea are the most common in this country; the three others, which are of lower incidence, are chancroid, lymphogranuloma venereum, and granuloma inguinale. There are a number of other diseases which are transmitted by sexual contact, such as venereal warts; monilial infections; trichomonal, crab, and lice infestations; and a few others. However, these diseases are not considered to be classic examples of venereal disease and are not serious social problems.

Syphilis, in recorded history, is notably absent until Columbus' crew introduced it into Europe upon returning from the New World. As syphilis was propagated through the Old World, principally by migrant armies, millions of people lost their lives. For centuries, it was not recognized that there was a correlation between a history of early syphilis in a patient and his subsequent death many years later owing to organic complications of the disease. Columbus himself died psychotic and paralyzed, the victim of late syphilis.

Gonorrhea smoldered along at apparently a high incidence in Europe, and somehow a confusion arose as an effort was made to understand the pathogenesis of the venereal diseases. Since gonorrhea and syphilis were often contracted at the same time, the diseases came to be considered as one. Hunter "proved" this in the eighteenth century by infecting himself with pus from a patient with gonorrhea (who also had syphilis). He developed both diseases and proclaimed them to be one and the same. This error was not finally untangled until Neisser discovered the gonococcus in 1879, and Schaudin and Hoffman identified *Treponema pallidum* in 1905.

Syphilis

As seen in temperate climates, syphilis is a sexually transmitted treponemal disease related to other sexually and asexually spread treponematoses. Biologically related treponemal organisms produce different symptoms in infected individuals living in warmer climates from those produced in colder climates. The causative organism of venereal syphilis is *Treponema pallidum*. It is a spirochete and is classified with the bacteria for lack of a better category in which to place it. The organism is great in length, averaging 7 microns, though so narrow in width that it cannot be visualized satisfactorily without the use of a dark-field microscope. It is found in skin lesions of early syphilis; this fact is responsible for the relatively short communicable period which exists in this disease.

The incubation period in syphilis is about three to six weeks. In order to acquire the disease, it is necessary to have warm, moist, prolonged contact (essentially sexual intercourse) with another human being who has accessible syphilis lesions containing the causative organism. The organism is capable of invading several kinds of tissues. A lesion will usually develop at the site where original entry of the causative organism occurred after the incubation period. This is *primary syphilis* and the lesion is referred to as a chancre. The lesion is usually single, elevated, ulcerated, indurated, and painless. The commonest site in the male is the glans penis, and in the female frequently on the cervix, where it may go unnoticed. This lesion vanishes spontaneously in around two weeks as *Treponema pallidum*, which have proliferated at this site, leave to enter the circulatory and lymphatic systems. At this time, syphilis is no longer a local disease, but becomes systemic; the entire body is now infected and the manifestations of *secondary syphilis* begin to appear. The skin usually will provide visual evidence of total body involvement with the appearance of a rash typically maculopapular in nature. Each small skin lesion in the rash represents a colony of multiplying *Treponema pallidum*. Other signs of bodywide spread also occur, such as fever, malaise, lymphadenopathy, pharyngitis, and alopecia. Secondary lesions occurring in moist areas of the body such as the genitals, anus, and mouth are considered most communicable. The duration of secondary syphilis varies, but the symptoms commonly vanish spontaneously in less than a month; occasionally, relapsing secondary syphilis will occur with periodic recrudescent lesions up to two years.

From this point syphilis loses its communicability and may never be symptomatic again; it is now said to be "latent." Infections of less than two years' duration are referred to as *early latent* syphilis, and those of longer than two years' duration are termed *late latent* syphilis. Although the disease may never become noticeable to the patient again, if he is not adequately treated his longevity will be reduced to a 14 per cent probability of his reaching age 65. About 12 per cent of untreated syphilitics will develop symptoms again any time within one year or even much later.[6] If syphilis causes sufficient organ damage, these cases are reclassified as *late syphilis*, and reference is made to the organ so damaged. Late syphilis involves the cardiovascular system, the central nervous system, the skin, and the gastrointestinal system.

Congenital syphilis is a special biologic situation and the mechanism is poorly understood. It represents asexual transmission of the disease from an untreated or inadequately treated, infected mother to the unborn fetus. After the seventeenth week of pregnancy, it is considered possible for live *Treponema pallidum* circulating in maternal blood to cross the placental barrier and infect the fetus. The father need not have syphilis. Congenital syphilis is not hereditary, but it is a familial disease occurring in one family unit. Congenital syphilis is amenable to prevention through premarital and prenatal examinations for possible syphilis. However, six states still have no laws requiring a test for syphilis as part of the prenatal examination, and six states have no premarital examination laws. Of this number, two states and, in addition, the District of Columbia have neither premarital nor prenatal examination laws.

The diagnosis of syphilis is relatively easier than that of gonorrhea. While the disease is in its incubation stage, a probable diagnosis can be made on the basis of exposure to another known infected case. Since skin lesions of the disease contain the causative organisms, the diagnosis can be made on dark-field examination of serum taken from a suspected lesion. The commonly used reagin tests for syphilis will begin to become reactive late in primary syphilis, increasing to the point where, in secondary syphilis, 100 per cent of patients are considered to have a reactive serology, or a positive blood test for syphilis. In cases of syphilis of long standing, when the physician doubts the diagnosis, special tests of a treponemal nature (TPI and FTA)[7] will confirm that the patient has previously had syphilis, but they offer little assistance in determining whether treatment has been adequate. Special diagnostic techniques exist for determining the presence of syphilitic involvement in the cardiovascular, central nervous, skin, and visceral systems, but these require comprehensive professional study and evaluation.

The patient with syphilis whose treatment has been neglected will eventually produce a large amount of antisyphilitic antibody resulting in partial protection against reinfection. This is one reason the long-term professional prostitute is not materially responsible for the spread of syphilis in society. However, treatment in a very early stage of primary or secondary syphilis results in the immediate death of *Treponema pallidum*. This cancels any further antigenic response and results in minimal production of antisyphilitic antibody. Thus, patients who are diagnosed and treated early may become reinfected.

In the 1800's, mercury, principally in the form of ointments, became widely used in the treatment of syphilis. Such treatment was highly toxic, in fact so toxic that research studies began to report the morbidity produced by treatment versus a "control group" of syphilitic patients who were allowed to undergo an undisturbed pathogenesis of the disease. Ehrlich searched for a preparation to be given intravenously, which would kill the spirochete of syphilis and not affect the host. His 606th try produced Salvarsan ("606"), which was effective, but so toxic it had to be given in small repeated doses over a two-year treatment course.

The most significant development in finding a cure for syphilis came in 1943 when Mahoney found that penicillin (first discovered in 1926) seemed to cure several male volunteers. Penicillin is now the drug of choice and is successful in almost 100 per cent of cases under proper management. Penicillin G in various forms is relatively innocuous and can cure syphilis with as little as one injection. Patients who are allergic to penicillin can be successfully treated with tetracycline or erythromycin. Mercury, bismuth, and arsenic, with their uncertain results, long treatment course, and disastrous physical effects, are no longer used in the treatment of syphilis. Syphilis has been transmitted to a number of laboratory animals, and virulent organisms can be cultured. This has resulted in attempts to produce a vaccine for syphilis,[8] and the eventual development of an effective preventive is within the realm of possibility.

Gonorrhea

The most pressing venereal disease problem at present is gonorrhea because of its incidence, complications, and lack of good diagnostic techniques. This disease has never been transmitted to laboratory animals, although the causative organism, *Neisseria gonorrhoeae*, may be grown in artificial media. The bacterium proliferates anaerobically, usually on columnar epithelium. It is, therefore, found primarily in the urinary tract (especially in males), the reproductive system (especially in females), rectum, pharynx, and conjuctiva. In a few cases, it mimics its close relative, the meningococcus, and becomes invasive producing septicemia, meningitis, endocarditis, and arthritis.

The incubation period is short, from three to ten days. Usually the male is symptomatic and communicable three days after exposure. Therefore, case finding must be immediate in gonorrhea. The male who waits until he has been symptomatic for five days before seeking treatment can have had contacts who, in turn, have been capable of spreading the disease for two days. Gonorrhea is communicable as long as the patient remains infected; in the female particularly, this may last for years. She will by no means infect every sex partner but only an occasional one. It is not unusual for males to acquire several infections in one year.

Unfortunately, gonorrhea is really two different diseases, according to the sex of the infected patient. Males usually develop an anterior urethritis and are symptomatic from penile discharge and dysuria. They can usually be counted on to appear for treatment. If treatment is not prompt, the organism may by mechanical means spread over the urinary lining, involve the remainder of the male urinary tract, and produce a descending infection involving the testicles. Testicular infection results quite often in sterility.

The primary complication in the male, however, is urinary obstruction, which is seldom recognized early. Healing in the urethra results in scar tissue formation, which, over many years, results in scar proliferation and ultimate urinary obstruction.

The female receives her infection most often deep in the vagina. Her urinary system is usually spared. The prime site of female infection is in the deep secretory glands of the cervical os, i.e., the opening to the uterus. Here the gonococcus finds its ideal environment. A problem of early recognition is that the cervix is insensitive to pain, and the physiologic manifestations, such as discharge produced, are minimal. The female almost completely lacks symptomatology in gonorrhea; hence she does not seek medical assistance voluntarily. Therefore, she serves as reservoir for the disease. About 25 per cent of females, by mechanical means, will develop an inflammation of one or both fallopian tubes (salpingitis) and thus will risk sterility, surgical removal of her organs of reproduction, and tubal pregnancy.

A fetus leaving an infected mother on delivery will obviously subject its eyes to infection. Gonorrheal conjunctivitis at one time was the leading cause of blindness of the newborn but may be prevented by instillation of silver nitrate solution or penicillin ointment directly into the infant's conjunctiva at time of birth. This prophylactic procedure is now required in 47 of the 50 states.

The diagnosis of gonorrhea is based on the likelihood of individual exposure and on symptomatology, since the diagnostic laboratory tests generally used are not the most specific, especially for female infections. A serologic test for gonorrhea exists but is insensitive and inaccurate, therefore of little use in the average case. Although reported effectiveness varies, laboratory smear and culture confirm the disease with about 80 per cent effectiveness in the male and about 50 per cent effectiveness in the female. Thus, if diagnosis and treatment of the female are based on positive laboratory findings alone, only half the reservoir of the disease can ever be eliminated.

It has been alleged that young females and sometimes males have acquired gonorrhea from towels, toilet seats, and other inanimate objects. This is practically impossible. A recent study[9] showed that not one child over the age of one year acquired gonorrhea asexually. Young children, especially females, may develop discharges resembling gonorrhea which are due to other organisms. This may be the origin of some of the myths regarding asexually acquired venereal disease. At any rate, although treatment should be administered, a diagnosis of gonorrhea in a young child is not considered justified without positive laboratory findings confirmed by special laboratory techniques.

Infection with the gonococcus results in the production of minimal, fleeting, or ineffective antibody, thus facilitating frequent reinfection. At present, no preventive vaccine seems possible. Treatment of gonorrhea has varied as the organism has become resistant to each newly available chemotherapeutic agent. Local therapy with potassium and silver salts was at one time effective. The organism has become relatively resistant to sulfa drugs, and resistance to penicillin is increasing.[10] However, penicillin given in large amounts is still the drug of choice because of its low cost and its availability as an intramuscular injection with prolonged absorption. As resistance to penicillin increases, tetracyclines may become the drugs of choice in spite of their cost and the requirement of patient responsibility to take medication as prescribed.

As a result of the increase in the incidence of gonorrhea during recent years, an old technique has been updated and will be effective if conscientiously used. Patients known to have been exposed, who are presently asymptomatic, and for whom laboratory work is noncontributory are treated for the disease and diagnosed as being "epidemiologically treated for gonorrhea." "Epi treatment" [11] arises from past prophylactic experience and is now justified and used more frequently for the treatment of both gonorrhea and syphilis.

Chancroid

Chancroid is caused by infection with the bacillus *Hemophilus ducreyi*. The incubation period is usually from three to five days. One or more lesions will occur on the genital organs and are characteristically unclean-looking, painful ulcerations. The initial lesion usually vanishes spontaneously. In about 50 per cent of those infected, the lymphatic glands in the inguinal area become enlarged and may possibly break down producing a draining sinus to the skin. The causative organism can be identified on smear or culture of exudate from the ulcer or aspiration from an inguinal bubo. A skin test for this disease exists but is little used. Treatment with tetracycline is effective.

Lymphogranuloma Venereum

Lymphogranuloma venereum is caused by a filtrable virus. The incubation period is from about 5 to 21 days, and the initial symptom is usually an insignificant small papule which is evanescent and frequently undetected. This disease also produces enlargement of lymphatic glands and drainage through fistulous openings. The causative virus presumably exists in the initial lesion, and inclusion bodies produced by the virus are demonstrable in the cytoplasm of lymphatic tissue cells. Diagnosis is often not made until it becomes necessary to perform surgery for removal of matted lymph nodes that have produced symptoms such as rectal stricture. A complement fixation test exists for the diagnosis of lymphogranuloma venereum, and a skin test is also available. Therapy of choice at present is tetracycline for a period of approximately 30 days.

Granuloma Inguinale

Granuloma inguinale is caused by *Donovania granulomatis*. The incubation period is extremely variable and may be quite long, from 8 to 12 weeks or more. An initial lesion appears which is at first papular, then breaks down to become ulcerated, and continues to spread producing large, disfiguring, granulomatous ulcerations, usually confined to the genital areas. The lesions heal and produce scars while spreading continues. The patient has a characteristic sour and pungent odor. The causative organism may be demonstrated on smear or biopsy from a local lesion; the organisms group themselves together intracytoplasmically in what is known as Donovan bodies. Tetracycline is effective therapy.

PATTERN OF SPREAD OF VENEREAL DISEASES

Every person infected with venereal disease (the primary case) has acquired his infection from another individual (his source case) and probably has infected others (his spread cases). Failure to seek immediate treatment for the primary case, the source, and spread cases increases the community reservoir and therefore increases the risk of infection spread. The identification of each source of infection and of all those exposed is a responsibility of the infected patient and his personal physician. It becomes the responsibility of public health agencies to protect the public by case finding, that is, identifying the source and spread cases and treating them to prevent further spread of infection.

If undetected, venereal disease can become epidemic. In 1965, the American Social Health Association[5] identified 69 venereal disease outbreaks which involved a chain of infection of ten or more cases epidemiologically related. These outbreaks occurred in 28 states and involved 9715 people. Figure 9-1 shows the pattern of infection during an outbreak of syphilis in one midwestern urban area during 1965. The figure shows how one man infected with syphilis initiated the ultimate exposure of 274 other persons, resulting in 42 additional cases of infectious syphilis within a relative short period of time before the health officials finally eliminated the epidemic.

PROBLEMS OF PREVENTION AND CONTROL

The venereal diseases are not associated with sudden death or immediate dramatic complications. As a consequence, they are less likely than some other diseases to command public attention. The fact that their transmission is primarily dependent on sexual activity interferes with open discussion, public and professional education, implementation of legislation, and effective control. Social taboos and related attitudes influence the individual in practicing prophylaxis, seeking medical care, and providing cooperation in

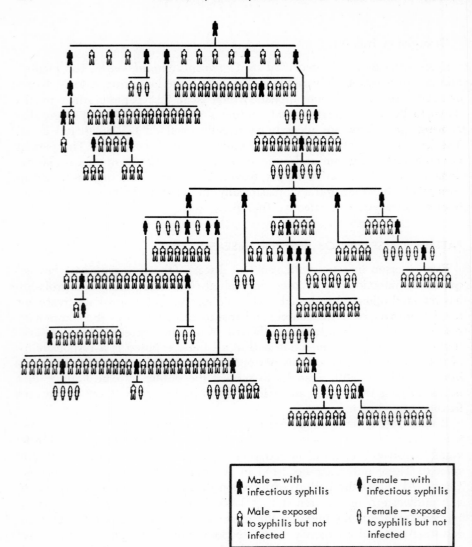

FIGURE 9-1. Infectious syphilis outbreak in a Midwestern urban area, 1965. (Source: The Association of State and Territorial Health Officers, The American Venereal Disease Association, and The American Social Health Association: A Joint Statement. *Today's VD Control Problem*. American Social Health Association, New York, 1966.)

the identification of sources and potential cases of venereal diseases. Prevailing attitudes toward promiscuity and discrepancies between society's mores and behavior also confuse the efforts to prevent these diseases. These are all problems of social ideology and behavior, and they cannot be ignored in efforts of public and professional education, prevention, and control.

Prophylactic measures (such as condoms, soap and water, and douches) may minimize the risk of venereal disease. However, public acceptance of prophylaxis is not universal because some consider that it is offensive and interferes with sexual satisfaction. Since promiscuity increases the probability of acquiring venereal disease, there has been a tendency for some cultural groups to rely on sexual abstinence as the major means of control. However, it is not likely that universal prevention could be achieved through this or any other method which requires significant modification or restriction of sexual activity.

There has been little interest in or public support for research for the production of immunizing agents against the venereal diseases. If a vaccine is ever produced, public acceptance could be a problem because of the moral issues. Although there has been recent favorable experience with public acceptance of birth control pills, the issues are not necessarily comparable because use of the pills is within the context of a stable family. The use of immunizations for protection against venereal diseases, on the other hand, may be viewed by the public as licensing planned, protected promiscuity.

Community programs in venereal disease education have lagged because of the point of view that the problem is individual and not social, that contracting a disease merely reflects irresponsible social behavior, and that good moral practice prevents risk of exposure. However, such views do not take into account the tendency toward more casual and informal sexual relationships that has developed in modern life. The individual who is denied knowledge regarding the existence of venereal diseases and their causes, methods of transmission, symptoms, and effects is at a distinct disadvantage. In a study conducted recently in Los Angeles, only 2 per cent of teen-agers admitted to any venereal disease education in the home. The subject can best be handled in the classroom where the trained teacher can impart accurate, objective knowledge and can serve as a continuous resource to young people whose questions require definite, factual answers free of evasiveness and mythology. Venereal disease education probably will neither prevent nor stimulate promiscuous sexual activity. However, it may result in more selectivity in sexual behavior, and it certainly will result in infected persons seeking early treatment and cooperating with physicians or health departments in bringing source and spread cases under treatment.

There has been a shift of responsibility for venereal as well as other communicable disease control to the private physician, so that his role in the identification and treatment of all source and spread cases has become of great importance. However, the private sector of medical practice usually does not have available the resources or facilities that are needed in order to meet the challenge universally to control venereal disease spread. Therefore, health agencies must be prepared to provide services of diagnosis, treatment, and contact follow-up in recognition of the reality that all patients will not seek private medical care, and all physicians will not accept such cases and, if they do, will not be able to undertake the complex and specialized task of identifying and treating source and spread cases.

SOCIAL CONTROL MEASURES

The prevention and control of venereal diseases are based on public and professional recognition of venereal disease as a social problem; on a sense of responsibility on the part of the individual and the practitioner; and on community organization and support for planned measures to minimize risk through education, case finding, reporting, diagnosis, and treatment. The community aspect involves legislation, the role of the physician, and the availability of clinical services and cooperative follow-up investigative services.

The Public Health Service Task Force on the Eradication of Syphilis [12] has recommended a broad program of prevention and control, most elements of which are applicable to the venereal diseases in general. Thus, it has been recommended, first, that an intensive effort be made to enlist the private physician and his professional societies and associations in the control effort. Second, a program should be established to ensure that all laboratories, including public, private, hospital, and blood banks processing blood tests for syphilis, cooperate in the control effort by notifying appropriate health departments of all reactive or suggestive specimens. Third, current patient interview-investigation services should be intensified and extended to cover all infectious cases. Regardless of reporting sources, every infectious case should be interviewed and reinterviewed for sex contacts and important associates so that contacts can be brought under medical supervision and treatment. Fourth, a comprehensive and dynamic education program should be developed for health workers as well as for the public. The public education efforts should be aimed at persons in younger age groups most likely to contract venereal diseases. Fifth, research in immunology, therapy, and laboratory procedures should be continued, and research in adolescent and young adult sex behavior should be greatly expanded. Sixth, even when incidence rates begin to decline, federal, state, and local efforts and budgets should continue.

Legislative Measures

Venereal disease prevention and control cannot be carried out effectively without public health laws and regulations requiring the prompt reporting of cases to the health department. This includes not only the newly discovered cases, but also cases in the communicable stage who discontinue treatment without notifying the physician or clinic that treatment is being obtained elsewhere. For effective prevention of new cases and in order to discover other source and spread cases, such reporting must be by name and address rather than by serial number or other subterfuge methods. While the law in some states permits or requires isolation of patients in the communicable stages who are not under treatment, this procedure usually is not invoked.

Some states already require the reporting of all positive blood specimens by public and private laboratories, including hospital laboratories and blood banks. There is some difference of opinion regarding this approach, since some public health and medical professionals believe that if practitioners and clinics met the requirements of reporting communicable diseases, laboratory reporting would be unnecessary. However, experience has shown that new, previously unknown or undiagnosed cases are discovered, and more conscientious reporting by physicians is stimulated by laboratory reporting.

As mentioned earlier, most states have adopted laws requiring premarital serologic tests for syphilis and a serologic test for all pregnant women under a physician's care. Routine blood testing of all hospital admissions was required by regulation at one time in some states and is practiced voluntarily by some hospitals today.

Educational Programs

Professional Education. The techniques of diagnosis and treatment of individual cases of the venereal diseases are included in medical school curricula. While the biology and the biologic factors in the natural history of the venereal diseases may be covered, the social aspects of the diseases' natural history usually are not included. Medical school curricula also have been deficient in the behavioral sciences, which, if offered, would contribute to an understanding of the attitudinal, behavioral, and cultural factors which underlie problems of venereal disease control. As medical schools become forced to provide the total spectrum of health care for a given population, in contrast to the traditional practice of selecting cases, the experience with venereal disease management by medical students, interns, and residents will be enhanced.

Professional schools for the training of personnel other than physicians must include appropriate consideration of the venereal diseases as a community problem. Dentists, nurses, social workers, teachers, ministers, and other community service personnel need some introduction to the identification and control problems of these diseases. The social factors are as important as the biologic problems, if not more so, especially from the standpoint of prevention and minimizing the risk of disabilities and future dependency.

Education of the Public. The professional groups can provide only some aspects of venereal disease prevention; other aspects are the responsibility of the public. Public understanding of the natural, social, and biologic course of these diseases as they occur in population groups is essential. The public is generally ignorant of the cause, the mechanisms of spread, the effects, and the incidence of venereal disease in the populace. Therefore, education beginning in high school with planned curricula, and carefully designed health education programs directed toward the general public, must be stimulated and promoted.

Sex education too frequently has been equated with venereal disease education. However, sex education involves much broader issues than just the risks of venereal diseases. Physiology, anatomy, psychology, and moral issues are basic elements in sex education, and the range of sexual behavior as influenced by cultural backgrounds, family attitudes, and changing environmental stresses are other factors to be considered. It is reasonable to expect that free and open discussion of human biology and sexual behavior would have a favorable influence on community programs for the prevention of sex-related diseases.

The facts about venereal diseases should be presented to young people in an unemotional manner, without defensiveness, insecurity, or fear—in contrast to the way in which too many parents tend to discuss the issues. The younger generations will listen to factual discussion and are impressed until moral and religious considerations become the obvious issue. The concept that venereal diseases need no longer be feared since they are so easily and conveniently treated is learned by the younger public by word of mouth from associates. In many instances this stimulates early diagnosis and treatment but not necessarily cooperation with physicians and health department personnel in the identification of source and possible spread cases.

Clinical Services and the
Role of the Physician

Treatment is an effective control measure for infectious venereal disease because modern therapy can promise a cure to all, and once treatment is instituted, it renders the patient noncommunicable within a few hours. Therefore, clinical services must be freely available to anyone with actual or suspected venereal diseases. These services must be provided either through private physicians or through public clinics for those who cannot afford private medical care. Furthermore, they must be available at hours convenient for the worker who cannot meet the 30-to-40-hour standard medical service schedule. The schedules of clinics operated by community agencies should be arranged to enhance the contact with source and spread cases who will otherwise serve as additional reservoirs of the venereal diseases.

The physician in private practice optimally follows several procedures with respect to venereal disease prevention and control. These include being alert to the venereal diseases in the differential diagnosis; taking an exhaustive history; providing a complete examination, including all body orifices and mucocutaneous junctions, and dark-field examination of exudate from lesions; obtaining appropriate laboratory tests in support of the differential diagnosis; adequately treating the patient and contacts willing to submit to treatment; and reporting other contacts to the health department for diagnosis and treatment. The safe and modern treatment of venereal diseases affords the medical profession the opportunity to treat on the basis of exposure contact and presumptive infection. The physician and the public health investigator should use the acute stage of a venereal disease as an opportunity for health education and patient motivation for the practice of prevention.

Conscientious case reporting, effective epidemiologic investigation and follow-up, and early treatment are the methods of preventing venereal disease epidemics or of bringing them under control. This requires cooperation between the private physician and the health officials. In some areas, the apparent rise in venereal disease rates is merely the result of systematic reporting of source cases by physicians and diligent follow-up by the local health department. The reporting of the source case may cause some retaliatory reaction of patients and others on occasions; however, with physician-patient shared understanding of the importance of the prevention of infections, these adverse reactions can be minimized.

Follow-up Investigative Services

Follow-up investigative services can be provided by a health agency with well-trained investigators who can maintain the physician's cooperation and acquire the confidence and cooperation of the patient. In addition to the venereal disease investigator, the public health nurse, social worker, and health educator all have a role in community venereal disease control programs.

The physician initiates follow-up investigation by a telephone call to the local health department, arranging for an investigator to interview the patient in the physician's office, preferably at the time of diagnosis. The interview averages about 45 minutes and requires special skills in obtaining the names of all the patient's contacts. Special techniques are particularly needed to obtain homosexual contacts. The health department venereal disease investigators, public health nurses, and social workers locate the contacts and persuade them to obtain treatment. They also obtain the names of additional contacts who are, in turn, located and brought under treatment. When the source or spread cases live in other cities or states, the information is telephoned to the health department having jurisdiction over the address. All follow-up activities are confidential, and no names are released to anyone. Speed of action in reporting, interviewing, locating contacts, and initiating treatment reduces the number of new infections. Reporting by mail, and location of the patient by mail for interview in his home or in the health department office, cause delays which provide more time for additional contacts and spread cases.

Some state codes provide that the attending physician, in every case of venereal disease coming to him for treatment, shall endeavor to discover the source of infection as well as other sexual contacts. These efforts are time consuming, and there is risk of delay in follow-up. Some physicians are uneasy in contacting people who are not known to them and tend to rely on the primary case to persuade his contacts to come in for examination. It is faster and more efficient in most situations to report the case to the health department and leave the follow-up to that agency. This is especially true in the large metropolitan areas.

FUTURE NEEDS IN VENEREAL DISEASE CONTROL

The single greatest need in the future control of venereal diseases is, of course, the development of means to ensure that all infected persons receive treatment, and that they receive it early. The various kinds of inhibitions to seeking such treatment must be systematically identified and removed. Of almost equal importance, is the development by private practitioners of an awareness of the serious nature of the venereal disease problem generally, and the potential seriousness of each diagnosed case, no matter how minor the symptoms. Private physicians must become aware of the importance of reporting cases to health authorities and of the potential danger to the population if they fail to do so. A marked reduction in the presently estimated high rate of nonreported cases of venereal disease is a tangible goal that could be achieved through means already at hand.

The physician in private practice and physicians in community health agencies, especially official health departments, must all think in terms of the prevention of venereal disease in the population as a whole, rather than in terms of single case situations. They must recognize the fact that venereal diseases are pervasive and not confined to any particular socioeconomic, ethnic, or cultural group. Society, on the other hand, must resolve the moral and religious issues associated with sexual behavior and venereal disease, so that professional health workers can develop and carry out more effective programs to prevent and control these diseases.

Financial support and organizational provisions have lagged in the maintenance of previously high levels of community venereal disease programs. The consequences of waning public interest and diminished governmental assistance have become all too apparent in recent years. Even today, in the face of rising incidence of venereal diseases and their sequelae, financial support and organization at the federal, state, and local levels do not begin to meet the challenge. New and more effective organizational patterns must be established, and federal, state, and local appropriations must be increased in order to reattain the previous gains and to establish additional control of the venereal diseases.

SUMMARY

The venereal diseases are communicable, preventable, and likely to have serious consequences if not diagnosed and treated early. Untreated infections may lead to severe chronic conditions in the individual and to epidemics in the population. Unlike most of the other communicable diseases, human beings only are the reservoirs and vectors; sexual intercourse is almost the sole mode of transmission.

There are five major types of venereal disease: syphilis, gonorrhea, chancroid, lymphogranuloma venereum, and granuloma inguinale. Each has its characteristic causative organism, incubation period, symptoms, developmental pattern, diagnostic techniques, and modes of treatment.

Earlier in the present century, syphilis occurred the most frequently, but since the late 1940's, gonorrhea has had the highest rate of reported cases in the general population. In 1943, the discovery of penicillin as an effective therapy for both syphilis and gonorrhea caused the incidence of reported cases to decline, but this trend has been maintained only for latent and late syphilis. For gonorrhea and for primary and secondary syphilis, the incidence has been generally increasing since the late 1950's. There is some evidence that certain segments of the population are at special risk of venereal disease infection, including younger age groups, homosexuals, migrant workers, and several others.

Although incidence data—which are based on the number of *reported* cases of infection—provide some indication of general trends over a period of time, the true extent of the venereal disease problem is not known because of substantial underreporting of infected cases. Underreporting occurs because some persons may have a venereal disease but do not know it, because some may suspect they are infected but do not seek treatment, and because an estimated large proportion of private physicians do not report diagnosed cases to public health authorities.

The reversal of what was previously a downward trend in the incidence of gonorrhea and infectious syphilis is of particular concern to health workers because it indicates that venereal disease has again become a serious threat to the population. The resurgence of the problem has occurred because too much reliance has been placed on treatment alone; community control programs have been allowed to diminish; and federal, state, and local support has been permitted to decline.

Elements in the pattern of spread of venereal diseases are the primary case, the source case, and the spread cases. The key to prevention and control is early identification, diagnosis, and treatment of all these cases in order to forestall increases in the community reservoir of infection. Problems in the prevention and control of venereal diseases include impediments arising from society's attitudes toward sexual behavior and venereal disease infection, public reluctance to use prophylactic measures, lack of public support of research in the production of immunizing agents, lag in venereal disease education, and shift of responsibility for venereal disease control to the private sector of medical practice which lacks the resources for the complex and specialized task of identifying and treating source and spread cases.

Measures for the control of the venereal diseases include public health laws and regulations, educational programs for professional persons and the public, clinical services provided by private physicians and public clinics, and follow-up investigative services provided by local health departments. Considerable expansion of these measures is needed, and federal, state, and local organizational provisions and financial support must be increased if the venereal diseases are to be controlled and prevented.

REFERENCES

1. KETTERER, W. A., and CONDIT, PHILIP K. Syphilis eradication—the task ahead. *Calif Med*, **102**:306–9, April 1965.

2. SAN JOSE CITY HEALTH DEPARTMENT. *The Role of Private Physicians in the Epidemiology and Reporting of Venereal Diseases*. The Department, San Jose, California, 1961.

3. CURTIS, A. C. National survey of venereal disease treatment. *JAMA*, **186**:46–49, 1963.

4. LERNER, M., and ANDERSON, O. W. *Health Progress in the United States, 1900–1960*. The University of Chicago Press, Chicago, 1963.

5. THE ASSOCIATION OF STATE AND TERRITORIAL HEALTH OFFICERS, The American Public Health Association, The American Venereal Disease Association, and The American Social Health Association: A Joint Statement. *Today's VD Control Problem*. American Social Health Association, New York, 1967.

6. ROCKWELL, D. H., YOBS, A. R., and MOORE, M. B. The Tuskegee study of untreated syphilis. *Arch Intern Med*, **114**:792–98, December 1964.

7. MOORE, M. B., and KNOX, J. M. Sensitivity and specificity in syphilis serology: clinical implications. *Southern Med J*, **58**:963–68, August 1965.

8. MAGNUSON, H. J., THOMAS, E. W., OLANSKY, S., KAPLAN, B. I., DEMELLO, L., and CUTLER, J. C. Inoculation syphilis in human volunteers. *Medicine*, **35**:33–82, February 1956.

9. BRANCH, G., and PAXTON, R. A. A study of gonococcal infections among infants and children. *Public Health Rep*, **80**:347–52, April 1965.

10. THAYER, J. D., and MOORE, M. B. Gonorrhea: present knowledge, research and control efforts. *Med Clin N Amer*, **48**:755–65, May 1964.

11. MOORE, M. B., PRICE, E. V., KNOX, J. M., and ELGIN, L. W. Epidemiologic treatment of contacts to infectious syphilis. *Public Health Rep*, **78**:966–70, November 1963.

12. U.S. DEPARTMENT OF HEALTH, EDUCATION, AND WELFARE, Public Health Service. *Eradication of Syphilis: Task Force Report to the Surgeon General*. Public Health Service Publication No. 918, U.S. Government Printing Office, Washington, D.C., 1962.

CHAPTER 10

CHRONIC DISEASES

The significance of the chronic diseases as health problems and the challenges that are emerging regarding their control are discussed in this chapter. The first section of the chapter reviews the general magnitude of the problem, which is then described specifically in terms of mortality in the following section. The third section discusses various aspects of chronic disease morbidity, including the possible factors that influence onset and course of these diseases and the sources of information on their incidence and prevalence. The status of chronic disease programs is reviewed in the next section from the standpoint of the provision of community services, the role of the health department, and the activities of the federal government. The remaining sections of the chapter are devoted to descriptions of selected categories of chronic diseases with particular attention to significant specific disease conditions within the categories.

PERSPECTIVE CONCERNING THE
MAJOR CHRONIC DISEASES

Chronic diseases, viewed either from the standpoint of the provision of care for long-term illness or the sequelae of disability, are emerging as major scientific, medical, public health, and socioeconomic problems to be faced in the United States and throughout the world. Particularly in the United States, these problems have stimulated recent governmental concern as well as an overwhelming amount of legislative, professional, voluntary-organization, and community debate.

Concern over mounting chronic disease and disability has been expressed periodically since the early 1920's. However, recognition of a need for a national program to reduce the cost of these diseases is of more recent origin. Initially, it was the economic depression of the 1930's and, subsequently, World War II which stimulated chronic disease rehabilitation on a mass scale. Industry found ways to use many handicapped persons in providing essential services during the war effort. Beginning in the 1940's, many persons returning from military service with service-connected impairment received the benefit of modern methods of rehabilitation. In 1947, a joint committee of the American Hospital Association, the American Medical Association, the American Public Health Association, and the American Public Welfare Association issued a statement urging that prevention be considered the basic approach to chronic illness.[1] The joint statement also focused on the need for diagnostic and treatment facilities for chronic illness and set as an objective the availability of high-quality services to all income groups. When the statement was written, it was recognized that home care, care in nursing homes, rehabilitation teamwork, and the coordinated efforts of many groups in the community would be required in order to make a chronic disease control program effective.

As a result of the joint committee statement, the National Commission on Chronic Illness was organized in 1949. The commission conducted studies, served as a clearinghouse for information, and prepared a four-volume series of reports to establish guidelines for program planning. The commission defined chronic illnesses as comprising all health impairments or deviations from normal which have one or more of the following characteristics: permanency of residual disability caused by nonreversible pathologic alterations; a requirement of special patient training for rehabilitation; and a long period of medical supervision, observation, or care.[2]

Long-term care is a sensitive topic in the United States today and a matter of national concern because of the demands that it makes on the economy. It has been recognized that long-term illnesses occur in all age groups and in all ethnic and socioeconomic groups, and all demand a strenuous application of the principles of prevention, diagnosis, treatment, and management. Even though the young in the population are affected to some extent, it is the older population that incurs the bulk of suffering from chronic conditions. In the past, however, the problems of chronic diseases probably have tended to stimulate more social action directed toward the younger than toward the older age group.

Chronic illness cannot be viewed in isolation; rather, it must be considered as part of the problem of general medical care. In planning for the care of the chronically ill, consideration must be given to the entire spectrum of illnesses and to the appropriate care provided for all gradations of patient need, from the acute exacerbation, or flare-up, to the stable chronic condition. Care for the chronically ill must be viewed in the context of comprehensive care, wherein three settings are specified: (1) inpatient care,

(2) home care, and (3) outpatient care. Each of these categories has been extended to include specialized settings for the chronically ill. In 1963, the Association of State and Territorial Health Officers observed two problems pertinent to the medical care of the long-term patient: (1) an increasing fragmentation in the delivery of services, such as a separation between preventive and curative services, and (2) a pervading emphasis on categorical disease. The Association noted that official health departments have primary responsibility for the general health of all the people and outlined some of the governmental functions that would lead to improving the health of those with chronic disease. With the passage of significant legislation which deals with many of the problems noted by the Association, the public health and welfare agencies are being joined together in defining practical methods for chronic disease control.

CHANGING MORTALITY AND CHRONIC DISEASES

Chronic diseases are not new in occurrence, but there has been an improvement in the diagnostic methods and a recognition of the social importance of these diseases. Environmental factors have influenced the etiology, early detection, management, and acceptance of social responsibility related to these conditions. Changing infectious disease patterns, a shifting age distribution of the population and longevity, and a rising standard of living generally are considered interrelative factors which have affected the trend toward chronic disease as a major cause of death and disability.

The over-all downward trend in the mortality rate in the United States probably began during the early nineteenth century and accelerated during the latter half of that century. A consistent mortality rate decline occurred between 1900 and 1954, and the rate has exhibited a slower, uneven decline since then. By the turn of the century, control over certain of the infectious diseases was underway, and as early as 1900, the deaths from chronic diseases were already proportionately higher than those from acute diseases. By 1955, the chronic diseases accounted for more than 80 per cent of all deaths.

The three leading causes of death in 1900 (pneumonia and acute respiratory diseases, tuberculosis, and gastrointestinal conditions) amounted to only one twentieth of all deaths in 1960. The diseases which could be influenced through environmental control, such as water, food, general sanitation, hygienic practices, and medical care, demonstrated the greatest decline. Table 10-1, which shows the ten leading causes of death in 1963, reveals that three categories of chronic diseases head the list. Diseases of the heart have the highest death rate—about 375 deaths per 100,000 population—followed by malignant neoplasms and vascular lesions affecting the central nervous system (i.e., cerebrovascular diseases).

A reduction in death rates has occurred in the younger age groups, which

TABLE 10-1   The Ten Leading Causes of Death, United States, 1963 *

	Death Rate per 100,000 Population
Diseases of heart	375.4
Malignant neoplasms †	151.4
Vascular lesions affecting central nervous system, i.e., cerebrovascular diseases	106.7
Accidents	53.4
Influenza and pneumonia ‡	37.5
Certain diseases of early infancy	33.3
General arteriosclerosis	19.9
Diabetes mellitus	17.2
Other diseases of circulatory system	12.9
Other bronchopulmonic diseases	12.3

Source: Adapted from U.S. Bureau of the Census. *Statistical Abstract of the United States, 1965*, p. 60.
* For method of selecting the leading causes of death, see U.S. Department of Health, Education, and Welfare, Public Health Service, *Vital Statistics of the United States, 1960*, Vol. II, Part A.
† Includes neoplasms of lymphatic and hematopoietic tissues.
‡ Except pneumonia of the newborn.

permits a higher percentage of the population to reach the age of greater risk from chronic diseases. In 1960, 59 per cent of all deaths were among persons 65 years of age and over. In that year, also, the mortality rate for the broad category of major cardiovascular-renal diseases was six times as great for persons over age 65 as it was for those between the ages of 45 and 64. In contrast to this, deaths from malignant neoplasms were not so concentrated in the older age groups. Similarly, deaths due to other chronic disease causes have become relatively more important in the younger age groups. Thus, from middle age onward, chronic diseases are the most frequent causes of deaths, but these diseases are also not insignificant at earlier ages.

Marked changes in life expectancy have accompanied these changes in mortality and causes of death. In 1900, the expectation of life at birth was about 50 years. By 1960, it approached 70 years. The rate of this gain, however, appears now to be decreasing. In 1900, the expectation of life at birth for females was greater than that of males, and the trend has been a continuing spread in this differential. Thus, longevity was two years greater for females at the turn of the century and is more than six years greater at the present time. On the other hand, the life expectancy of ethnic groups has been converging over time. In 1900, the average expectancy was almost 15 years greater for whites compared to nonwhites, whereas in 1960, this difference was only seven years.

It would be fallacious to attribute increased impact of chronic disease solely to the aging of the population. Only until 1940 was the proportion of the total population in the older age groups increasing. Past, as well as current, levels of fertility are responsible for this recent reversal of the general aging trend in the United States population. In the past two decades, there has been an *increase* in the relative proportion of persons under 20 years of age, with a corresponding *decrease* in the major wage-earning groups of 20 to 44 years. Thus, rather than observing an increase in prevalence or mortality *rates* owing to the chronic diseases, it is more likely that with the population growth, little change will occur. However, the *absolute numbers* of persons affected and disabled by chronic diseases and the numbers of deaths from these diseases will be observed to increase over the latter half of this century.

MORBIDITY ATTRIBUTED TO CHRONIC DISEASES

It is possible that the natural history of a chronic disease may involve a time scale in which there is a critical point, prior to recognizable pathologic change, when symptoms or signs of the disease could be detected.[3] Therapy which is instituted prior to this critical point is more effective than when it is instituted afterward. For most chronic diseases, the critical point would usually represent not a cure but a significant delay in the progress of a disease and a limitation on the severity of disability during the protracted period from onset to final outcome. For example, in carcinoma of the cervix, there appears to be such a critical point *after* the development of a positive diagnostic test (Pap smear) and *before* distant metastasis (spread) occurs or before the malignancy is inoperable because of local extension.

This hypothetical time scale is difficult to validate in any specific chronic disease, and the scheme may not apply in many instances. It requires the development of methods for identification of the stages of the disease and the duration at each level. Information of this type comes from several sources. These sources include chronic disease reporting by physicians, chronic disease surveys involving household interviews of a probability sample of the population, chronic disease examination surveys, industrial periodic examinations, health record surveys, and multiphasic screening procedures.

Possible Factors Influencing
Chronic Diseases

Knowledge of the natural history of many chronic diseases is very fragmented and tenuous and is under accelerated research and study. There is hope for prevention and control resulting from basic research in genetics and research on the influence of the environment as a cause or aggravation of chronic disease. Social habits and attitudes may have major influence,

such as the use of tobacco, alcohol, and drugs, as well as the stressful ac-
companiments of the competition for excellence, economic status, or superiority. The stresses of the urban environment, of increasing population
density, noise, tightly scheduled living, 60-to-80-hour "portal-to-portal" work
weeks for many persons, environmental pollutions, reduced physical and
mental recreation, and the increasing pressures of conformity are among the
many sociophysical stresses believed to have some influence on changing
patterns of disease.

Both life-span and the chronologic period of potential contribution to
society have been extended. However, for many, impairment and a dependency status drain community resources and force society to face the
ethical issues in social planning and such matters as priority for utilization
of health facilities. Prevention of chronic disease often requires the development by the *patient* of responsibility in matters such as diet or the
alteration of smoking habits, and *society's* role in prevention includes the
responsibility for broad programs such as improvement of the standard
of living, slum clearance, and occupational hygiene. The task confronting
behavioral scientists is to establish a framework through which personal
habits can be influenced, but until this level of competence is reached,
case finding and early detection are the best hope for reduction of disability and premature death from chronic diseases. No simple solution is
evident for assuring the early detection of incipient chronic disease. Periodic health examinations offer only a dim hope in this regard. Educational
campaigns directed toward the general public are needed in order that
medical attention be sought promptly before the individual becomes aware
of symptoms.

Problems in Measuring Incidence and Prevalence of Chronic Disease

The chronic diseases, with the exception of a few which are infectious
(e.g., tuberculosis), are not reportable conditions as are the communicable
diseases. Therefore, it has been difficult to establish reliable trends of incidence and prevalence. Nevertheless, several methods have been used to
establish rough estimates of the incidence and prevalence rates of some
chronic diseases in recent years. There seems to be no question of general
increase in these rates, with some identification of risks for specific age, sex,
ethnic, occupational, and other groups.

Incidence rates are conjectures in many instances and are not as useful
at this time because they require data related to onset, early signs, and
initial symptoms of disease, whereas most of the chronic diseases have an
undeterminable incubation period, variable biologic and psychologic host
response, and a delayed diagnosis. These factors also influence the validity
of surveys for determining prevalence. The prevalence of the major chronic
diseases, derived from many reports, parallels the rank order of mortality.

However, there are also other disorders of frequent occurrence which primarily interfere with normal function and social adjustment. Such conditions include peptic ulcer, arthritis and rheumatism, hernia, allergies, chronic bronchitis and sinusitis, blindness, deafness, neurologic and sensory diseases, and sundry female conditions.

Sources of Information on
Chronic Disease Morbidity

There are a few readily available sources of morbidity information on a limited number of specific chronic diseases. For example, tuberculosis case histories have been useful as an adjunct to the chronic disease control program. Also, cancer case registries have provided useful information when broadened into longitudinal studies. With the introduction of recent federal legislation providing a government-supported health insurance program for certain segments of the population, new opportunities for chronic disease reporting by physicians may be evidenced in many states.

Household Interview Surveys of Chronic Disease. Periodic household interviews have been used over the past 40 years as a means of obtaining information on chronic disease morbidity. Usually a sample is drawn wherein the family selected is representative of a large number of families in a given area. One member or more of each household is interviewed about social characteristics, illnesses, and disability of a specified severity and occurrence, and within a specified period of time. Also inherent in the methodology is the development of a structured interview with careful controls on both respondent and interviewer errors.

The Health Interview Survey, which is one of the three activities of the National Health Survey, has been in operation since 1957. Annual modifications of the questionnaire permit collection of data on a large number of topics, more topics than could be included in a single-visit interview. As shown in Table 10-2, the National Health Survey disclosed that 44 per cent of the population of all ages reported one or more chronic disease conditions in the period 1961–1963. The percentage of persons with chronic conditions increased markedly with age—up to 81 per cent of those aged 65 and over —but even in the 17-to-44 age group, about half reported at least one condition. Table 10-2 also shows the degree of severity associated with the chronic conditions reported.

Chronic Disease Examination Surveys. A health examination morbidity survey is a clinical examination of a well-defined sample of a population. This examination includes a physician-administered interview, physical examination, and review of all available laboratory results. In many situations, a physician-administered examination is repeated on the same population, thereby providing information as to the number of new cases of chronic disease which have occurred during the intervening period of time.

TABLE 10-2   Persons with Limitation of Activity Due to Chronic Conditions, by Degree of Limitation According to Age, United States, July 1961– June 1963

	Age (Years)				
	All Ages	Under 17	17–44	45–64	65 and Older
			Per Cent		
Persons with one or more chronic conditions	44.1	19.9	47.5	64.1	81.0
With no limitation of activity	31.9	17.8	39.3	43.7	32.3
With limitation, but not in major activity *	3.4	1.1	3.1	5.9	7.3
With limitation in amount or kind of major activity *	6.6	0.8	4.5	11.6	25.9
Unable to carry on major activity *	2.3	0.2	0.6	2.8	15.5
Persons with no chronic conditions	55.9	80.1	52.5	35.9	19.0

Source: Adapted from U.S. Department of Health, Education, and Welfare, Public Health Service, National Center for Health Statistics. *Chronic Conditions and Activity Limitation, United States, July 1961–June 1963* (Data from the National Health Survey). Public Health Service Publication No. 1000—Series 10, No. 17, May 1965, p. 12.
* Major activity refers to ability to work, keep house, or engage in school or preschool activities.

Multiphasic Screening Procedures. Multiphasic screening involves the administration of a battery of tests by health and medical personnel. The tests are for the purpose of detecting signs of disease, and they provide information specifying the probability that a follow-up physician examination would validate a given diagnostic condition. For example, a positive test finding on tonometry (the measurement of intraocular tension) should properly be the basis for a referral for follow-up diagnostic procedures which would lead to the final step of a physician diagnosis of, for instance, wide-angle glaucoma.[4]

Physician services are often utilized in the interpretation of suspicious findings obtained by mass-screening procedures and for performing follow-up diagnostic studies of suspects. Since the screening is done for several diseases simultaneously, the procedures can lead to the discovery of a considerable number of cases of incipient diseases which might be overlooked in routine checkups. Multiphasic screening is not a substitute for a comprehensive health examination, but it does assist in organizing an economical follow-up service.

One of the tools frequently used in household surveys which has been applied to the multiphasic screening procedure is the questionnaire. There are many difficulties inherent in the use of a screening questionnaire, as was found in the Baltimore Survey of 1953, when questionnaire information and the results of a clinical evaluation were compared. The comparison showed that very high rates of both false-positive and false-negative reports applied to the many diseases toward which the screening procedure was directed.[3] In a more recent study in Nashville, Tennessee, questionnaire response was compared with physician history, and inconsistent answers were reported in more than two thirds of the cases.[5]

One important concept in considering a screening test is that of the screening level. Whether one is dealing with a series of questions, a biochemical analysis of serum, or an interpretation of an x-ray, there should be a definition of what level of response, what concentration of a given metabolite, or what type of observation on the film will be considered as having an acceptable probability of leading to diagnostic confirmation. This defines the level of "abnormality" which is appropriate to the screening procedure and is to be considered a *"positive test."* Consideration in assigning this "positive" screening level must be based on a composite formula which estimates the over-all health value to the community of screening at each given level. This formula is composed of balancing the value of true-positives and true-negatives, as opposed to the detriment of false-positives and false-negatives. The potential for improving the health of those screened as "positive" must be considered in terms of the cost to patients' families and to the community, as well as from the standpoint of facilities existing for treatment (following the necessary diagnostic follow-up) and the physicians available for such services.

Current Status of Measuring Chronic Disease Morbidity. Of the various approaches to measuring chronic disease morbidity that have been described, none is entirely satisfactory. However, each provides useful information that will, in some sense, lead toward data relative to ultimate prevention, although at the present time, the chief utility is in early detection of disease. This entire facet of the problem has come into focus under proposed legislation entitled "Preventicare," which would set up a nationwide network of mass screening centers for adults over 50 years of age. The program has not been described in detail but probably would involve a combination of multiphasic screening procedures and periodic health examinations. Many experts are inclined to feel that it will take several decades to establish effectiveness of various methods of case detection of the multiple types of chronic diseases now under attack.

CHRONIC DISEASE PROGRAMS

Concepts of Care and Provision of Community Services

Effort directed toward the control of chronic disease and the provision of treatment facilities requires special attention to the unique characteristics of each of the diseases in this heterogeneous group. For example, a program of prevention, early detection, and treatment aimed at cerebrovascular disease must take into account all the many causes as well as all known means for restoration and improvement of function. Community services, such as a rehabilitation center, home care, visiting-nurse service, or long-term hospital care, can be organized to serve persons with all types of chronic disease, but each specific program must be tailored to the individual patient with suitable recognition of the unique characteristics of his disease. Pessimistic attitudes about many of the chronic diseases, such as cerebrovascular disease, are now giving way to more realistic expectations that many individuals with this condition can recover a substantial amount of function through intensive diagnostic and therapeutic efforts, coupled with the utilization of recent developments in physical medicine and other aspects of rehabilitation. It is now recommended that many such patients live at home rather than in hospitals or nursing homes. Rehabilitative services have been directed toward job re-employment of such impaired adults.

There is a gradual assumption of responsibility for the care of the chronically ill in general hospitals and a deceleration in the growth of separate chronic disease institutions. In many instances, the large public hospital has served as a focus for organized medical home care programs, utilizing extensive outpatient facilities and a carefully developed visiting nurse service. Many community agencies, including health departments, have participated in the development of chronic disease home care programs. In view of the relatively large proportion of the population in this country which is afflicted with chronic disease conditions, it is easily seen that one cannot isolate care of patients with long-term illnesses from the general medical care of the community. A dream, as yet unachieved, is true continuity of care wherein the general hospital conducts community-based programs which are integrated with nursing home-care programs and community agency activities to provide comprehensive care.

Comprehensive care can be viewed as a galaxy of services that can be called upon when needed. The first step in effecting such a service is the periodic re-evaluation of a patient's physical status, his psychosocial state, and the economic resources available to him and his family. A setting wherein comprehensive care is given has a full spectrum of organizational patterns. Outpatient care includes not only an outpatient department of a hospital but also programs such as the ambulatory service of a rehabilitation center and visits of chronic disease patients to their family physician in their own community.

Probably one of the most significant developments in long-term care has been the interest in the area of *continuity of care*. Many hospitals have developed services wherein the follow-up care plan was made during the course of confinement as an inpatient and extends beyond discharge as a follow-up procedure in the community. Frequently, a public health nurse in the patient's community and a medical social worker play important roles in linking the hospital staff and resources to the patient in his home. A very carefully planned discharge and periodic re-evaluation of the individual's rehabilitation status form the nucleus for this type of comprehensive service.

One obstacle to full rehabilitation is the lack of continuity in providing social and vocational service at the time and place of need. It does little good to restore a person with medical services and subsequently fail to provide him with the vocational training or the social work counseling which he needs to prepare himself for work or for a life situation suitable to his impairment. The programs of public and voluntary agencies in the health or welfare fields have benefited from the work of rehabilitation coordinators, who provide an understanding of the importance of sequence and continuity in all types of services. Medical services only form the platform from which the other rehabilitative services are launched. Significant aspects of the activities of the public health and social welfare fields are aimed at preventing the progress of disease, evaluating disability, and restoring the handicapped to optimum usefulness. A lesson learned long ago in the care and treatment of tuberculosis was the need for community planning in order to complete the rehabilitation process.

Role of the Health Department

Despite a considerable growth of activity in the area of public health concern with chronic disease control, many state and local public health departments have not undertaken an extensive program such as that recommended by the American Public Health Association.[1] Reasons for the lag include shortages of funds and personnel, opposition of local medical societies, interagency conflicts, and many others. Usually, the health officer with a direct interest in chronic diseases will find ways to circumvent this opposition. To most informed local health officers, the chronic disease field will represent a constellation of activities which extend from community surveys to early detection of disease, rehabilitation, planning for patient care (particularly for the indigent and other special groups), nursing-home supervision, and activities in mental hygiene. The local health officer frequently has assumed leadership in coordinating community facilities for rehabilitation of the handicapped in cooperation with social agencies, health councils, official vocational rehabilitation groups, and professional organizations in the community.

The health department usually cannot provide the totality of chronic disease services, but it can make its resources available in developing a comprehensive community plan. The health officer can provide tools and equipment within his own organization or persuade other agencies to do so. Moreover, he may perform a vital role by augmenting community medical efforts directed to physical restoration, laboratory tests for rehabilitation patients, bedside nursing services, mental hygiene services, re-examinations of the handicapped, and instruction of patients in self-care and maintenance. The health department can promulgate administrative regulations to provide support for programs of other groups and agencies, for example, the establishment of standards of care in various types of facilities such as nursing homes, convalescent homes, hospitals, and homes for the aged. Even a small health department can undertake many types of services for chronic conditions that might be integrated with the general community health programs.[2]

Programs of the Federal Government

Public Health Service. The Public Health Service engages in two general areas of activities in the field of chronic disease: research and training and the application of research through a variety of service programs. Several institutes of the National Institutes of Health have responsibilities for research and training activities. The *National Cancer Institute* conducts research relating to the cause, prevention, and methods of diagnosis and treatment of cancer. It also supports such research, as well as training programs, in universities, hospitals, laboratories, and other public or private nonprofit institutions. The Institute cooperates with many state and local agencies, organizations, and institutions engaged in cancer activities and collects information on cancer for dissemination through publications and other media. The *National Heart Institute* has a similar series of responsibilities with regard to diseases of the heart, lungs, and blood vessels, as does the *National Institute of Neurological Diseases and Blindness* in connection with neurologic and sensory diseases. The *National Institute of Allergy and Infectious Diseases* has responsibilities pertaining to chronic diseases with an allergic or infectious component. The *National Institute of Arthritis and Metabolic Diseases* is concerned with arthritis, rheumatism, and metabolic diseases and conducts and supports research in these and related fields. Among its activities, the Institute conducts a research and development program in the improvement of artificial kidneys and related treatment modalities for the maintenance of patients with chronic kidney failures.

Service programs of the Public Health Service related to chronic disease include the development and coordination of community health measures to remedy and alleviate problems of the chronically ill and aged and the provision of consultation on nursing-home and noninstitutional care services. The Service is also responsible for programs in particular chronic diseases such as heart disease, cancer, emphysema, diabetes, and arthritis and for the dissemination of information on the hazards of smoking. Responsibility for the conduct of chronic disease programs is vested in the newly established National Center for Chronic Disease Control within the Bureau of Disease Prevention and Environmental Control.

Vocational Rehabilitation Administration. The administration of programs to increase the vocational rehabilitation of disabled persons and their greater utilization in gainful and suitable employment is the responsibility of the Vocational Rehabilitation Administration (U.S. Department of

Health, Education, and Welfare). The basic program of vocational rehabilitation services is carried out cooperatively between the states and the
federal government. Under this program, disabled persons apply or are
referred to the state vocational rehabilitation agency to receive whatever
combination of services they require. Provision is made for medical, surgical,
hospital, and psychological services, as well as vocational and other educational training, job placement, follow-up in employment, and several other
related services. While some services may be provided directly by the state
agency, most services are obtained by purchase from physicians, hospitals,
rehabilitation centers, clinics, schools, sheltered workshops, and other
sources. The Vocational Rehabilitation Administration is responsible for
the establishment of standards in the various areas of services, for the approval of state plans and amendments, for technical and professional assistance to the states, and for various other activities. In the rehabilitation
program, federal funds are matched by state and other public funds and
under certain conditions by private sources. Under the Social Security
Amendments of 1965, specified sums have been made available from Social
Security Trust Funds to pay for the cost of providing rehabilitation services
for selected recipients of social security disability benefits. All such beneficiaries are referred to the state vocational rehabilitation agency for necessary vocational rehabilitation services.

In addition to the basic program just described, the Vocational Rehabilitation Administration is responsible for a program of training for professional personnel through training grants to public and voluntary educational
institutions and agencies and to individuals. The Administration supports
research and demonstration projects to advance knowledge of ways of overcoming handicapping conditions and to seek solutions to vocational rehabilitation problems. It is also responsible for an international rehabilitation
research program.

The Heart Disease, Cancer, and Stroke Program. As indicated in Chapter 2, one of the significant actions of the Eighty-ninth United States Congress was the passage of legislation to enable a concerted attack on the
problems of heart disease, cancer, and stroke. The legislation was based on
recommendations made in 1964 by the President's Commission on Heart
Disease, Cancer, and Stroke. In a comprehensive report, the Commission
made some 35 recommendations covering several different areas of concern.[6]

The Commission's first set of recommendations pertained to the establishment of a national network for patient care, research, and teaching in
heart disease, cancer, and stroke. Part of the network is to consist of *regional centers*—25 are recommended for heart disease, 20 for cancer, and
15 for stroke—to carry out clinical investigation, teaching, and patient care
in universities, hospitals, research institutes, and other institutions throughout the United States. Thus, the centers are to be established where possible
in conjunction with a major existing medical institution, and they are to

be staffed by specialists from the clinical disciplines and basic medical sciences that are necessary for a comprehensive attack on problems of the particular disease of concern to the center. Each center is to have both inpatient and outpatient facilities. The remainder of the national network is to consist of *diagnostic and treatment stations*—a recommended 150 for heart disease, 200 for cancer, and 100 for stroke—with 100 *rehabilitation units* to be established in association with many of the stations. In general, the stations are to provide emergency care, diagnostic facilities, and out-patient services; they would also provide consultation to physicians in the community and would develop systems of professional and public educa-tional programs. The various kinds of facilities would be created over a five-year period.

In a series of recommendations regarding the application of medical knowledge in the community, the Commission advocated a special program of incentive grants to communities to stimulate the development of a system for planning and coordinating health activities. It also recommended a number of specific supportive activities to be undertaken by the Public Health Service and the Vocational Rehabilitation Administration.

In connection with the development of new knowledge, the Commission recommended the establishment of 25 *noncategorical biomedical research institutes* at qualified institutions throughout the country, and the creation of at least 30 *specialized research centers* for intensive study of specific aspects of heart disease, cancer, and stroke in order to supplement the research and training efforts of the regional centers. Other recommenda-tions of the Commission covered the education and training of health man-power and the expansion and utilization of certain facilities and resources.

CARDIOVASCULAR-RENAL DISEASES

The cardiovascular-renal diseases consist of a broad heterogeneous group-ing of conditions primarily involving the heart and blood vessels. Table 10-3 shows the principal subdivisions of disease categories within this grouping (according to the International Statistical Classification of Dis-eases, Injuries and Causes of Death, seventh revision), and provides an indication of the relative importance of the categories in terms of death rates. The table indicates that the major cardiovascular-renal diseases are subdivided into two categories: *diseases of the cardiovascular system* (heart and blood vessels), with by far the higher death rate—about 522 per 100,000 population in 1963; and *chronic and unspecified nephritis and other renal sclerosis* (diseases of the kidney and kidney blood vessels), with a relatively low death rate—6 per 100,000 population. As a cause of death, the cardiovascular-renal diseases as a whole (keeping in mind that the far largest contribution is from cardiovascular diseases) appear to have in-creased in recent decades; this is attributable largely to the increasing percentage of older persons in the population. With regard to morbidity, the 1959–1962 Health Examination Survey of the National Health Survey showed that among adults of age 18 to 79, 13.2 per cent (an estimated 14.6 million persons) had definite cardiovascular diseases and 11.7 per cent (about 12.9 million persons) had suspected cases of these diseases.[6]

The diseases of the cardiovascular system are, in turn, subdivided into several categories, as shown in Table 10-3. The principal category, as

TABLE 10-3   Classification of Major Cardiovascular-Renal Diseases and Deaths Due to These Diseases, United States, 1963

	Death Rate per 100,000 Population
Major cardiovascular-renal diseases	527.6
Diseases of cardiovascular system	521.7
Vascular lesions affecting central nervous system, i.e., cerebrovascular diseases	106.7
Diseases of heart	375.4
Arteriosclerotic heart disease, incl. coronary disease	290.0
Rheumatic fever and chronic rheumatic heart disease	8.8
Nonrheumatic chronic endocarditis and other myocardial degeneration	29.7
Other diseases of heart	14.5
Hypertensive heart disease	32.4
Other hypertensive diseases	6.7
General arteriosclerosis	19.9
Other diseases of circulatory system	12.9
Chronic and unspecified nephritis and other renal sclerosis	6.0

Source: Adapted from U.S. Bureau of the Census. *Statistical Abstract of the United States, 1965,* p. 59.

measured by mortality, consists of *diseases of the heart*, with a death rate of about 375 per 100,000 population in 1963. Next, are the *cerebrovascular diseases* (vascular lesions affecting the central nervous system, commonly known as stroke), with a death rate of about 107 per 100,000 population. It will be recalled from Table 10-1 that diseases of the heart and cerebrovascular diseases were the first and third leading causes of death, respectively, in 1963. These two categories of diseases will be discussed in the remainder of this section.

Diseases of the Heart

Table 10-3 shows that among the various diseases of the heart, two groups are most prominent as causes of death: *arteriosclerotic heart disease, including coronary disease* (accounting for 290 deaths per 100,000 population in 1963) and *hypertensive heart disease* (about 32 deaths per 100,000 population). Rheumatic fever and chronic rheumatic heart disease account for about nine deaths per 100,000 population (Table 10-3). Table 10-4 shows the upward trend in death rates which has occurred over a 64-

TABLE 10-4   Deaths Due to Diseases
of the Heart, United
States, Selected Years

	Death Rate per 100,000 Population
1900	137.4
1905	161.9
1910	158.9
1915	163.9
1920	159.6
1925	184.8
1930	214.2
1935	245.4
1940	291.9
1945	321.5
1950	356.8
1955	356.5
1960	369.0
1963	375.4

Source: Adapted from U.S. Department of
Health, Education, and Welfare, Public Health Service. *Vital Statistics of
the United States, 1945.* Part 1 (p.
xxxii). Also, U.S. Bureau of the Census.
*Statistical Abstract of the United States,
1965,* p. 59.

year period—1900 to 1963—for all conditions that are classified as diseases
of the heart.

Arteriosclerotic Heart Disease, Including Coronary Disease. This group
of diseases includes a number of different conditions which, in one way
or another, cause narrowing or occlusion of the arteries, commonly known
as "hardening of the arteries." Certifications of death show that the number
of persons succumbing to arteriosclerotic heart disease has been increasing
in the past 15 years. White males have the highest death rates, nonwhite
males have the next highest, and women (both white and nonwhite) have
the lowest.[6] The risk of death from these diseases increases markedly with
age.

Most of the cases that are classified under arteriosclerotic heart disease
consist of *coronary heart disease.* In 1960–1962, the National Health Survey
estimated that 3.1 million adults in the United States had definite coronary
heart disease, and 2.4 million had suspected cases.[6] This disease not only
affects the elderly, but also takes a toll of many persons who are in the
prime of life.

Prevalence and incidence studies have identified several factors associated with an increased risk of developing coronary heart disease, although
(as has been pointed out in Chap. 4) such associations do not necessarily

mean that the factors cause the disease. The risk factors that have been found to be associated with coronary heart disease include an elevated serum cholesterol level, elevated blood pressure levels, cigarette smoking, and obesity. Investigations of possible social influences have shown some indication that incidence of coronary heart disease among males is related to factors such as urban background and frequent changes of residence or occupation, but such findings provide only inklings, and the role of social, psychologic, personality, and stress factors still remains to be determined. The same is true for genetic and environmental factors, although evidence regarding the influence of the environment on coronary heart disease is beginning to grow.

Prevention is a particularly urgent need in coronary heart disease because the mortality from an acute heart attack is so high (one third of those who suffer an attack die within three weeks, a large percentage of these within 48 hours), and even survivors have a shortened life expectancy. Since optimal prevention and control measures depend on knowledge of the etiology of disease, expanded research efforts in many different aspects of coronary heart disease are of primary importance. In order to provide a program for preventing disability and premature death, it is recommended that physicians assist in the early recognition of the disease and educate their patients on the risk factors. Screening efforts frequently include chest x-ray to detect enlargement of the heart, pulse check for regularity of rhythm, measurement of the blood pressure, review of symptoms referrable to cardiorespiratory function, and examination of the electrocardiographic tracing. Unfortunately, as a screening effort, these tests are not very specific. In one screening project, only 32 per cent of the persons subsequently diagnosed as normal were screened as negative. The sensitivity of any one of the tests is generally of the order of only 50 per cent.[7]

Hypertensive Heart Disease. Hypertension is the elevation of arterial blood pressure above the range encountered generally in the population. With respect to prevalence, hypertensive heart disease is the most commonly encountered specific form of heart disease. In 1960–1962, the National Health Survey estimated there were 10.5 million adults in the United States with definite hypertensive heart disease and about 4.8 million adults who had suspected cases.

Hypertension is classified as primary (essential) or as one of the many categories of secondary hypertension. It is very difficult to define a given blood pressure, which is the clear indication of hypertension in a particular individual or a population. Although an effective array of hypotensive agents exists, the cause of essential hypertension remains unclear, and there is no known cure for the condition.

Factors found to be associated with hypertension include a familial tendency, use of salt in the diet, and obesity. Elevated blood pressure levels tend to exist among people moving from rural to urban environments and among people who have experienced upward social mobility. There has been recent interest in the relationship of hypertension to ingested cadmium and hard water, but no conclusive evidence has been obtained in this regard.

The male-female mortality ratio for persons under 50 years of age has been increasing over the past two decades for hypertensive heart disease. It is noteworthy that after age 50, the female rates exceed the male rates. Hypertensive heart disease is slightly more prevalent in the female for both races, whereas definite hypertension is twice as great for Negro adults.[8] The mortality rate for nonwhites is three times that of whites. Hypertensive heart disease accounts for only about 6 per cent of all deaths due to cardiac disease, but it is prevalent in the adult population at a rate of almost 10 per cent.

Cerebrovascular Diseases

There has been an over-all secular decrease in the age-adjusted death rate due to strokes, principally as the result of a drop in mortality due to cerebral hemorrhage. Of the various kinds of strokes, cerebral hemorrhage is most intimately associated with hypertension. Other causes of stroke, such as cerebral thrombosis and embolism, probably have been increasing over the last several decades and, probably, are not so closely related to the risk factor of high blood pressure.

The prevalence of cerebrovascular disease is difficult to estimate. Household interviews suggested that three tenths of 1 per cent of the adult population noted paralysis due to stroke; a clinical study suggested over 2 per cent of adults over age 65.[9] Clearly, the age-adjusted death rates have shown a decrease in recent years for both sexes.

One of the greatest challenges in medicine today is identifying the transient cerebral ischemia (diminished blood supply) that occurs in many persons over 45 years of age. This premonitory sign of early cerebrovascular disease generally consists of repeated episodes, lasting several minutes or for as long as an hour, with weakness, visual disturbances, and, occasionally, difficulty in swallowing, confusion, and vertigo. A careful examination may reveal a decrease in carotid pulsation in the neck or a decrease in blood pressure in the ophthalmic artery, as measured by ophthalmodynamometry.

CANCER

The term cancer, or malignant neoplasms, includes a group of diseases characterized by the transformation of normal body cells into abnormally growing parasitic cells. From the standpoint of both treatment and research, cancer presents one of the most complex and difficult medical problems because of the nature of the biologic change involved and the fact that it can occur in any part of the body. Malignant neoplasms have certain biologic features in common, but they differ widely with respect to known etiology, diagnostic and treatment methods, clinical course, and curability.

The more common kinds of cancer involving various biologic systems and sites include: (1) gastrointestinal malignancy—colon, stomach, pancreas, rectum, liver, and biliary tract; (2) respiratory malignancy—lung, larynx, nasopharynx; (3) breast malignancy; (4) genital malignancy—prostate, uterus, ovary; and (5) leukemia and lymphomas. There are also many types of skin cancer, thyroid cancer, and the more uncommon malignancies of various organs in the body.

Mortality Due to Cancer

Mortality from malignant neoplasms, as shown in Table 10-5, has been increasing steadily over the past several decades, from 64 deaths per 100,000 population in 1900 to about 151 in 1963. It will be recalled from

TABLE 10-5   Deaths Due to Malignant Neoplasms, United States, Selected Years *

	Death Rate per 100,000 Population
1900	64.0
1905	73.4
1910	76.2
1915	80.7
1920	83.4
1925	92.0
1930	97.4
1935	108.2
1940	120.3
1945	134.0
1950	139.8
1955	146.5
1960	149.2
1963	151.4

Source: Adapted from U.S. Bureau of the Census. *Historical Statistics of the United States, Colonial Times to 1957.* Washington, D.C., 1960, p. 26. Also, *Statistical Abstract of the United States, 1965,* p. 59.
* Includes neoplasms of lymphatic and hematopoietic tissues.

Table 10-1 that malignant neoplasms were the second leading cause of death in 1963. Age is a prominent consideration, with the percentage of deaths due to cancer having two peaks: one peak is between 5 and 14 years of age and the other between 50 and 59 years of age.[6]

There are also differences in mortality from cancer according to sex and race as shown by Table 10-6 for the period 1930–1960. The table shows

TABLE 10-6   Deaths Due to Malignant Neoplasms, by Race and Sex (Age-Adjusted Rates), United States, Selected Years *

| | Death Rate per 100,000 Population | | | |
| | White | | Nonwhite | |
	Male	Female	Male	Female
1930	104.6	126.6	57.3	110.9
1935	110.4	128.5	67.9	117.2
1940	117.7	125.5	83.7	119.5
1945	120.7	121.1	92.1	116.6
1950	130.9	119.4	125.8	131.0
1955	138.4	114.9	145.0	129.8
1960	141.6	109.5	154.8	125.0

Source: The President's Commission on Heart Disease, Cancer and Stroke. A National Program to Conquer Heart Disease, Cancer and Stroke: Report to the President, Vol. II, p. 118.
* Includes neoplasms of lymphatic and hematopoietic tissues.

an increase in death rates for males, both white and nonwhite; a decrease for white females; and a somewhat variable pattern for nonwhite females. In 1960, mortality rates per 100,000 population from highest to lowest for these groups were as follows: nonwhite males (154.8), white males (141.6), nonwhite females (125.0), and white females (109.5).

The sexes differ according to the site of the malignancy that causes death. Table 10-7 shows that in 1962, the most frequent single site among males

TABLE 10-7   Deaths Due to Cancer of Ten Major Sites, by Sex, United States, 1962

Male	Per Cent of All Cancer Deaths	Female	Per Cent of All Cancer Deaths
Lung	23	Breast	19
Prostate	10	Colon *	13
Colon *	9	Uterus †	11
Stomach	8	Ovary ‡	6
Pancreas	6	Stomach	6
Lymphomas §	5	Pancreas	5
Leukemia	5	Lung	5
Rectum	4	Lymphomas §	5
Bladder and urethra	4	Leukemia	4
Buccal cavity and pharynx	3	Liver and biliary passages	3
Total of 10 major sites	78		76

Source: Adapted from the President's Commission on Heart Disease, Cancer and Stroke. A National Program to Conquer Heart Disease, Cancer and Stroke: Report to the President, Vol. II, p. 119.
* Excluding rectum.
† Corpus and cervix.
‡ Including fallopian tube and broad ligament.
§ Including lymphosarcoma, Hodgkin's disease, and multiple myeloma.

was the lung, accounting for 23 per cent of all cancer deaths (the mortality *rate* having increased fivefold over the past 30 years). Among females, the most common site of malignancy was the breast (19 per cent). For both males and females, neoplasms within the gastrointestinal system accounted for at least 27 per cent of the cancer deaths in 1962.

Morbidity Due to Cancer

Morbidity methods have yielded certain information about the number of new cases of cancer in this country during a given year. One estimate is that approximately one-half million new cases occur each year, and the prevalence of cases treated in one year is over three quarters of a million. With present methods of treatment, an over-all five-year survival is achieved in approximately one third of cancer cases.

This type of information does not come from the typical household survey but rather from the special type of cancer morbidity surveys performed by the Public Health Service, plus the cancer case registry data provided by several state health departments and by many large hospitals. The Public Health Service Metropolitan Center Survey in 1957 involved careful studies of physician and hospital records. Thorough canvassing of these records has yielded information about the number of new cases occurring in a given area over a specified period of time. Registry data are generally considered better for providing survival information but are more liable to underreporting problems.[10] It has been recognized that registry information which is collected in a valid and useful fashion is expensive and is not feasible for all state and local health departments.

Factors Associated with Cancer

Some oncologists believe that cancer exhibits some genetic or hereditary influence, but most studies of the natural history of the different forms of cancer indicate that the changing environment has the major influence. Familial factors have been found particularly with respect to breast cancer, wherein an incidence twice that expected occurred in members of families with breast cancer histories. The same kind of association, but to a lesser extent, has been observed with respect to stomach, colon, and cervical cancers. However, the only form of cancer with a recognized hereditary etiology is retinoblastoma, a relatively rare childhood malignancy of the retina of the eye. Thus, the search for environmental agents has been directed toward the familial and host associations which the epidemiologist has uncovered. For example, marital status has been noted to display certain patterns with respect to cancers of genital origin; this applies to both the cervix and the prostate, where the rate is higher among married people compared with single persons. For breast cancer in the female, a higher rate has been observed among single women. Early marriage seems to favor cancer of the cervix but may be a protective factor with respect to breast cancer in the female. The oncologists are attempting to untangle the riddle of these kinds of associations in terms of a specific virus, a specific carcinogenic chemical, or exposure to some physical agent, such as ionizing radiation.

Recent epidemiologic studies of Burkitt's lymphoma in Africa have pointed toward a viral etiology for this endemic malignancy. Chemical inhalants from cigarette smoke have been implicated not only in cancer of the lung, but also in cancer of the larynx, bladder, and oral cavity. There is some epidemiologic evidence that not only does cigarette smoke play a role, but also air pollution should be considered as a factor in lung cancer.[11] The epidemiologist has presented data establishing that relatively high doses of radiation can be leukemogenic. However, the isolation of each specific carcinogenic agent and laboratory validation remain formidable tasks. Traditional toxicologic methods used to identify and quantitate a chemical agent in causing a pathologic effect and the microbiologic techniques used for establishing an infectious disease etiology are not easily applied to the problem of providing laboratory confirmation of these epidemiologic inferences.

Specific problems have been encountered thus far in solving this puzzle. Many suspect environmental carcinogens do produce a similar cancerous lesion in one or more laboratory animals. However, the species variation in this carcinogenic response has been shown to be large. Moreover, the corresponding human cancer found in exposed groups cannot be distinguished pathologically from the less frequent cancer of that organ which occurs in the nonexposed population. Also, the observed frequency of induced cancer is usually low, irrespective of the dose of even a potent carcinogen or the duration of exposure. The susceptibility factors involved are not clear, but certain "cocarcinogens" or promoters have been identified in laboratory animals. The induction time (the time from exposure to onset of a lesion) is usually a matter of many years. This requires making observations on exposed groups over a long period in order to accumulate even the small expected yield and requires an adjustment in attack rate calculations to account for competing causes of death. In addition, the dose-response curve for laboratory cancer induction experiments usually is nonlinear. Radiation leukemia and radiation lung cancer probably are noteworthy exceptions to this. Some agents become carcinogenic only after metabolic alteration in the host. Since metabolic processes differ between species, and to some extent within a given species, it is difficult to quantitate exposure; e.g., the carcinogen for human "aniline dye bladder cancer" is a chemical reactant not present in the primary dye.

Cancer Detection and Prevention

Prevention of most cancers is obscure and in many cases impossible. Early diagnosis and treatment seem to influence disability and longevity for some types of cancer, whereas in many others little effect can be expected; the reasons for these differences are not understood.

Various screening centers or cancer detection centers have been established throughout the United States, and the effectiveness of screening procedure varies considerably among the types of cancer. Several surveys have been performed to establish the prevalence of "cancer-suspect" abnormalities of cells examined under the microscope. These usually relate to examination of tissue which is derived from the cervix of the female. This kind of procedure of obtaining cells representative of the lining cells of a specific organ has offered a challenge to public health to demonstrate that periodic observations can lead to early detection and significantly alter the course of the disease in various population groups. A related detection study is that of sputum cytology, which has suggested that even with a negative x-ray, positive or suspicious cells can be indicative of a marked increase in lung cancer risk.

Chest x-ray programs are another method of cancer detection. Analysis of one major chest x-ray program, involving 1,870,000 residents of a large metropolitan area, yielded approximately 3500 suspect lung cancers, from which 244 were found to be substantiated bronchiogenic carcinoma. Of these, only 24 were in the survival group indicative of cure, namely, five-year survival. A sober evaluation of these data has led to the conclusion that a chest x-ray every six months would be the absolute minimum necessary for an adequate program, and that probably for most of the population, such a program would not be suitable as a method for early detection.

In spite of a major effort in this country to encourage women to examine themselves for early lesions in their breasts, a careful evaluation of mortality experience has indicated little effectiveness of this program. A recent development which points toward some possibility of success in detection of breast cancer is that of mammography, or diagnostic x-ray of the breast, as an early screening procedure for nodules which are not palpable by either the patient or the physician.

CHRONIC METABOLIC DISEASES

Diabetes

Diabetes is a hereditary, metabolic disease resulting from malfunction of the pancreas, pituitary, or other endocrine glands. These glands are interrelated in their hormonal influence on carbohydrate metabolism. Imbalance of glandular function and metabolism not only contributes to the etiology of diabetes, but also to the long-term complicating diseases of the neurologic, cardiovascular, and other biologic systems.

One form of diabetes, diabetes mellitus, ranked eighth among the ten leading causes of death in 1963 (as shown earlier in Table 10-1). In one year, recently, diabetes caused an estimated 31,000 deaths, and it was probably a contributing factor in another 33,000 deaths. Female nonwhite mortality is considerably higher than the female white death rate, which in turn slightly exceeds the male rate for both races.[8]

It is estimated that over 3 million people in the United States have diabetes, and that approximately half of them are not aware of it. There are an estimated 70,000 new cases of diabetes per year which, in view of approximately 60,000 deaths a year, result in a net gain of 10,000 new cases annually. The diabetic has a life expectancy ranging from 6 to 20 years less than the nondiabetic, but this is not as startling a difference as it might seem when one considers that the life expectancy of a ten-year-old diabetic in 1914 was only a little more than one year. Even at the age of 50, there has been a doubling in life expectancy.[12]

Since diabetes is a metabolic disease characterized by a high blood sugar level and excretion of sugar in the urine, its etiology is clearly more hereditary than environmental. For identical twins, where one has diabetes, the frequency of diabetes in the paired sibling is about 50 per cent, whereas a fraternal twin or a nontwin sibling has a risk of about 5 to 10 per cent. However, this does not imply that factors other than heredity are unimportant. Thus, although heredity determines diabetes susceptibility in most cases, the occurrence of the disease among adults is closely correlated with obesity. It has been estimated that more than half of all diabetics sometime during their life are 20 per cent or more above average weight. If one considers that diabetes involves genetic recessive type of heredity, the occurrence of this disease in succeeding generations could at least be reduced by family counseling. The usefulness of this method, however, is mitigated by the fact that diabetes generally is not detected until the adult years.

The beta cells of the pancreas are probably involved in the etiology of most cases of diabetes, although there are some indications that the intracellular movement of insulin or the dissociation of the active hormone may be involved, rather than a simple hereditary deficiency. In some cases, it appears that antibodies to insulin are present, or that abnormalities in the destruction of insulin or the transport of sugar play a role. In certain forms of diabetes, the pancreas does not appear to be involved, but diabetogenic substances occur, which are derived from other hormonal origins.

In most instances, the control of diabetes consists of early detection, which is important because diabetics with minimal complications at the time of diagnosis have a death rate one third less than patients who are not diagnosed before they have serious complications. Short-term complications are diabetic coma and various types of infections. The long-term complications are cataract, neuritis, retinitis, and glomerulonephritis, as well as risk for coronary heart disease, cardiovascular disease, and peripheral arteriosclerosis.

The principal means for the detection of diabetes are urine tests and blood tests. About 4 per cent of the population in the United States has glucose in the urine, which is almost double the true prevalence of diabetes.

This false positivity is influenced by stress and pregnancy. Given a presence of glycosuria, it is important that a follow-up blood-sugar test be performed. The blood-sugar test usually is taken two hours after a regular meal or a glucose test meal. Approximately 140 mg of true glucose per 100 ml blood is generally accepted as the cutoff point for indication of an abnormality. The condition called "prediabetes" is defined by an absence of any abnormality of glucose level in blood or urine following the administration of a glucose test dose, but it is recognizable, however, by the occurrence of certain complications of pregnancy, such as prenatal wastage, toxemia, congenital anomalies, or large babies (over 10 lb at birth).

Screening programs frequently concentrate on members of families where a diabetic has been identified, persons who are overweight, or persons over 40 years of age. This will yield the greatest return in screening tests. Once diabetes is established by diagnosis, it becomes important that both diet and drugs be regulated. This often requires a long period of time.

The discovery and almost universal use of insulin, oral hypoglycemic agents, and nutritional management all have contributed to a significant control of diabetes during the past several decades. In many cases, medical control can be achieved without insulin. For example, weight reduction and weight control are effective in almost half of adult-onset diabetics.[12] In many cases, the oral hypoglycemic agents can be used rather than necessitating the injection of insulin. Another item of considerable importance is the re-education of the individual to control his physical and psychosocial stress. Special emphasis must be placed on long-term avoidance of infection with its associated complications. Giving detailed instructions in hygiene and diet for diabetics can be very time-consuming, and efforts have been made to organize such teachings in group classes.

Despite substantial progress, diabetes remains a major health problem in the United States, particularly for the middle- and old-age groups. The focal point of the attack must be on early detection, because management of the disease from its incipiency not only reduces disability, but also offers the hope of some restoration of pancreatic function and the obviation of long-term complications of the disease.

Obesity

Obesity is a bodily condition marked by excessive deposition and storage of fat. No scientific quantitative definition exists for this condition, either in terms of a specific method of measuring the fat or in terms of the pathogenesis of the condition. It has been demonstrated that weight and height alone are not good indicators of "fatness," and that as a practical matter one must view obesity with a composite picture of the sex, weight, age, body type, state of health, and specific measurements such as skinfold thickness.[13]

Almost all prevalence data relative to obesity are based on the height-adjusted weight, or the deviation of observed weight from a "desirable" weight estimate. Despite the inadequacy of this incomplete measure, the figures suggest that a high proportion of the population of the United States weighs more than is "desirable." Table 10-8 shows that a considerable increase in

TABLE 10-8   Persons Deviating from Best Weight, United States

	Per Cent of Persons Who Were 20 Per Cent or More Above Best Weight	
Age (Years)	Men	Women
20–29	12	12
30–39	25	25
40–49	32	40
50–59	34	46
60–69	29	45

Source: Adapted from Metropolitan Life Insurance Company, New York. Frequency of overweight and underweight. *Statist Bull Metrop Life Insur Co,* 41:4, January 1960.

overweight occurs with advancing years. Thus, the percentage of men who are overweight is fairly constant after 39 years of age, whereas women over 40 tend to be even more frequently overweight.

Since a large proportion of this overweight is due to excessive fat, one could presume to associate this prevalent condition with an increased risk to disease and increased mortality. However, an unequivocal answer to the question of obesity as a health hazard is not easily attained. There have been many large-scale studies conducted by insurance companies which seem to support the contention that obesity carries with it a high risk of heart and circulatory disease and shortened longevity, with mortality experience being apparently most unfavorable for the young, obese adult. In another study, not only was an association with mortality from all causes reported, but also an increase in death attributable specifically to diabetes, heart and circulatory diseases, and digestive diseases. This, of course, does not mean that obesity was the cause of the increased mortality, and in addition, one can question what might have been observed in an uninsured population in this regard. Moreover, there was no standardization in the method of measuring the overweight or in the reporting of causes of death in the insured population.

A study conducted by the Public Health Service in Framingham, Massachusetts, suggested that relative weight did not appear to be associated with an increased risk of developing coronary heart disease unless both hypertension and elevated serum lipids were present. Whether or not obesity is causal relative to adult-onset diabetes is controversial; however, many obese diabetics appear to benefit by a weight-reduction program.

The many psychologic disturbances frequently found in obese patients pose a special health problem. It has been suggested that psychologic processes are responsible for overeating and play a factor in maintaining the individual in his obese state. It is difficult to describe and measure this disturbance and document its implications from an epidemiologic point of view.

The past decade has witnessed a research interest in the neurophysiologic and biochemical basis for obesity. Recent twin studies have strongly suggested the existence of a hereditary factor. Also, the prevalence of obesity in children has been shown to be four times higher if one parent is obese, and eight times higher if both parents are obese. However, the fact that the nature of the diet in the United States tends to be high in calories and that there is limited exercise expenditure of these calories raises a question regarding the importance of genetic influence and highlights the difficulty of segregating hereditary factors from the environmental milieu.

It is apparent that the mechanism for regulating food intake is vulnerable to many neurologic, metabolic, and psychologic disturbances. The relative importance of each of these etiologic factors in the various types of obesity is not clear, and hence the question of disease risk remains obscure. One study seems to show clearly that obesity in childhood tends to persist into adulthood, and that the degree of overweight is directly proportional to the adult attainment. Obese children in adolescence constitute a major reservoir for obesity in adult life. As a consequence, the importance of controlling obesity in childhood has gained a significant amount of recognition.

In spite of the lack of knowledge as to the causes of obesity, prevention and treatment can be undertaken and can be strongly recommended. Obese persons have been observed to have a higher prevalence of serum lipids, fasting blood sugar, and blood pressure, all of which can be more or less reversed by a weight-reduction program. These changes accompany the psychologic benefits often reported by patients undergoing weight reduction. Until more is known about the mechanism of the early development of obesity, preventive measures will be based essentially on action to curtail food intake and increase energy expenditure. The evidence relative to the health problems and treatment failures in this method of control clearly points toward a need for early obesity prevention. Health education, particularly as part of a school health program, should include information about the caloric value of food and the caloric cost of exercise.

CHRONIC RESPIRATORY DISEASES

Chronic respiratory diseases may be subdivided into several categories as follows: (1) chronic nonspecific lung diseases, often referred to as "chronic obstructive lung diseases"—chronic bronchitis, chronic asthmatic bronchitis, and emphysema; (2) chronic lung diseases in which an infectious agent plays a prominent role—tuberculosis and several other infectious diseases affecting the lungs, such as histoplasmosis and brucellosis, which have been described in Chapter 8; (3) sensitivity diseases including recurrent acute asthma and chronic granulomatous diseases associated with sensitivity to inhalants; (4) predominantly occupational diseases in which the agent is a pneumoconiosis-producing dust or a chemical irritant; and (5) various other conditions, including diseases of the pulmonary vascular tissue and neoplasms of the lung.

This section will give particular attention to the "chronic obstructive lung diseases" and tuberculosis, which are the conditions that account for the bulk of potentially disabling lung disease. *Chronic bronchitis* is a long-continued inflammation of the bronchial tubes, often with a tendency to recurrence after stages of quiescence. It is characterized by attacks of coughing, expectoration, and secondary changes in the lungs. One of these is *chronic asthmatic bronchitis* wherein airway obstruction occurs with wheezing and episodic dyspnea in addition to coughing and expectoration. This may or may not be an allergic reaction in hypersensitive individuals. When it is an allergic reaction with or without persistent bronchitis, it is known as asthma. *Emphysema* is a pathologic enlargement or overdistention of the lung alveoli or smaller bronchioles, which may be chronic or acute, diffuse or local, of varying etiology, and which often may result in secondary changes in the lung. *Tuberculosis* is a chronic communicable disease caused by a bacterium and characterized pathologically by inflammatory infiltrations, caseation, tubercle formation, and fibrosis. Cough, fatigue, fever, weight loss, hoarseness, chest pain, and blood-stained sputum may occur, often not until advanced stages.

Basic Considerations in Chronic Respiratory Diseases

Physiology of the Respiratory System. In order to understand the chronic respiratory disease problem, it is important to review the present physiologic concepts pertaining to the respiratory system. Inspired air passes into the two main-stem bronchi, which branch out into a system of 23 major bronchi. As these tubes stretch out peripherally, the small-caliber tubes, called bronchioles, lead into tiny microscopic air sacs called alveoli. There are approximately 750 million alveoli, each of which is surrounded by a network of tiny capillaries. It is at this membrane interface that oxygen passes into the blood stream and carbon dioxide passes outward to the air sac.

In advanced obstructive disease, breathing becomes labored and a definite shortness of breath is noticed. In the bronchitic type of emphysema, a chronic cough is prominent. Usually such an individual has a long history of chronic bronchial "infections" and heavy cigarette smoking. Over a period of years his bronchial tubes have narrowed and become thickened with mucus. The unusually narrow passages tend to trap air in the lungs and put some air tension on alveolar walls, which "rupture" and become functionless. In other types of emphysema, cough is not prominent and the individual may exhibit wheezing or simply the gradual onset of increasing dyspnea.[14]

When ventilation of air in and out of the respiratory tree is impaired, the disease process is considered to be *obstructive*. Various tests for ventilation are used to detect the disease and to follow its progress. This is not to imply that the basic or initial lesion is necessarily one of ventilatory impairment. There is some evidence to support alternative interpretations; e.g., emphysema may involve a primary event of a capillary injury and minute diffusion or perfusion defects. These latter two physiologic measures pertain to the function of the alveolar membrane. Many diseases such as sarcoidosis, berylliosis, and malignant pneumoconiosis affect the alveolar membrane. It is generally agreed that a combination of all factors can contribute to the abnormal distribution of gases and gas exchange within the emphysematous lung tissue; that is, in certain alveoli good ventilation is not occurring, whereas in others the capillary perfusion function is impaired.

Many of the chronic diseases of the lung result in the appearance of some degree of fibrosis. This type of tissue is relatively inelastic and leads toward what is called a *restrictive* lung function; i.e., the vital capacity is reduced. This latter measure of pulmonary function consists of measurement of the total volume the person can force out of his lungs from deepest inspiration to maximal expiration. This predicted total volume varies in the normal individual depending on height and age. As the individual incurs progressive restrictive lung disease, whether due to specific or nonspecific pulmonary diseases, the total lung volume is distributed with a smaller vital capacity and a larger residual volume. In advanced obstructive emphysema, however, the total lung volume exhibits marked increase, the residual volume increases to greater extent, and vital capacity is thereby compromised. The hallmark of obstruction is a reduced flow rate of air on forced expiration.

Factors in Chronic Respiratory Disease. Principal *agent factors* in chronic respiratory diseases are dust and chemicals. Larger dust particles in inspired air tend to be deposited in the bronchi and bronchioles, while the smaller-sized particles affect the alveoli. A similar pattern tends to occur for other particulate matter such as organic material, including infectious agents. Chemical agents have unique effects when absorbed onto particles which are capable of reaching the bronchioles and alveoli.

There may be acute exposure to high levels of dust, chemicals, and other particulate matter which may produce an immediate reaction, or there may be long-term exposure to low concentrations of chemicals or other airborne materials which may produce insidious disease and disability. Some of the airborne materials may produce an allergic reaction, which may be acute or anaphylactic owing to hypersensitivity of the host; other reactions may be insidious, arising from long-term exposure and less positive sensitivity.

In addition to the agent factors which can produce chronic lung disease, there are host and environmental factors which determine susceptibility and modify the exposure to specific agents in the population. Examples of *host factors* are age, sex, race, genetic endowment, nutritional state, and immunologic experience. The *environmental factors* which impinge on certain individuals of the population and increase or decrease risk include: crowding, place of residence, occupation, climate, and many undefined psychosocial elements. The interaction of each of these primary or accessory factors in determining the prevalence of emphysema or chronic bronchitis has not been well studied. For example, it is well known to clinicians that atopic conditions, such as asthma, are familial, but the genetic mechanism is not clear.

Chronic Obstructive Lung Diseases

During the decade from 1950 to 1960, there occurred a dramatic change in the distribution of deaths due to respiratory diseases. The male mortality rates due to acute and chronic infectious diseases of the lungs dropped from 82 per 100,000 population to 30 per 100,000, whereas "chronic obstructive lung diseases" rose from 5 to 12 per 100,000 population. This increasing mortality ascribed to emphysema, chronic bronchitis, and chronic asthma has had its impact primarily in individuals over 50 years of age. It may also be noted that the increase largely occurred in the *adult male* population where it became a frequent cause of disability and sickness absence.[15] One might question whether the increase in frequency was related to a shift in diagnostic methods or awareness, or whether it was related to changing environmental risk factors. Whatever the explanation, in 1960 the "chronic obstructive lung diseases" had been catapulted to the foreground in public health and now challenge the tuberculosis problem in public health programming.

The Social Security Administration reported that 8 per cent (12,000) of its total cases of disability were due to chronic obstructive pulmonary diseases. The bulk of these cases during 1960 occurred in the age group 50 to 64, the same bracket where a sharply increasing mortality was noted. It is difficult to estimate the incidence or prevalence of chronic bronchitis, chronic asthmatic bronchitis, and emphysema in the general population at this time. Part of the difficulty in this estimate is the lack of a definition of early disease and a suitable yardstick to measure stages of disease.

Since the "chronic obstructive lung diseases" are the prevalent chronic respiratory diseases, a major national effort is taking shape to define their incidence, identify areas vulnerable to control, and provide for early treatment and/or rehabilitation. In some sense this challenge is shared by organizations oriented toward combating the parallel menace, lung cancer. Moreover, clinicians are making inroads in defining preventive programs for special-risk groups.

Programs to detect early "chronic obstructive lung disease" generally have utilized a questionnaire to elicit symptomatology referrable to one of the diseases and/or a spirometry test to assess the probability of *obstructive* or *restrictive* abnormality. Leadership in this area has been demonstrated by the National Tuberculosis Association and its many local associations. For example, the Tuberculosis and Health Association of Los Angeles County has launched a major project which combines mass detection with household sampling and longitudinal epidemiologic studies. Commonly referred to as the "Breathmobile Project," the new project features a mobile laboratory with electronic data-processing equipment, permitting the analysis of the mass of spirometry data by a computer. Community detection programs can be expected to expand along the lines charted by the many tuberculosis associations now pioneering in this area, particularly because of the emergence of a national concern for air pollution and the hazards of cigarette smoking.

Tuberculosis

The causative organism or infectious agent in tuberculosis is the *Mycobacterium tuberculosis* (tubercle bacillus), which begins its pathology in the alveoli. Man is primarily the reservoir, although in some areas diseased cattle are reservoirs. The source of infection is the respiratory secretions of persons with bacillary-positive pulmonary tuberculosis. The airborne route may be a frequent mode of spread; indirect contact through contaminated articles or dust is less important. The disease is communicable as long as tubercle bacilli are discharged. Prolonged household exposure to an active case usually leads to infection of contacts and frequently to active disease. What constitutes susceptibility, in terms of genetic mechanisms and specific environmental elements, remains an enigma. Certain age groups have increased tendency for infection, and others for progression of the disease following infection. Moreover, silicosis and diabetes are accepted as predisposing independent diseases.

Current Status of the Tuberculosis Problem.   Mortality from tuberculosis in the United States is given in Table 10-9, which shows a marked regular decline from about 194 deaths per 100,000 population in 1900 to a rate of about 5 per 100,000 in 1963. Many factors have undoubtedly contributed to the decline in tuberculosis mortality in the United States since 1900. These include: (1) a rise in the standard of living, including improved housing (lessened crowding and improvement in general household cleanliness), shorter working hours and lessened physical exhaustion, and better and more wholesome nutrition; (2) social legislation and social services affecting residents of urban and rural slums; (3) general improvements in community sanitation; (4) dissemination of public information regarding cause and control of tuberculosis; and (5) improvement in scientific knowledge regarding treatment of the disease.

TABLE 10-9   Deaths Due to Tuberculosis, United States, Se-
lected Years *

	Death Rate per 100,000 Population
1900	194.4
1905	179.9
1910	153.8
1915	140.1
1920	113.1
1925	84.8
1930	71.1
1935	55.1
1940	45.9
1945	39.9
1950	22.5
1955	9.1
1960	6.1
1963	4.9

Source: Adapted from U.S. Bureau of the Census. *Historical Statistics of the United
States, Colonial Times to 1957.* Washington, D.C., 1960, p. 26. Also, *Statistical Abstract of the United States, 1965,*
p. 59.
* All forms of tuberculosis.

Although the tuberculosis mortality picture has improved significantly in
the United States, it still persists as a public health problem in urban areas,
especially among the poor and among certain other high-risk groups. Mortality rates increase with age, are higher among males than females, and
are much higher in nonwhite than white groups. Although females generally have lower mortality rates from tuberculosis, they die earlier.

With regard to morbidity from tuberculosis, reported case incidence and
prevalence are declining in the United States. In 1962, the reported incidence of new cases was 29 per 100,000 population. Prevalence of pulmonary
tuberculosis is low under 20 years of age and rises with age, being highest
in males over 50. Thus, youth and early adult life are the periods when
infection is most likely to occur; adult life is the age at which the more
common forms of the *disease* manifest themselves; and old age is the period
in which the *death rate* is highest.

Although it is of considerably lesser significance in the United States
relative, for example, to several noninfectious chronic diseases, the tuberculosis problem in other parts of the world remains staggering and may account for as many as 100 deaths or more per 100,000 population per year.
In 1962, Burma and the colored population of South Africa each had a
death rate of about 75 per 100,000, and about the same time, India had a
death rate of around 61 per 100,000. Peru's death rate from tuberculosis was

about 45 per 100,000 in 1959, and Chile reported approximately 41 per 100,000 in 1964.

Prevention and Control of Tuberculosis. Adequate machinery for the control of tuberculosis consists of systems for early case detection and reporting; thorough examination of contacts and follow-up of suspects; provision of prompt, effective, and continuous medical treatment and other needed care; supervision of relapse and reinfection cases at risk; reduction of environmental and social factors which contribute to and complicate the disease; maintenance of records and data-retrieval apparatus for sequential effectiveness rating; and finally, coordination of community resources and regulatory agencies in order to ascertain responsibilities and to channel resources toward defined goals. Such goals could include the targeting of the community toward a 10 per cent decline in new active case rates over a succeeding decade.

Principal methods for the detection of tuberculosis are the tuberculin test and chest x-ray. The purpose of the *tuberculin test* is to identify individuals who have been infected with the tubercle bacillus at some time in the immediate or distant past, and the testing procedure can be easily adapted to mass screening. In many communities, a 1 per cent tuberculin-positive rate among 14-year-olds is a long-term goal to be established by periodic cross-sectional tuberculin surveys of children at various school ages. The *chest x-ray* has been discarded for most screening purposes because of its high false-positive rate and low yield of new active cases. However, it does have utility in the screening of adult populations in communities where the prevalence of tuberculosis is excessive and in the examination of certain groups at special risk of infection. Contacts of active cases, both familial and otherwise, deserve consideration as part of a community detection program.

Among the measures designed for the prevention of tuberculosis infection, *BCG vaccination* (a living culture of bovine tubercle bacilli) is to some extent effective in providing resistance. Mass vaccination has little role in areas where the risk of infection is low, but it may be used for household contacts of active cases or for special-risk groups. *Chemoprophylaxis*, consisting of the administration of isoniazid, has also been tried with promising results as a preventive measure for contacts and special-risk groups and under certain other circumstances. The most general method of prevention consists of *health education* of the public regarding the importance, mode of spread, and methods of control of tuberculosis.

Advances in the treatment of tuberculosis have occurred in connection with new drug therapy and surgical techniques. Whereas in 1900, the sanitaria were used for protracted confinement of tuberculosis patients, today the hospital stay serves as a useful introduction to drug therapy and rehabilitation. Surgical intervention is reserved principally for cases of advanced cavitation. With drug treatment, the sputum test can be expected to become negative within a period of a few months, and a chemotherapy surveillance program maintained over the next few years averts relapse. The antimicrobial drugs used in the treatment of tuberculosis are isoniazid, para-amino-salicylic acid, and streptomycin, administered for one or more years.

Certain patterns in the control and treatment of tuberculosis are now generally accepted. For the *active cases* of tuberculosis, in addition to the x-ray and sputum examinations at monthly intervals, hospitalization is advisable to initiate uninterrupted chemotherapy. Reporting of active cases to the local health authority is required in most states, and it is recommended that health departments maintain a current register of such cases. *Probable active cases* should also be hospitalized and have a complete medical work-up. For *inactive cases,* the periodic sputum examination should be done as long as chemotherapy is given, or for at least one year. For those individuals who are only *quiescent cases,* chemotherapy should be continued indefinitely and sputum examinations repeated at quarterly intervals. *Casual contacts of active cases* should be examined at least once.

SUMMARY

In the United States, and elsewhere in the world as well, the chronic diseases are becoming major scientific, medical, public health, and socioeconomic problems; they have been gaining particular attention in this country since World War II. Chronic illness is especially significant because it is likely to require long-term care and is likely to be characterized by some degree of disability. All ethnic and socioeconomic groups are affected, as well as all ages, although the greatest impact is on the older age groups.

A large majority of the deaths that occur in the United States are due to chronic diseases. In recent years in the United States, the three leading causes of death have been *diseases of the heart, malignant neoplasms,* and *cerebrovascular diseases. Diabetes,* another serious chronic disease, is the eighth leading cause of death. *Tuberculosis,* a chronic infectious disease, has been steadily declining as a cause of death, but the death rate due to *"chronic obstructive lung diseases"* (emphysema, chronic bronchitis, and chronic asthmatic bronchitis) is increasing dramatically.

Knowledge of the natural history of the chronic diseases—describing the interaction of agent, host, and environmental factors—is fragmentary in most instances. As yet there is no universal, systematic means for assembling information on the incidence and prevalence of chronic diseases; the most commonly used methods at present consist of household interview surveys, chronic-disease examination surveys, and screening programs which are sometimes of a multiphasic nature.

The general goals of chronic-disease programs include prevention, early detection of disease, prompt treatment, and rehabilitation. The provision of comprehensive care and the concept of continuity of care are also guiding principles. Although local health departments usually cannot provide the full array of services needed for full-scale chronic-disease programs, they can play a significant role in the community in stimulating and maintaining such programs. The federal government is participating in the fight against chronic disease through several of its agencies, including the Public Health Service, which conducts research, training, and service programs related to chronic disease; and the Vocational Rehabilitation Administration. Plans for the federally sponsored heart disease, cancer, and stroke program provide promise of significant accomplishments in the attack on these diseases.

REFERENCES

1. PROGRAM AREA COMMITTEE ON CHRONIC DISEASE AND REHABILITATION. *Chronic Disease and Rehabilitation—A Program Guide for State and Local Health Agencies.* The American Public Health Association, New York, 1960.

2. THE AMERICAN PUBLIC HEALTH ASSOCIATION. *Control of Chronic Diseases in Man.* The Association, New York, 1966.

3. LILIENFELD, ABRAHAM M., and GIFFORD, ALICE J., eds. *Chronic Diseases and Public Health.* The Johns Hopkins Press, Baltimore, 1966.

4. THORNER, R. M., and REMEIN, Q. R. *Principles and Procedures in the Evaluation of Screening for Disease.* Public Health Monograph No. 67 (PHS Pub. No. 846). U.S. Government Printing Office, Washington, D.C., 1961.

5. ZEIDBERG, L. D., SCHUENEMEW, J. J., HUMPHREY, P. A., and PRINDLE, R. A. Air pollution and health: general description of a study in Nashville, Tennessee. *Air Pollut Control Assoc J,* 11:289–97, June 1961.

6. THE PRESIDENT'S COMMISSION ON HEART DISEASE, CANCER AND STROKE. *A National Program to Conquer Heart Disease, Cancer and Stroke: Report to the President,* Vol. I and Vol. II. U.S. Government Printing Office, Washington, D.C., December 1964.

7. Conquering Heart Disease. *Med Clin N Amer,* 50, January 1966.

8. LERNER, MONROE, and ANDERSON, ODIN W. *Health Progress in the United States, 1900–1960.* The University of Chicago Press, Chicago, 1963.

9. U.S. DEPARTMENT OF HEALTH, EDUCATION, AND WELFARE. *Cerebrovascular Disease Epidemiology—A Workshop.* Public Health Monograph No. 76. U.S. Government Printing Office, Washington, D.C., 1966.

10. AMERICAN CANCER SOCIETY, INC., AND NATIONAL CANCER INSTITUTE, U.S. Public Health Service. *Proceedings of the Fourth National Cancer Conference (University of Minnesota, Minneapolis, September 13 to 15, 1960).* J. B. Lippincott Company, Philadelphia, 1961.

11. Medical advances in cancer. *Med Clin N Amer,* 50, May 1966.

12. Diabetes. *Med Clin N Amer,* 49, July 1965.

13. U.S. DEPARTMENT OF HEALTH, EDUCATION, AND WELFARE. *Obesity and Health—A Source Book of Current Information for Professional Health Personnel.* Public Health Service Publication No. 1485. U.S. Government Printing Office, Washington, D.C., 1966.

14. Modern management of respiratory diseases. *Med Clin N Amer,* 51, March 1967.

15. BRESLOW, LESTER. Chronic disease and disability in adults. In: Sartwell, P. E., ed. *Maxcy-Rosenau Preventive Medicine and Public Health,* 9th ed. Appleton-Century-Crofts, New York, 1965.

CHAPTER 11

MATERNAL AND CHILD HEALTH

This chapter focuses on the health of mothers, infants, and preschool children. The first section of the chapter reviews the primary reasons why the health of mothers and children is of public concern. In the second section, the principal maternal and child developmental periods are enumerated and defined; the next three sections provide a more detailed discussion of these periods, including mortality trends, major health needs, and ways of providing for the needs. Several categories of high-risk mothers and children are described in the sixth section of the chapter, followed by a discussion of the special problems and needs of handicapped children. The next section provides a brief review of some of the federal legislation which affects maternal and child health, and the section that follows gives an account of the major responsibilities of local, state, and national public and voluntary agencies. The last section of the chapter describes several important problems of mothers and children in other countries, with emphasis on those nations that are in the early stages of economic development.

PUBLIC HEALTH CONCERNS IN
MATERNAL AND CHILD HEALTH

Maternal and child health includes all efforts to promote health and prevent illness in mothers and their children. In this context, health includes physical, mental, and social well-being. The goal of these efforts is a healthy child, delivered and cared for by a healthy mother.

There are several factors which have played a role in making maternal and child health a matter of public health concern. First, childbearing women and growing infants and children are, in general, the more dependent members of a society. As a society evolves, there is a trend toward greater concern for these dependent members, and public efforts develop in their behalf. Second, there is the economic significance of childbearing and rearing to the future of any civilization. Some community activity to ensure healthy arrival in the production of its members is essential to the maintenance of the society's future. A third reason stems from the fact that at the turn of the century, deaths of mothers and children were major contributors to mortality in every community in the United States. Approximately 60 mothers died for every 10,000 pregnancies which produced liveborn infants. Out of every 1000 of these liveborn infants, 100 babies did not survive their first year of life. Improving community health, which is the primary purpose of public health, meant preventing the diseases that led to maternal and infant deaths. Thus, maternal and child health became, and continues to be, a major focus of public health attention. The fourth reason for the role of public health in maternal and child health is the ever-increasing complexity of organizing and meeting the high cost of the services necessary to provide the best solution for many of the health problems of mothers and their children. Only through organized community efforts can the necessary services be made available to all citizens who are in need.

The size of the population affected by maternal and child health activities is large, although it varies somewhat from community to community and from country to country. At the present time in the United States, children from birth through 14 years of age constitute 31 per cent of the total population, and women in the childbearing years from age 15 through 44 constitute an additional 20 per cent of the population.[1] Thus, maternal and child health programs potentially affect half of the nation's population. Obviously not every mother and child receives direct services from public programs. However, the well-being of mothers and children is significantly influenced by the recommendations and standards established by public maternal and child health programs throughout the nation.

From the monetary standpoint, maternal and child health programs in the United States constitute one of the largest segments of ongoing public health programs. In New York City in 1963, for example, maternal and child health was the largest single item in the budget. Clearly, maternal and child health is of major importance to any community from the point of view of both the number of persons affected and the amount of money involved.

PRINCIPAL DEVELOPMENTAL PERIODS

For descriptive purposes, the development of mothers, infants, and young children may be divided into several periods. These developmental periods are enumerated and defined below and are presented schematically in Figure 11-1.

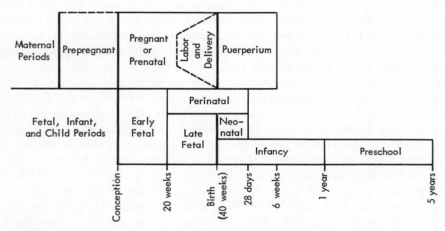

FIGURE 11-1. Principal developmental periods of the maternal, infant, and preschool years.

The maternal periods include the following:

Prepregnant: all nonpregnant time during the mother's reproductive years;
Pregnant or Prenatal: from conception until the delivery of all products of conception, including the placenta;
Labor and Delivery: that portion of the prenatal period from the beginning of true labor until the delivery of all products of conception including the placenta;
Puerperium: the six weeks following delivery.

The periods related to infants and children include:

Fetal: from conception until delivery—
    Early: from conception through the twentieth week,
    Late: from the twentieth week to delivery;
Neonatal: from birth through 28 days of life—
    Early: from birth through the first seven days of life,
    Late: from the eighth day of life through the twenty-eighth day;

Perinatal: from the twentieth week after conception through the first 28
days after birth, thus combining the late fetal and neonatal periods;
Infancy: from birth to the first birthday;
Preschool: from the first birthday to the fifth birthday.

It is important to keep in mind that while developmental periods are
convenient descriptive devices, they are artificial. Growth and development
are continuous processes which proceed at all times, rather than in a series
of arbitrary periods.

MATERNAL HEALTH

Maternal Mortality

The primary vital statistic which public health has traditionally used to
follow the degree of health of pregnant women has been the maternal mortality rate. This rate is defined as follows:

$$\frac{\begin{array}{c}\text{All mothers dying}\\ \text{while pregnant}\end{array} + \begin{array}{c}\text{all women dying within 90 days of}\\ \text{having delivered an infant}\end{array}}{\text{All live births}} \times 10,000.$$

The numerator is considered to include all women who die from causes
related to the pregnant state. While the denominator is actually a measure
of birth, it will, at least in theory, include most women who have been pregnant. The resulting fraction is multiplied by 10,000 because in recent years
in the United States, the maternal mortality rate has fallen to less than 1 per
1000 and it is desirable to have the statistic expressed in a whole number.

From Figure 11-2, it is apparent that between 1922 and 1935, the maternal
mortality rate in the United States was fairly stable at about 60 per 10,000
live births among white mothers and 100 per 10,000 in the nonwhite group.
By the 1960's, this figure had dropped to approximately 3.3 per 10,000 in
the white group and 13 per 10,000 in the nonwhite group. Thus, while
there has been a twentyfold decrease in the mortality of white mothers,
there has been only a fivefold decrease in the mortality of nonwhite mothers.
In addition to this racial variation, there is also considerable variation from
state to state and from urban to rural areas. It is now felt by many that a
maternal mortality of two deaths per 10,000 live births is not an unreasonable goal for all population groups throughout the nation.

The most direct causes of maternal deaths include toxemia of pregnancy
(a poorly understood condition which includes swelling, elevated blood
pressure, and protein in the urine), as well as hemorrhage, abortion, death
due to anesthesia, and sepsis (infection of the blood stream). Approximately
three quarters of these deaths are judged to have been avoidable and thus
can be considered to be the result of inadequate quality or quantity of
maternal care.

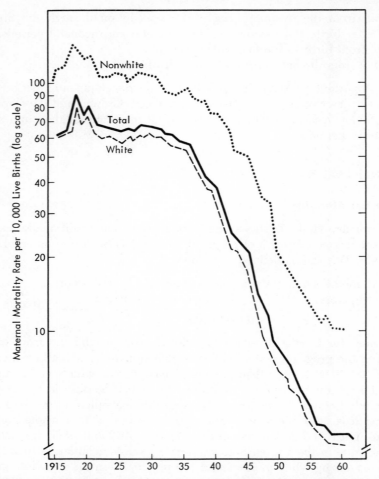

FIGURE 11-2. Maternal mortality by color, United States birth registration area, 1915–1963. (Source: Adapted from National Center for Health Statistics, Public Health Service, U.S. Department of Health, Education, and Welfare. *Vital Statistics of the United States,* 1965.)

In the various states in this country, maternal mortality committees investigate the causes of maternal deaths. These committees consist of experts in all fields germane to maternal health and are usually appointed by state departments of public health. The committees carefully investigate in detail the events surrounding each maternal death reported in their state. This investigation includes a survey of all the records of each case and an interview with all the individuals involved with the case. The committee then submits a report summarizing the events surrounding the death and includes a judgment as to whether or not the death was avoidable.

Prepregnancy Period

Whether or not a woman will survive a pregnancy and provide an adequate environment for the growing child depends to an enormous extent on her health prior to and at the time of conception. Any chronic disease in the mother which alters her normal physiologic homeostasis can profoundly affect both the mother's health and that of the developing child.

Good mental health is also essential for a satisfactory pregnancy. Pregnancy may be a time of stress for the mother, both psychologically and physiologically. If the mother enters pregnancy with any serious emotional problems, these may become exaggerated. Sometimes, however, the opposite may occur: on occasion, an emotionally unstable woman will have fewer adjustment problems during pregnancy.

Closely intertwined with the mental health of the mother is the quality of her social environment. While a marriage certificate prior to the onset of pregnancy does not in any way guarantee a better pregnancy, a stable social environment for the mother is very important during pregnancy. The value of emotional support during this period cannot be overestimated. The important consideration is not that the mother meet any arbitrary social standards of marriage or family constellation, but rather that she be comfortable and happy with her social environment and receive support from others during the pregnancy.

Because all the above factors have become increasingly recognized as being important to the outcome of pregnancy, a new field known as preventive obstetrics is developing. The purpose of preventive obstetrics is to ensure that physical, emotional, and social factors are as satisfactory as possible prior to the onset of pregnancy. Thus, a woman who has reached childbearing age or who has recently married will receive a careful history and physical examination to discover any health problem which might increase her risk during pregnancy. Any problems which are identified are corrected to the maximum possible extent prior to conception so that conditions during pregnancy may be optimal. Family planning is, of course, an important part of preventive obstetrics so that the children will be wanted and the pregnancy will occur when desired and when conditions are optimal for the outcome.

Pregnancy Period and Prenatal Care

Purpose and Nature of Prenatal Care. Pregnancy involves profound physiologic and biochemical changes in the mother. Therefore, it is essential to diagnose pregnancy as soon as possible in order that health supervision can be provided which will assure maintenance of good maternal health and will help to minimize the chance of pregnancy wastage. The phrase "pregnancy wastage" has been coined in recent years to refer to unfavorable results of pregnancy with regard to the fetus or infant. This includes the entire spectrum from fetal and infant death through all degrees of sub-lethal damage which can cause lifelong handicapping conditions such as cerebral palsy, mental retardation, or congenital malformations. While at present a definitive diagnosis of pregnancy is not usually possible before approximately 10 to 12 weeks after conception, there are new chemical tests on the horizon which show great promise of making detection possible within the first several weeks.

Proper health supervision during pregnancy, or prenatal care, is now accepted as an important part of public health. There are several essential phases of prenatal care. At the first prenatal visit, which should be as early in pregnancy as possible, a complete medical history is taken and a complete physical examination is performed. Laboratory examinations always include blood-typing of the mother, a serologic test for syphilis, a hemo-globin test, and a routine urinalysis. Advice and guidance are given at this time on such matters as desirable activities and exercise, nutrition, and danger signals to watch for; emotional support is also provided. Subsequent visits are usually monthly through the sixth month of pregnancy, every other week through the seventh and eighth months, and weekly during the ninth month of pregnancy. At each of these visits, a brief physical examina-tion is done which includes assessment of fetal growth and development, determination of blood pressure, and urinalysis; advice and guidance con-tinue to be offered. Because much of the advice and guidance are common to all pregnant women, it has become frequent practice for this information to be given in group classes.

In most parts of the United States, prenatal care is provided by private physicians. Nearly all counties, however, also provide public prenatal clinics for those who cannot afford this service privately. These public prenatal clinics may be administered through a county hospital or through the health department. The quality of medical care provided by the professional staff in public clinics is in general quite high.

Obstacles to Providing Prenatal Care to the Individual. In spite of the availability of good prenatal care, large numbers of women are known to go through all or much of their pregnancy without such care. There are a number of reasons for this. Since prenatal care is primarily preventive in nature, the pregnant mother must present herself for this care when she may not feel ill in any way. While the value of preventive health care is understood by many people in the United States, there are still large groups of individuals who would never consider going to a doctor unless they felt sick. Hence, for a number of women, going for a checkup during pregnancy when they feel fine is unthought of. While health education would help overcome this negligence, it is difficult to locate these women so that the health education may be applied. There is no system in the United States, as there is in many countries, for ensuring the case finding of new pregnancies in the population. At the present time, the only system is for public health nurses to be observant while working in the districts they serve. When an expectant mother is discovered, the nurse can explain the value of care and make an appropriate referral. Unfortunately, many expectant mothers go undiscovered.

Even if a pregnant woman is persuaded to attend a prenatal clinic for the first time, she may not maintain the desired schedule of subsequent visits. The rate of broken appointments is high in clinics for a number of reasons, including long waiting periods, long distances to travel, and often lack of provision for the care of children at home.

Another obstacle in providing public prenatal care to the individual is that large numbers of pregnant women may find themselves ineligible for such care, while at the same time they cannot afford the optimal amount of private care. Many counties have eligibility requirements for county health care, which may include one or two years of residency in the county or the establishment of financial need through a means test that may be too stringent.

Other Problems in the Provision of Prenatal Care. In the provision of public prenatal care in the United States, the mother often receives care in a clinic far removed from the hospital where she will deliver her child. One disadvantage of this arrangement is that it is often difficult to get her prenatal records to the hospital in time for her delivery. It also frequently means that she will see one physician for prenatal visits and subsequently will be delivered by a different physician. This, of course, has psychological as well as medical disadvantages.

The shortage of trained personnel in the United States is also a significant problem in providing prenatal health care. Even if all pregnant women should present themselves early in pregnancy for prenatal care either to private physicians or to public clinics, it would be impossible for these women to be cared for adequately. At present, there are not enough obstetricians, general practitioners, or clinics; and even with the rapidly growing number of medical schools it will be a long time before there are enough physicians to provide a sufficient quantity of prenatal care.

Other nations, such as England and the Scandinavian countries, have at least partly solved the problem of the personnel shortage through the use of nurse obstetric assistants (nurse midwives). After the prenatal patient has been examined on the first visit by the physician, she is placed in a high-risk or low-risk category depending on her medical history. If she is unlikely to have any complications, she is considered low risk and may be followed on subsequent visits by a nurse obstetric assistant and subsequently may even be delivered by this assistant. The high-risk pregnancy and any mother followed by nurse midwives who develops complications are referred to the physicians for follow-up and delivery.

There has been considerable resistance in the United States to the use of nurse obstetric assistants in spite of the fact that several of the major medical centers in the country, including Johns Hopkins University and Columbia University, train such individuals. The fear is that these individuals may not be sufficiently trained for some of the unanticipated complications of pregnancy and delivery. Such fears are unfounded when one considers the training and qualifications of these assistants. They have all received at least two years of training and experience in midwifery beyond their regular nurses' training. There is no doubt that these nurses start off with much more experience in the management of pregnancy and delivery than the average general practitioner who enters practice after his internship. There are serious variations in the quality of prenatal care and delivery care provided in this country, and most professional persons who have studied the feasibility of nurse midwifery agree that the use of such nurses could only improve the quality of services.

Labor and Delivery Period

While pregnancy lasts nine months, labor and delivery usually last less than 24 hours. This 24-hour period is, however, by far the most critical time for the health and survival of both the mother and the infant. The physiologic stresses on both these individuals are high.

The risks for the mother at this time include hemorrhage, complications of anesthesia, and the introduction of infectious agents into her uterus. Because of such risks there has been a trend in the United States over the past 50 years toward more and more deliveries to be performed in the hospitals. In 1964, 97.5 per cent of the deliveries in the United States occurred in a hospital.[1] Hospital delivery has the advantage of having all facilities to handle sudden problems as they arise during these critical hours. It has the disadvantage of having the mother out of the familiar surroundings of her home and the familiar comforts of her family. In England, where there is a serious shortage of hospital beds, a system has been devised whereby all low-risk mothers with uncomplicated pregnancies may be delivered at home by nurse obstetric assistants. There is always available, on immediate call, an ambulance from the nearest hospital which contains all the necessary equipment for any obstetric emergencies.

Obviously the fact of being in the hospital does not in itself guarantee good supervision of labor and delivery. For example, the mother may be delivered by a hospital staff nurse because the busy physician did not arrive in time, or the baby may be held back until the physician can arrive. In order to correct and forestall these and other unsatisfactory procedures, many cities, counties, and states have developed standards of hospital practice of obstetrics. In New York City, for example, a team of experts from the health department surveys the hospital charts and studies the practices in the labor rooms, delivery rooms, and newborn nurseries before any hospital can receive a license. Many private hospitals have their own appointed committees to conduct a similar surveillance of practices. It is difficult, however, for one physician in a private hospital to criticize a fellow physician in the same hospital. For this reason, there are distinct advantages in having an independent, outside agency such as the health department provide such surveillance. It is also beneficial to be able to use licensing as a means of ensuring good practices.

Puerperium Period

The puerperium is a period of important physiologic and psychologic readjustment for the mother. Because of the shortage of hospital beds and because of the importance of early ambulation, most mothers are now discharged from the hospital within three days of delivery. In some busy county hospitals they may be discharged within 24 hours of delivery. A subsequent checkup by a physician (postpartum checkup) thus becomes a very important procedure. Again, however, this is primarily a preventive measure, and large groups of women will not return for such checkups. Public health nurse follow-up of recently discharged new mothers is of considerable help in getting these women back to their doctors.

Abortion

The medical definition of abortion is any interruption of pregnancy during the first half of the pregnancy. There are two types of abortions, spontaneous (commonly called "miscarriage") and induced. Spontaneous abortion will be discussed in a later section of this chapter dealing with the "early fetal period."

Induced abortions are divided into legal and illegal. Most states in the United States have laws which allow physicians to interrupt pregnancy legally for certain health reasons. These reasons vary from state to state, but in general they pertain to health considerations which would endanger the life of the expectant mother, such as serious heart disease. Some of the laws also allow physicians to interrupt pregnancy if there is an extremely high risk of a malformed infant, as in the case of a mother who contracts rubella (German measles) very early in pregnancy.

The major health problem, however, is not the legally induced abortions but the illegal procedures. There is absolutely no way of knowing what the incidence of such illegally induced abortions is in the United States today, but it is thought to be extremely high. Estimates run between 6 and 12 per cent of all pregnancies. As has already been mentioned, abortion is listed as one of the major causes of maternal mortality, and in almost every case, this is an illegally induced abortion. Illegal abortions are very frequently self-induced or performed by a nonmedical person using techniques or agents which are extremely dangerous. Furthermore, a large but unknown number of attempted illegal abortions which fail undoubtedly damage the progress of the pregnancy and result in a deformed child. This is particularly likely when drugs or chemicals are used. Not to be underestimated also is the emotional trauma which the mother must suffer for having performed an illegal act. Because of these problems, there are many medical and public health people who feel strongly that provisions for legal abortion should be broadened. There are several countries where this has been done, and the experience of these nations needs be given serious consideration in an effort to find guidelines which will lead to prevention of needless deaths of a large number of women in the United States.

FETAL AND PERINATAL HEALTH

In addition to having effects on the mother, pregnancy, of course, also has effects on the developing child. The normal nine-month pregnancy is actually 40 weeks long. For research and statistical purposes, these 40 weeks are usually divided into two equal periods. The first 20 weeks is the period of early fetal development and takes place before the developing child is capable of survival outside the uterine environment. The second 20 weeks, the late fetal period, is the time when a child is, at least theoretically, capable of surviving in the outside world.

The problems of the late fetal period and those of the first 28 days after birth (the neonatal period) are intertwined inexorably. Any attempt to study these problems must include both periods in order to be meaningful. It is for this reason that the concept of the perinatal period has been developed, which, it will be recalled from an earlier section, combines the late fetal and the neonatal periods.

Early Fetal Period

Information about the health needs and problems of the fetus during the first 20 weeks of gestation is still very limited. Even the number of deaths which occur during this period can only be estimated. Only a few states require the reporting of a fetal death prior to 20 weeks of gestation, and even in these states the reporting of such deaths is very poor. Many pregnant women will miss one or two menstrual periods and then spontaneously abort ("miscarry") a very small fetus without even realizing they have been pregnant. Many early fetal deaths may be the result of illegal interruption of pregnancy and, of course, will not be reported. It is estimated that more than 10 per cent of all human pregnancies spontaneously abort prior to 20 weeks of gestation. Many investigators feel spontaneous abortion represents nature's way of taking care of imperfectly formed fetuses. Eastman,[2] however, believes that a significant proportion of the women are aborting unnecessarily. This group includes mothers who have a characteristic tendency to lose their pregnancy spontaneously in the early weeks. Many authorities believe that such women could and should be amenable to preventive obstetrics.

Factors which influence early fetal development are very poorly understood. The fetus and the inside of the uterus where it is developing (the intrauterine environment), while only a few inches from the outside world, have, until recently, been unavailable for scientific study. Attempts to enter this environment, even in experimental animals, have so profoundly altered it as to make any findings of questionable significance. Newer research tools and methods are now beginning to solve some of the technical problems, and before long many of the mysteries of this period of life will no doubt be solved.

It is known that the first 20 weeks is the critical period in the development of all major organ systems of the body. This is the period when insults such as infections, drugs, or an adverse environment may cause congenital malformations or even fetal death. The discovery of the relationship between an undesirable outcome of pregnancy and German measles infection in early pregnancy, or thalidimide taken in these early weeks, has brought widespread attention to such problems. There has also been a great deal of discovery recently in the area of the genetic causes of congenital abnormalities, but it is still not possible to state whether the genetic components of the developing fetus or the intrauterine environmental factors are more important in the production of defects. It is perhaps most likely that there is an interaction between the environment (including infectious agents and drugs) and the genetic components which determines the development of many congenital abnormalities. As more is learned about genetics, the fetus, and the intrauterine environment, it will be possible to prevent some of this pregnancy wastage.

Perinatal Period

The perinatal period is one of great importance with respect to the survival and future well-being of the child. During the last weeks of pregnancy, the fetus becomes capable of independent existence outside the uterus, and during the first weeks after birth numerous complex changes necessary for physiologic independence take place.

Perinatal Mortality. The risk of death is greater during the perinatal period than at any other time until after age 60. Perinatal mortality is defined as death after 20 weeks of gestation but prior to delivery ("stillbirth"), plus death in the first 28 days of life. To determine a perinatal mortality rate, this figure is used as the numerator; the denominator consists of all infants at risk and therefore includes all live births plus all stillbirths. Thus, the perinatal mortality rate is computed as follows:

$$\frac{\text{Deaths after 20 weeks' gestation} + \text{deaths in the first 28 days of life}}{\text{Stillbirths} + \text{live births}} \times 1000.$$

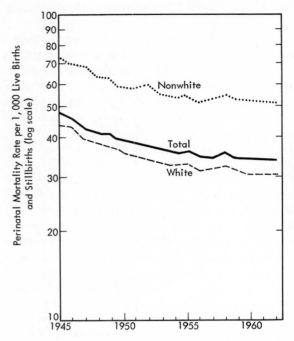

FIGURE 11-3. Perinatal mortality rates by color, United States, 1945–1962. (Source: Adapted from National Center for Health Statistics, Public Health Service, U.S. Department of Health, Education, and Welfare. *Infant and Perinatal Mortality in the United States.* Series 3, No. 4, 1965.)

Figure 11-3 shows perinatal mortality trends in the United States for the period 1945 through 1962. A rapid decline occurred in the total perinatal mortality rate until 1956, when it began to level off. Thus, there were 47.2 deaths per 1000 live and stillbirths in 1945 compared to 35.6 deaths in 1955, with only a very slight further reduction to 33.7 deaths in 1962. The nonwhite perinatal mortality rate has consistently exceeded the white rate, as shown in Figure 11-3; in 1962, there were 51.4 and 30.4 deaths per 1000 live and stillbirths in the nonwhite and white groups, respectively.

The single most common *cause of death before birth* is anoxia, or lack of oxygen. Anoxia is usually related to a cutoff of the supply of oxygen from the mother's blood by a too early separation of the placenta from the uterus, but sometimes it is the result of pressure on the umbilical cord. Another common cause of stillbirths is toxemia in the mother. A similar increased incidence of sudden death of the fetus late in pregnancy is found in diabetic mothers. When all known causes of stillbirths are added together, there are still from one quarter to one third which remain unexplained.

The most common *cause of death during the first seven days after birth* is "prematurity," which accounts for somewhere between one quarter and one third of these deaths. The next most common cause is asphyxia, or lack of oxygen, which accounts for approximately one quarter of the deaths. Asphyxia is usually secondary to some disease of the lungs or the part of the brain which controls respiration. The other two major causes of neonatal mortality are birth injuries, which are estimated to cause approximately 15 per cent of the deaths, and congenital malformations, which cause approximately another 15 per cent.

Premature or Low-Birth-Weight Infants. Many authorities agree that little headway will be made in the reduction of perinatal mortality until something can be done about prematurity. The problem with prematurity is that it is a phenomenon and not a specific disease. It is also difficult to define. Ideally, prematurity would mean an infant born too early. However, there are as yet no reliable means of determining the gestational age (age from conception) of an infant at birth and therefore no reliable means of determining the length of pregnancy. Since body weight in general increases with increasing length of pregnancy, and since this measurement is easily obtained internationally, the World Health Assembly defined prematurity in 1948 as an infant weighing less than 2500 gm (5 lb, 8 oz). This definition was not totally satisfactory because birth weight *normally* varies with sex of the infant, with race, and from place to place. Thus, girls have average birth weights lower than boys, and nonwhite infants tend to be smaller than white. Birth weight also declines as land altitude rises.

More recent investigation has suggested that there may be at least two separate subgroups among infants under 2500 gm. Infants with birth weights between 1500 and 2500 gm in general have a much lower mortality rate and seem to have much less difficulty in later life. It is this group which is associated with the sex, race, and geographic factors just mentioned. On the other hand, infants weighing less than 1500 gm at birth may represent a different phenomenon. Seventy-five to eighty per cent of these infants die in the first week of life, while only 10 to 15 per cent of the larger babies succumb. In addition, longitudinal follow-up studies have demonstrated conclusively that even if the smaller infants survive the neonatal period, they carry a definitely increased risk of mental retardation, neurologic handicaps, eye defects, and other medical problems. Recent studies have also indicated that perhaps a significant number of the smaller infants may not have had as short a gestation as their weight would indicate, but rather are so-called "small-for-dates" infants. By this is meant that their birth weight is smaller than one would expect for the calculated length of their gestation. It is hypothesized that this growth retardation is part of a pathologic process which is associated with the increased risk these infants have been shown to have.

Because of the studies demonstrating the discrepancy between birth weight and length of gestation, the World Health Organization in 1961 changed the term applied to infants weighing less than 2500 gm at birth from "premature" to infants of "low birth weight." Regardless of the term used, however, the fact still remains that a child whose birth weight is significantly below 2500 gm is at considerably greater risk than a larger infant.

The incidence of low birth weight in a given population varies with a wide number of factors. One of the most important factors is socioeconomic status. As socioeconomic status declines, the rate of low birth weight rises and, secondarily of course, the perinatal mortality rate also rises. In addition, the incidence of low birth weight increases with the following factors: multiple birth, young mothers (under 16), older mothers (over 35), first pregnancy, fifth or greater pregnancy, smoking by the mother, illegitimacy, history of previous premature delivery by the mother, and poor prenatal care. At the present time, the over-all incidence in the United States of infants with birth weights below 2500 gm is approximately 7 per cent. Much more study is needed to understand both the physiologic and the sociologic factors involved in early delivery and low birth weight if this proportion is to be lowered.

Prevention of Perinatal Mortality. The need for improved programs to combat perinatal mortality is indicated by the magnitude of the prevailing death rates. Many studies have shown a high correlation between perinatal mortality and the provision of quality prenatal care. An epidemiologic study of perinatal mortality in England [3] demonstrated that it was possible to identify situations rather early in pregnancy where the risk of perinatal mortality was extremely high. When such identification was made, special, more intensive care could be provided for this high-risk group. The results of such studies have led to recent legislation in the United States which provides federal funds to support special programs to identifying high-risk mothers and to offer them the necessary intensive prenatal care.

Another group of programs directed toward the prevention of perinatal mortality are those which attempt to improve the quality of care during labor and delivery. The maternal mortality committees assist in this effort by pointing to the failures and attempting to identify the mistakes so that they may be rectified in the future. Many health departments are also involved in surveillance of standards of care in obstetric and newborn units in hospitals, both public and private.

Programs directed toward the management of recognized high-risk newborn infants also prevent perinatal mortality. For example, the medical management of the very small low-weight infant is a highly technical task. Because of this, many "premature" centers have been set up in larger municipalities where such high-risk infants may be transferred shortly after birth for intensive care. Some of these centers, with the support of public health funds, have provided special training programs for physicians and nurses from outlying hospitals to improve the management of similar infants in these hospitals. Equally important has been the role of public health nurses in the follow-up of the high-risk newborn infants. Many health departments have developed systems whereby any infant who is considered in the high-risk group is identified by the hospital, and the name of the infant is forwarded to the health department. The public health nurse then visits the home prior to the infant's discharge from the hospital to assist the family in preparing for the care of the baby. The public health nurse thereafter continues to make home visits frequently to help in the management of the infant and also to assure that the infant is returning for proper medical care.

Serious problems remain in providing an optimal program for the prevention of perinatal mortality. A major concern is the previously discussed large group of mothers who do not present themselves for prenatal care and who do not present their infants after birth for proper medical prevention and treatment. In addition to the problem of properly motivating the individual to seek preventive health care, another problem in providing such programs is to erase all roadblocks in the path of the individual seeking such care. When the individual has not sought prenatal care, the finger of blame should not simply be pointed at the individual, but rather, consideration should be given to how the program could be modified or changed so that the individual would be more likely to seek proper care.

INFANT AND PRESCHOOL HEALTH

Infancy, it will be recalled from an earlier section of this chapter, is defined as the period of life from birth to the first birthday; the preschool period extends from the first to the fifth birthday. Infancy is a time of particularly rapid rate of growth and development. At birth, many organs have yet to reach their maximum efficiency in carrying out their essential physiologic and biochemical functions. By the end of the first year, these organ functions have matured considerably. In addition, numerous outwardly visible evidences of physical and psychologic growth and development occur in infancy and continue throughout the preschool period.

Infant and Preschool Mortality

The infant mortality rate is the number of liveborn babies under one year of age who die during a calendar year, per 1000 live births during the same time period. The method of computation and the general utility of this rate have been described in Chapter 3. Figure 11-4 shows a reasonably steady decline in the infant mortality rate in the United States over a 48-year period, from about 100 infant deaths for every 1000 live births in 1915 to 25.3 deaths in 1962. However, there has been a leveling off of the downward trend since 1950. Most of the long-range decline in the infant mortality rate has been due to the control of infectious diseases through a combination of improved environmental control, immunization, and antibiotics. In view of these medical accomplishments and the generally high standard of living in the United States, it might appear that the infant mortality rates which have prevailed over the last several years reflect a biologic lower limit precluding further significant improvement. However, when comparisons are made with other nations of similar economic and social development, the error of this conclusion is apparent. Thus, as shown by Table

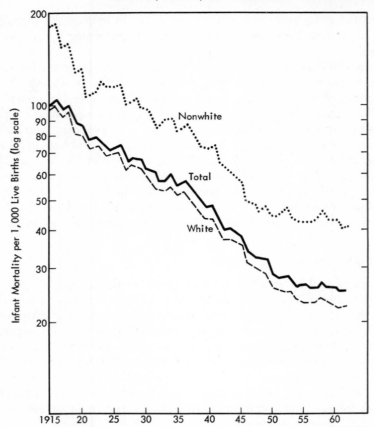

FIGURE 11-4. Infant mortality by color, United States birth registration area, 1915–1962. (Source: Adapted from National Center for Health Statistics, Public Health Service, U.S. Department of Health, Education, and Welfare. *Infant and Perinatal Mortality in the United States*. Series 3, No. 4, 1965.)

11-1, the United States had the highest infant mortality rate among a list of ten nations during the period 1959 through 1961. Three of the nations had fewer than 19 infant deaths per 1000 live births.

Excessive deaths among the nonwhite infants in the United States are a major source of the higher over-all infant mortality rate. Figure 11-4 indicates that, although nonwhite infant mortality has dropped over the years, it still remains at about 40 deaths per 1000 live births. White infant mortality fell below that point about 25 years ago. Numerous workers in the field believe this racial differential to be the result of socioeconomic factors rather than due to biologic differences. Poverty is no doubt one of the nation's major maternal and child health problems. It should not be assumed, however, that infant mortality in the United States is entirely the result of the unfortunate socioeconomic status of the nonwhite population. By 1962, only two states had reported white infant mortality rates of less than 20 per

TABLE 11-1   Infant Mortality, Selected Countries, 1959–1961

	Infant Mortality per 1000 Live Births
Sweden	16.3
Netherlands	17.7
Norway	18.5
Australia	20.4
Switzerland	21.4
Finland	21.8
Denmark	21.9
United Kingdom	22.6
New Zealand	23.1
United States	25.9

Source: Hunt, E. P., and Goldstein, S. M. *Trends in Infant and Childhood Mortality, 1961.* Welfare Administration, U.S. Department of Health, Education, and Welfare. Children's Bureau Statistical Series No. 76, 1964.

1000 live births: Delaware with 19.8, and Utah with 19.4.[4] Thus, even if the status of the nonwhite population were on a par with that of the white population, further improvement in conditions affecting all mothers and children, white and nonwhite alike, would still be needed in order to match the accomplishments of certain other nations in the world.

Risk of death among infants declines with age, the most critical period being the first month of life. In 1961, 71 per cent of infant deaths had occurred before these babies were one month old,[4] and hence the problems and causes of death are those previously discussed in connection with the perinatal period. For the infant who survives the first 28 days of life, congenital malformations continue to take their toll, and environmental hazards become more prominent; first, infectious diseases and later, as mobility improves, accidents become the major cause of mortality.

After a child has reached his first birthday, the risk of death drops sharply to about 4 per cent of what it was in the first year. At present, one child out of every 1000 in the preschool age group dies each year in the United States. This represents a striking improvement over the rate of about 20 deaths per 1000 at the turn of the century. Similar to the downward trend in infant mortality, the decline in deaths of the one-to-four-year age group is due primarily to the control of infectious diseases through environmental sanitation, immunization, and antibiotics. The mortality rate of nonwhite children during the preschool years continues to be about twice that of white children, or about two deaths per 1000 nonwhite children of preschool age.

Accidents are the number-one enemy of today's preschooler, accounting for 30 per cent of the deaths between one and four years of age. The percentage distribution of causes of accidental deaths for one-to-four-year-olds in 1959 is given in Table 11-2. It is also important to keep in mind that for

TABLE 11-2 Percentage of Accidental Deaths by Cause, Preschool-Age Children, United States, 1959

	Per Cent
Motor vehicles	31 *
Burns	23
Drowning	14
Poison	9
Falls	6
Suffocation	5
Firearms	2
Others	10

Source: Adapted from National Office of Vital Statistics, Public Health Service, U.S. Department of Health, Education, and Welfare. *Accident Fatalities: United States and Each State.* Vital Statistics, Special Reports, Vol. 54, No. 8, 1961.
* In half of the cases, the child was struck by a motor vehicle.

every accidental death, there are several hundred nonlethal events, many of which cause lifelong disability. The remaining 70 per cent of preschool deaths are divided primarily among pneumonia and influenza, malignant neoplasms, congenital malformation, diarrhea, and tuberculosis in decreasing order of frequency.

Health Needs of the Infant and Preschool Child

Infant and preschool years are a time of building foundations which will provide good support for a long, productive, and enjoyable life. Because of the very rapid rate of physical and psychologic growth and development, insults which might be minor at a later stage in life may cause lifetime deviations from normal when they occur in these early years. Basic health needs can be divided into three groups: environmental, physical, and emotional.

Environmental Health Needs. The child's environment should be comfortable, clean, and safe. The water, milk, and food supply must be free of harmful toxins or infectious agents. Disease-carrying insects must be excluded. Accident hazards need to be removed or controlled in accord with the ability of the infant and child, in order to prevent the much too frequent tragedy of accidental death or permanent disability. This is of major importance for preschoolers.

From age one through four years, children are very active and develop greatly in their gross motor abilities. These motor abilities of the preschool child far exceed his understanding of the possible injuries which may result from his actions. While a child needs to have some exposure to hazards in order to learn how to protect himself, the environment must be somewhat modified to match the combination of his developmental stage and the amount of supervision which can be provided. Some hazards can be partly controlled by laws, but the most significant measure for the prevention of childhood accidents is for those responsible for supervision of young children to understand the basic principles of growth and development and thereby anticipate what can be expected at various age levels.

Physical Health Needs. Physical needs include being kept reasonably clean and appropriately dressed. Nutrition must be adequate for good physical growth. Children's teeth should have attention during preschool years. Preventive dental appointments should begin at about two years, or earlier if any pathology is suspected. Fluoride has been shown to be a significant deterrent to the development of dental caries. In areas where the water supply is considered low in fluoride (less than 1 ppm), dental problems can be avoided by topical applications of fluoride at regular intervals during the preschool and school years or by use of daily supplemental fluoride.

Immunization is another of the physical needs of the infant and preschool child. It should be started as early as the infant's immune mechanism can respond. Currently this is considered to be about two months of age. At the present stage of medical achievement in immunology, diphtheria, tetanus, poliomyelitis, smallpox, and measles (rubeola) can probably be eliminated as causes of morbidity and mortality. Whooping cough (pertussis) vaccine, while quite helpful, is less effective than the other agents. This should not, however, detract from its regular utilization, since whooping cough is a deadly disease in the young infant. With the rapid developments in immunology, it is likely that further improvements will be made in this agent. Current research reports also indicate that other contagious diseases of childhood (chickenpox, mumps, German measles, etc.) will soon be on the list of health problems which can be eliminated through immunization. With regard to a recommended immunizing schedule, it should be noted that because of increase in knowledge and available agents, routines are in a state of change at this time. It is therefore advisable to obtain current recommendations from a knowledgeable source such as a health department, the American Medical Association, the American Public Health Association, or the American Academy of Pediatrics.

Regular physical examinations to detect any deviations from normal as soon as possible are also among the physical health needs of infants and preschool children. Medical science does not yet offer primary prevention for many conditions, but much can be done to lower mortality and morbidity if appropriate treatment is begun before serious and irreversible damage has taken place. The tuberculin skin test is now considered one of the essential tools of the infant health evaluation. This initial test is done at about one year of age and repeated at yearly intervals thereafter. With increasing knowledge about the biochemical defects of certain metabolic diseases, laboratory tests for their early detection are becoming available. Prominent in this group is the disease phenylketonuria (PKU), a cause of mental retardation which can be diagnosed with urine and blood tests. The effects of this condition can be lessened with appropriate dietary restriction begun in early infancy. Public interest in phenylketonuria has recently reached a high enough level in many states to bring about the passage of laws requiring laboratory tests on all infants. It would seem likely that eventually a battery of laboratory tests may be required for early detection of other diseases caused by biochemical defects.

Emotional Health Needs. The emotional needs of the developing child are of major importance to his future well-being. Parental love of an unselfish and undemanding nature will help develop trust and confidence in the world and its people. Some regularity of surroundings and responses is necessary in order that security can be created through predictability, yet there must be enough variation to meet the need for diversity and thus help to avoid the development of an excessively rigid personality. Inadequate human contact and stimulation may result in disturbed behavior, a failure to thrive, and even death. It is not necessarily the presence of the infant's biologic mother that is important, but rather the fact that he receives "mothering" kinds of attention such as cuddling, being played with, and being talked to.

Secure, happy children are also those who have reasonable and consistent limits set throughout their lives. By expectations being established appropriate to their developmental ability, children are gradually able to internalize the limits and to develop a self-control which provides the security of knowing what to do and when to do it. The development of this self-control begins in infancy. Parents often need help in understanding that discipline is an important expression of love. They need guidance in learning what can be expected at certain developmental stages and often firm direction in being consistent in their demands. Helping parents learn what can be expected of their infant and child in growth and development has come to be known as anticipatory guidance.

Well-Child Supervision

Physical evaluations including an assessment of development, immunizations, dietary advice, and anticipatory guidance are best provided together in programs of well-child supervision. Such supervision begins in the hospital during the newborn period. It is recommended that an infant be seen at monthly intervals thereafter for the first six months, bimonthly for the next six months, every three or four months in the second year of life, and every six months until school age.[5]

Well-child supervision is most frequently provided by a private physician, commonly a general practitioner. Unfortunately, many families cannot afford to have their children cared for privately. For such children, the community usually provides well-child clinics. At the present time, health departments are the main, though not exclusive, provider of public, well-child supervision. In some communities, clinics are sponsored by voluntary organizations such as service clubs or churches, which provide funds for equipment and salaries and a convenient place for holding a clinic at regular intervals. The Visiting Nurses Association is another organization which is very active in providing well-child clinics.

Child health supervision provided in the clinics has certain advantages over privately provided care. The emphasis of the clinics is prevention, and clinic personnel are usually quite enthusiastic about this aspect of child health care. The clinic facility is also usually staffed by a physician, one or two public health nurses, a registered nurse, a social worker, and one or more volunteers. Some arrangement for consultation with various medical specialists is also provided. Through the public health nurse, the service may even extend into the home. This team approach offers a broad kind of service which is difficult to provide in private practice. In general, well-child clinics provide one of the best examples which public health has to offer of primary preventive medicine.

Public well-child supervision is, however, far from ideal. There are frequently problems concerning which children should be eligible. Some people feel financial screening should be carried out. Those who disagree believe that such screening would discourage a significant number of families from coming even though they would not be able to afford the service elsewhere. These critics of financial screening argue that if healthy children are for the good of the entire community, then the community should give every encouragement to have all the children seen.

With the increasing population since World War II, providing services for all those requesting them has become more and more difficult. Public agencies are always short of funds, but even if there were unlimited financial resources for establishing more clinics, the shortage of medical personnel would still be a problem. These financial and personnel problems have resulted in many clinics across the nation limiting their service to infants and children under two years of age in spite of the recommended visit every six months thereafter throughout the preschool years. Even when this age limit is set, clinics remain crowded, and there is not sufficient time to give a thorough evaluation. A visit very often lasts less than five minutes. Counseling of a mother is frequently impossible.

A number of suggestions regarding better use of available funds and personnel in public well-child clinics have been made in the past few years. Siegel and Bryson describe a demonstration clinic where public health nurses have been given considerably more responsibility. Infants and mothers were seen by the public health nurse, only, for four out of seven visits during their first year and five out of ten visits during their preschool years. A physician saw the baby at 1, 6, and 12 months, and at every other visit thereafter unless the nurse felt consultation was necessary.[6]

Another solution to relieve some of the patient load problem has been to develop high-risk infant clinics. Infants with suspicious factors in their early fetal, perinatal, or family history receive special, more intensive well-child supervision. Such an approach enables the more skilled but scarce personnel to focus on a smaller group which has a relatively greater need for health surveillance. A number of health departments in the United States have opened such clinics in recent months.

Another deficiency of public well-child supervision is the lack of dental care for preschool children. Provisions for dental care are a rare luxury offered by only a small percentage of well-child clinics. In 1958, the National Health Survey reported that the most common physical defect of school-age children was dental caries, and that 50 per cent of the children under 15 years of age had never been to a dentist.[7] Widespread provision of good preventive dental care beginning in the preschool years would assist significantly in controlling dental pathology.

The artificial separation of well-child care from sick-child care is probably the major weakness of clinic supervision. If an abnormality is found, the child must be referred elsewhere for treatment. Obtaining health services from a variety of resources is unsatisfying for both the provider and the recipient. In order to improve the continuity of care, several solutions have been proposed. Some clinics have affiliated with approved hospital pediatric services in order to provide a more direct referral system. Community health centers, which are being developed in some low-income areas, offer a full range of outpatient services. Another method has been for the health department to discontinue all well-child services and, instead, to pay for private care for all lower-income children. A public health nurse is assigned to the families and works with the private physician just as she would with a clinic physician. A social worker may also be utilized. While this solution has many attractive possibilities for providing comprehensive and continuous care, the current shortage and uneven distribution of physicians makes it impractical as a plan for all communities. At present each community must take stock of its own needs and resources and develop a design for comprehensive care within its own limits.

HIGH-RISK MOTHERS AND CHILDREN

There are several groups of mothers and children who are at especially great risk for having health problems. High-risk mothers also include those with an increased risk of pregnancy wastage.

Mothers of Particular Ages and Parity or with Abnormal Medical Histories

Women under 16 and over 35, women having their first child, and women having their sixth or greater child have been shown definitely to have an increased risk for their own health and for the health of the developing child during pregnancy. All such women should receive special attention and careful supervision of the progress of their pregnancy. Furthermore, any mother who has a history of previous pregnancy failure is at higher risk of having a succeeding pregnancy failure. A woman with such a history needs to be identified early in pregnancy and followed closely.

Mothers and Children of Low Socioeconomic Status

There is no doubt that women in the lowest socioeconomic groups are at high risk both for death and for having complications which lead to pregnancy wastage. Earlier in this chapter it was noted that maternal mortality in the United States was four times higher among nonwhite mothers than among white mothers. It is generally agreed that this is due to a socioeconomic rather than a racial difference. Low socioeconomic status offers, also, many obstacles to the infant and the young child. Both mortality and morbidity are higher among children of lower-income families. Some means must be found for providing more comprehensive and well-coordinated health care for mothers and children from low-income families.

Unwed Mothers and Their Children

In 1963, there were 259,400 babies born in the United States who were reported on their birth certificates as being born out of wedlock. Of these babies, 10,200 were born to mothers younger than 20 years of age, with 5400 younger than 15 years of age.[8] There is no doubt that these figures are minimum estimates; even so, the total represents a marked increase over 20 years ago, when about 100,000 infants were reported to be born out of wedlock.

These unwed and frequently very young mothers have more health problems but receive less prenatal care. Social customs and sometimes regulations in prenatal clinics discourage unwed mothers from seeking health care during pregnancy. For example, some prenatal clinics require that any girl under 18 years attending the clinic must be accompanied by her mother. On the other hand, some health departments are developing new and imaginative programs to provide for the special needs of unwed mothers. Thus, the school district and the health department of Los Angeles jointly sponsor a program for pregnant teenage girls, which provides instruction in child care and other aspects of health, in addition to the regular school curriculum. There are also many homes run by voluntary agencies and religious groups throughout the country where unmarried mothers may live during their pregnancy and receive both regular prenatal care and health education. There is still, however, an urgent need for many more programs, if the problems of this high-risk group are to be met.

Infants born out of wedlock have numerous difficulties to face in all spheres of their growth and developmental needs. A study conducted over a five-year period in New York City showed that infant mortality among illegitimate births was about twice that of legitimately born infants, 48.2 and 23.9 per 1000 live births, respectively.[9] Special attention must be provided for these illegitimate infants if they are to have an equal chance for a healthy life.

Working Mothers and Their Children

There is still some question as to whether or not a woman who must work during pregnancy is a high-risk mother. Everyone agrees, however, that if a woman is working during pregnancy and has an additional health problem, she should be relieved from work. In the United States, there are frequently many factors to discourage such a woman from seeking relief from employment. Foremost, of course, is the loss of income for the family. In addition, she may risk loss of seniority or even loss of the job itself. These considerations may deter an employed woman from seeking prenatal care for fear that a problem will be discovered and the doctor will insist that she stop working. Such fears are unfortunate because there is general agreement that working mothers urgently need prenatal care to determine whether or not they have a health problem for which work may be detrimental.

In 1964, there were 12.3 million children under 14 years of age whose mothers were employed full time or part time for 27 weeks or more. Of these children, 3.8 million were less than six years of age and 1.6 million were less than three years old.[10] The mere fact that a mother works is not necessarily harmful to a child. What is of vital concern is the arrangement made for child care while the mother is away. There is a real need for more and better arrangements. Most states have laws governing standards, inspection, and licensing of larger child care facilities. The responsibility for seeing that the requirements are met is most commonly given to the welfare department, with the health department providing for sanitary inspections, only. Meeting the legal standards of the state and providing for the total growth and developmental needs of a child are not necessarily synonymous. In addition, a great many children are cared for in situations which do not come under public jurisdiction. For example, there may be a neighbor who takes five or six local infants or children into her home every day. The environment may be crowded, unsanitary, unsafe, and inadequately supervised, but the enterprise is not large enough to be subject to existing laws. There is considerable urging from both child welfare workers and child health workers for closer and more cooperative action to bring better day-care services to all children in need.

Mothers and Children in Migrant Families

In 1960, the United States census indicated that there were 400,000 to 500,000 domestic migrant workers. These people are one of the most underprivileged groups in the nation. They have all the problems of low socioeconomic status plus the very significant added difficulties of separation from relatives, isolation from community life and resources, lack of legal residence status, and no protection by minimum wage laws and unemployment insurance.

Mothers in the migrant labor group are an extremely high-risk group. In addition to being low-income mothers, they are often ineligible for prenatal care because they do not live in one place long enough to establish residency. They also frequently work throughout their entire pregnancy whether or not they have additional health problems.

Approximately 300,000 children belong to migrant families. They are often malnourished and anemic, have severe dental problems, are plagued with intestinal parasites, and have frequent skin, respiratory, and gastrointestinal infections. Also, because father, mother, and older siblings may all work, young children and even infants may be left unsupervised for many hours of the day. Newer federal legislation is focusing some health care attention on the need of migrant families, but a great deal more is required.

Infants with Congenital Abnormalities

Infants with known cogenital abnormalities suffer from three major groups of problems. The first group of problems consist of the handicaps, impairments, or limitations that arise from the particular abnormality. The second results from the difficulties which parents and others responsible for day-to-day care have in providing for the child's normal emotional needs. Thus, the infant with a known abnormality may not receive enough essential loving care or may be so excessively responded to that he is never allowed to develop any independence. The third problem area is that of medical care. While the particular malformation may be well treated, the care is often so highly specialized that the over-all needs of the infant are totally neglected. All too frequently such infants progress through their entire first year without well-child supervision and reach their first birthday or even later with no immunization, with nutritional deficiences, and with a firm start toward lifetime behavior problems. Infants with congenital abnormalities should be included among those attending special clinics for high-risk infants.

The Child of Abusive Parents

The child of abusive parents has come to be known as the battered child. This problem has recently been brought to public attention as a significant cause of disability and death in children. The child is commonly under three years of age and too young to give any explanations for his multiple bruises, swellings, and recent and old fractures. Frequently, though not always, there is also evidence of general neglect, malnutrition, and poor hygiene.

Laws against child abuse exist in all states, but the situation must come to the attention of proper authorities before any legal action can be taken. Since most of the battering episodes do not occur in public, they are seldom reported. It is not uncommon, however, for the child to be brought to a clinic or hospital for treatment of the most recent injury. Parents usually attribute the injuries to accidents or place the blame on baby-sitters or siblings. Many medical personnel have found it difficult to believe that a parent could be responsible for the injuries to his own child and have tended to accept whatever story was provided. Others, who may have been suspicious, have been afraid of becoming liable in some way if they interfere.

Public concern for the abused child increased so greatly that in 1963 the Children's Bureau and the American Humane Association prepared model laws which would make reporting of suspect cases by a physician mandatory, but would at the same time protect against civil or criminal liability. By the first part of 1966, all except three states had passed such laws. Reporting of a case does not mean immediate court action will be taken, but only that a careful investigation by trained child welfare workers will be carried out. If the suspicions are found to be true, steps are taken to protect the child and to help the family, if possible.

HANDICAPPED CHILDREN

Definition and Prevalence

A handicapped child has been defined by the American Public Health Association as any child who "cannot within limits play, learn, work or do other things children of his own age can do." He is a child who "is hindered in achieving his full physical, mental and social potentialities." [11] This functional definition is extremely broad and can include numerous diagnostic categories from mild emotional disturbances to completely incapacitating, multiple congenital malformation. One group of handicapped children, namely, the mentally retarded, has been discussed in Chapter 6.

The number of children in the United States with problems falling within the broad definition of handicapped is unknown. One estimate comes from the National Health Survey, which reported in 1961 that there were 1,120,-000 children under 17 years of age who were limited in normal activity owing to chronic conditions (conditions lasting more than three months). Fifty-two per cent of these were able to go to school but were limited in other ways; 36 per cent were limited to certain types of school or in the amount of attendance; and 12 per cent were not able to go to school at all.[7] Other estimates in the current literature based on numbers of children with specific diagnoses report much higher figures ranging from 10 to 20 per cent of the United States population under 21 years of age, or 8 to 16 million children.

Complexities of Health Care

Modern medical and educational advances offer a handicapped child a far better opportunity to develop his full potentialities than he has ever had in the past. Many previously handicapping conditions have been nearly eliminated through preventive and early treatment measures. Diseases such as poliomyelitis, tuberculosis and other infections of the bone, and rickets due to vitamin D deficiency are rarely seen today. Surgery, medication, special appliances, and a variety of therapy techniques can now decrease the crippling effect of many other conditions. The care must begin early and be comprehensive and well-coordinated in order to get the best results. It involves the skills of a multidisciplinary team of highly trained medical and paramedical specialists.

Many conditions require care throughout childhood, and for some it must continue throughout life. A small percentage of handicapped children are able to receive care through private arrangements, but the cost of such long-term care is far beyond the means of most American families. Only through organized community effort and tax support is it possible to provide this complex care for all children who need it. While the cost to the nation runs in the millions of dollars every year ($62,344,000.00 for crippled children programs in 1960), it must be remembered that early diagnosis and comprehensive treatment will help a large number of children become partly or completely self-supporting adult citizens rather than welfare recipients.[12]

Crippled Children's Programs

Community interest in the needs of handicapped children in the United States began early in the twentieth century with small voluntary agencies. While a few were created to help all handicapped children regardless of their diagnosis (such as the National Society for Crippled Children and Adults), most were categorical in approach. They offered broad services but only for a single disease category such as blindness. There were a few local efforts supported by tax funds, but for the most part the handicapped child and his family received sympathy and little else until the Social Security Act was passed in 1935. Federal funds through grant-in-aid programs were appropriated at that time to help states to locate and provide services for crippled children (under 21 years of age) and those with conditions leading to crippling, as well as to support research and demonstration projects. This federal support has been continued over the years. The Children's Bureau was given and continues to have the administrative responsibility for reviewing and approving funding of all state proposals and for providing consultation to the states. The number of children accepted for care and served in crippled children's programs has risen sharply over the 30 years since it began. Beginning with slightly over 100,000 in 1937, the total number to receive service in 1963 was 396,184.[13] However, if the estimates given previously of the number of handicapped children are anywhere near correct, a large number of children are being cared for in some other fashion, or not at all. The latter is probably the case for many.

Administrative methods, services, and eligibility requirements of crippled children's programs vary from state to state. Administration can be through any designated state agency. Health, welfare, education, universities, and specially created agencies are all represented among the programs. All programs, of course, have some kind of arrangement for diagnostic services, hospitalization, and the provision of required appliances and any special therapy recommended. While eligibility requirements are somewhat different in each state, in general they include the condition and its treatment outlook, the estimated length of care and cost, the family income and family size in relation to income, and family resources and obligations. Diagnostic services are offered regardless of financial status. Only after a diagnosis is made is it possible to determine if the condition would be sufficiently aided by treatment, how long it would take, and what the cost would be. If a child is either medically or financially ineligible, the family will be referred to a private-care source.

Problems of Medical Eligibility

The definition of medical eligibility continues to be a problem. Even though the federal legislation did not limit the definition of a crippling condition, states found it financially necessary to take a narrower view because they were not able to meet the costs of serving all children with handicapping conditions as they have been defined by the American Public Health Association. Priorities had to be set, and these were generally determined on the basis of whether a particular condition could be significantly corrected. The approach was categorical from the very outset. In view of the available medical skills in 1935, it is understandable that the orthopedic conditions rated first place on the lists. As medical knowledge and skill have increased, other chronic diseases have become significantly responsive to treatment. Many children who would have succumbed quickly to their diseases in 1935 are now being saved. To maintain or develop to their fullest potential, these children require the same complex, long-term, multidisciplinary approach as needed by children with orthopedic problems, blindness, or hearing difficulties. The costs are equally high and impossible for most families to handle.

Under public pressure, the lists of eligible conditions have grown and come to include some of these other chronic conditions, but still remain far too limited and categorical in most states. In addition to ignoring the similarity of needs which all children with any long-term, complicated conditions have in common, the categorical approach tends to place primary emphasis on the disease rather than on the child. Every effort is usually made in crippled children's programs to focus on the total needs of the whole child no matter what his diagnosis may be, but the very fact that he has been accepted for care because he has this particular condition rather than some other gives the condition a special emphasis of its own.

The 1965 amendments to the Social Security Act have given major recognition to the need for wider medical eligibility. Appropriations for crippled children's services were increased in order to help states to extend these services to areas not already served and to broaden their definition of crippling to include any kind of handicapping condition or long-term illness. It is hoped that eventually, definitions and services will be uniform from state to state so that no child will be deprived of the best possible care simply because of what he has or where he lives.

Educational and Other Needs

Education for the handicapped child is as important as any other part of his care. Magnificent medical care will be of little significance if his intellectual ability is not helped to reach its fullest potential. Various educational arrangements have been developed throughout the nation depending on particular community needs and resources. Whatever educational resources are used, it is essential to have close cooperation and coordination in planning among all agencies concerned—educational institutions, crippled children's services, and any other organizations which may be involved.

One of the major problems for those concerned with the health of the crippled child is his long-range future. Even though he may need the services for many years to come, he is usually no longer eligible for school after 18, and crippled children's services end when a child becomes 21. Various federal, state, and local assistance programs such as Aid to the Totally and Permanently Disabled provide cash benefits and some services. Vocational rehabilitation offers some help in job training, but only if the predicted potential for gainful activity is fairly high. Medical care, if it cannot be afforded privately, is provided by public hospitals or clinics. All in all, the care is neither comprehensive nor well coordinated. There have been recent amendments to the Social Security Act which are anticipated by many as providing a solution at least to the lack of continuing comprehensive medical care. Additional solutions must be found for the continuing educational needs.

Another unsolved problem is that of long-term custodial care for the more severely handicapped. Because of the advances in medical care, many children are now living beyond an age when it is possible for their families to continue to provide the physical care which is necessary. At the present time, except for a few wealthier families who can afford to send their handicapped member to one of the private-care centers or to hire someone to live in and help, the only resources are institutions for the retarded or public nursing homes for the elderly. Neither are appropriate for many of these handicapped people who are neither retarded nor old.

FEDERAL LEGISLATION AFFECTING MATERNAL AND CHILD HEALTH

The support offered by the United States government for the improvement of maternal and child health is the result of congressional legislative action since the turn of the century. The Maternity and Infancy Act (Sheppard-Towner) of 1921 established the national policy of federal-state cooperation to assure better health for all mothers and children. Federal funds were appropriated to help states through grants-in-aid to improve their maternal and child health services. The responsibility for the administration of these funds was placed with the Children's Bureau. The act was allowed to die in 1929, and even though the funds had been primarily for demonstration projects rather than for support of permanent programs, the states definitely felt the loss.

The Social Security Act

The Social Security Act of 1935 renewed the precedent which had been established by the Sheppard-Towner Act and authorized Congress to appropriate funds to help states improve their maternal and child health services, crippled children's services, and child welfare services. Through the years, both the appropriations and the kind of activities supported have increased. Some of the changes regarding the crippled children's programs have already been mentioned. In addition, funds are now available for projects to provide special services for high-risk mothers and infants and for comprehensive health care programs for low-income preschool and school-age children. Matching funds have also been provided to help develop better day-care services under child welfare grants.

In addition to the provisions which directly affect the health of mothers and children, the Social Security Act also has provided benefits through the various categorical programs which were discussed in Chapter 5 in connection with public assistance medical care. Thus, the provision of federal matching funds have helped states develop programs to aid low-income families that have dependent children, as well as to assist aged, blind, and disabled persons. The latter programs either help handicapped children directly when they reach age 18, or indirectly assist children who are dependent on disabled or elderly persons. A 1965 amendment to the Social Security Act, as also described in Chapter 5, overcomes a number of the deficits which have characterized these categorical programs in the past, by consolidating the programs and expanding the care provided.

The Vaccination Assistance Act

The Vaccination Assistance Act was passed in 1962 and amended in 1965. The Act provides special funds to states and—with state approval—to local communities in order to cover a portion of the cost of an intensive vaccination program against poliomyelitis, diphtheria, whooping cough, tetanus, measles, and any other diseases considered to be major public health problems. The primary age group to receive attention has been the oft-neglected preschooler.

The Migrant Health Act

In 1962, the health problems of migrant workers received the attention of Congress, and funds were appropriated to assist state, local, and nonprofit agencies to develop ways of improving the health conditions of workers and their families. Money was made available on a grant-in-aid basis for setting up and operating clinics, developing special demonstration projects, and training necessary personnel. The resulting programs have in no sense solved the health problems of these citizens, but they are a major step in the right direction.

The Economic Opportunity Act

It has been estimated that one fourth of the 4 million children entering school each year come from families in poverty circumstances. These children have commonly received minimal intellectual stimulation, and they begin school in the lower third of their class. Poor adjustment is common, academic failure follows, and school dropout is nearly inevitable. Health, education, and welfare workers have for many years recognized the vital importance of breaking this chain of events, but it was not until Congress passed the Economic Opportunity Act of 1964 that sufficient funds became available to plan and carry out a significant attack. Included in the Act was an appropriation for preschool programs for children from economically deprived families. These programs became known as "Operation Head Start."

A proposal for a Head-Start program must include plans for preschool educational activities, social service to the families of the children, parent involvement in the daily activities of the program, and arrangements for health examination and follow-up care. The health care has been one of the more difficult parts to provide in an adequate and coordinated fashion. In spite of all of the problems, however, the Head-Start program, after only the first summer of activity (1965), demonstrated it had enormous potential worthy of all the funds and effort it requires.

ADMINISTRATION OF SERVICES FOR MOTHERS
AND CHILDREN IN THE UNITED STATES

The provision of health services by the community for mothers and children is the result of a network of activities carried on by local, state, and national public and voluntary agencies. City or county health departments, as well as hospitals, provide many of the primary services such as prenatal and well-child clinics. Crippled children's programs may fall within health department supervision or be administered by some other local agency such as a welfare department or an independent crippled children's agency. The quality and quantity of all services provided at present still vary considerably from place to place throughout the nation. It is hoped that the results of research on new methods of providing services, in combination with the recent increased financial aid made available under the Social Security amendments, will soon make existing inequalities a part of the past.

State health departments provide some direct service in the more rural areas, but for the most part their role is to administer funds, establish and maintain standards, consult with local agencies about current and future programs, provide professional educational activities and publications, and act as a central coordinating agency throughout the state and with neighboring states.

At the federal level, the Children's Bureau is the primary agency with interest in maternal and child health. The formation of the Children's Bureau by an act of Congress in 1912 marked the beginning of federal programs which aid mothers and children in the United States. The Bureau was established to investigate and report to Congress on all matters relating to the welfare of children in order that federal legislative action could be directed where it was most needed. As new laws were passed and old ones amended, the Bureau was given increasing responsibility for the actual administration of governmental appropriations, as well as continuing its investigative and reporting functions. In general, the Children's Bureau gathers information, provides consultation, and supervises the distribution of a number of funds allocated in the form of grants-in-aid for helping the states improve their services to mothers and children and for conducting pertinent research. The actual planning and administration of the resulting programs is a state and local responsibility.

The Public Health Service is active in the promotion of school health services, accident prevention, immunization programs, communicable disease surveillance and consultation, and Indian and migrant worker health programs. The Service administers grants-in-aid which help states to improve their general public health services, many of which affect mothers and children both directly and indirectly.

Other federal agencies of importance include the Bureau of Family

Services of the Welfare Administration, which administers federal programs for needy families and for the disabled and blind. The Vocational Rehabilitation Administration (as described in Chap. 10) supervises the planning and implementation of programs which help several hundred thousand handicapped individuals each year become or remain productive citizens. The Social Security Administration is the official federal agency created to administer the Old Age Survivors and Disability Insurance, which affects the families of widows and of disabled heads of households.

Local, state, and national voluntary agencies also play a major role in improving the health of mothers and children. A variety of direct services, research, lay and professional educational activities, legislative promotion, and fund raising to support their particular activities are among the programs of these agencies. Maternal and child health in the United States benefits greatly from the cooperative interaction of voluntary and public agencies, which share the common goal of achieving a higher level of health for all mothers and children.

MAJOR MATERNAL AND CHILD HEALTH
PROBLEMS IN OTHER COUNTRIES

Many of the maternal and child health problems in the highly developed countries in the world are held in common. Programs, however, vary widely because of the variety of administrative arrangements for the provision of health services from country to country. Much can be learned about the advantages and disadvantages of the various types of health services by making comparison between countries.

In the emerging or developing nations, the health problems of mothers and children are completely different from those in highly developed countries. A review of some of the relevant health statistics demonstrates this point. Thus, maternal mortality in South America is approximately that of the United States 50 years ago, and the maternal mortality of most of Africa is approximately the same as that in the United States 100 years ago. Similar disparities are found with respect to perinatal, infant, and preschool mortality. As a consequence, the World Health Organization has assigned maternal and child health next to highest priority—exceeded only by malaria control—in ranking of health problems of the world.

Maternal Health Problems

The primary cause of the high maternal mortality in the emerging nations is reported as hemorrhage. Inspection of health records, however, reveals that in many cases there was also a severe anemia which left the mother without an adequate reserve of blood, and that the anemia, in turn, resulted from chronic malnutrition. Thus, chronic malnutrition and profound anemia, rather than hemorrhage, per se, are considered to be the major basic cause of death of these mothers. The second major cause of death of pregnant women is infection, which is due to the use of nonsterile technique at the time of delivery and to the lack of normal resistance to infectious agents that occurs in a chronically malnourished woman.

With both of the major causes of death of pregnant women, two critical factors are involved. One is chronic malnutrition and the other is proper medical attention during birth. Chronic malnutrition, while a health problem, finds its source in the general socioeconomic problems of the developing nations and has no simple solution. The provision of adequate medical attention during labor and delivery has been the source of vigorous international maternal and child health programs. In many emerging nations, traditional midwives have been given training in proper techniques of delivery. In many of these same countries, nurse midwives are being trained along with other types of health assistants to aid in the prenatal and delivery care of the mothers. Because of a great shortage of health professionals, only the women at highest risk may be delivered by a physician. With proper training, however, auxiliary health personnel can conduct sterile deliveries and cope with minor hemorrhage.

The maternal depletion syndrome is widespread among the emerging nations. In many of these nations, cultural mores dictate a heavy work load for women during the childbearing years. In addition, the women deliver a large number of children in succession. The combination of nearly continuous pregnancies, heavy work, and a large number of children to care for gradually results over a period of years in the maternal depletion syndrome. Thus, a woman in her thirties may appear to be twice her age and may suffer from severe chronic malnutrition and general debilitation. These women usually die quite young, and the final insult is often childbirth.

Infant and Preschool Health Problems

The infant and preschool mortality statistics in developing countries indicate that the infectious diseases such as diarrhea, respiratory diseases, and common contagious diseases such as measles are the main killers. Here again, when the health records of children dying from these infectious diseases are studied, it is frequently apparent that the child contracted the acute illness with no ability to fight the infection because he suffered from chronic malnutrition. There is, therefore, general agreement that the major basic cause of death in infants and young children in these countries is nutritional in nature.

The main nutritional deficiency of young children is lack of protein. Chronic protein malnutrition in young children is called kwashiorkor, which is found with some local variations in most parts of the world. This disease develops when the child is weaned from the breast and placed on a diet high in carbohydrate but almost totally lacking in protein. The cultural mores regarding age of weaning and what is considered appropriate for young children to eat have produced this widespread protein malnutrition. Efforts have been made by international health organizations to eradicate the pattern by introducing into these countries high-protein foods which can be easily grown and prepared locally. Unfortunately, cultural acceptance of the new foods has been a serious problem in many places. Changing practices which have been handed down from generation to generation takes time and patience.

In addition to chronic malnutrition being a major cause of death among infants and young children, there is also strong evidence to suggest that chronic malnutrition during early childhood may significantly depress intellectual functioning, perhaps on a permanent basis. If this is true, it represents an enormous drain on human potential in a developing country at a time when the nation needs all the human resources it can muster to successfully emerge in the modern world.

Since its beginning, the World Health Organization together with such agencies as AID and UNESCO has contributed enormously to the health services, health knowledge, and better understanding of the health problems of mothers and children in developing countries. Fortunately, through the device of expert committees, these organizations discovered early that because the health problems of emerging countries were so vastly different from the highly developed nations, many of the methods of Western medicine were inappropriate. New methods, therefore, have been developed which are more appropriate to the problems and the local people. Many important lessons in maternal and child health have been learned through such innovations, and it is quite possible that maternal and child health programs in the more highly developed nations such as the United States will benefit from the study of some of the program innovations in the developing countries.

SUMMARY

Public concern with the health of mothers and children has resulted from an awareness of their dependent status, their economic significance, and the fact that maternal and infant deaths were major contributors to the over-all mortality rate at the turn of the century. These factors, plus the need for a preventive approach to health care which is both complex and costly to provide, have made maternal and child health a major concern of public health. Public efforts have played a significant role in helping to bring about a marked decline since the turn of the century in the number of mothers and children dying each year in the United States.

There is, however, much room for further progress throughout all the maternal and child developmental periods. High-quality, comprehensive care for all mothers and children regardless of socioeconomic status is important to this progress. Such problems as case finding, health education, eligibility, and personnel shortages require continuing efforts. Prevention of the high and steadily rising incidence of illegal abortions, which too often lead to maternal deaths or fetal damage, is a pressing need. The causes and methods of preventing perinatal mortality require further basic laboratory and epidemiologic research. Recognition of high-risk mothers and infants and some means of providing whatever special attention their particular problem demands can help to make pregnancy a safer experience for the mother, decrease pregnancy wastage, and assure that all children achieve and maintain the highest possible level of health.

The handicapped child needs an opportunity to develop to his fullest potential. The current trends toward the use of broader and more uniform definitions of medical eligibility along with the provision of more comprehensive care by crippled children's programs throughout the nation will be of much help in this regard. Improved means of meeting long-term care needs of these children after they reach their adult years must be tackled with greater vigor.

Through the cooperative efforts of local, state, federal, and voluntary agencies, numerous programs have been developed and continue to be improved to meet the multiple needs of mothers and children throughout the United States. Federal legislation has contributed major support to these activities.

Maternal and child health problems in the United States are very similar to those in other economically well-developed nations. Some of these nations have advanced significantly ahead of the United States, as reflected by their lower infant mortality rates. Their methods might well suggest ways and means which could be effectively used in this country. Maternal and child health problems of the less-developed nations are of quite a different nature at present and are intrinsically interwoven with their economic problems. Malnutrition and those conditions secondary to it, combined with the very limited availability of medical personnel and equipment, underlie most maternal and infant deaths. Through the intensive efforts of the World Health Organization, considerable progress has been and continues to be made in all parts of the world.

REFERENCES

1. U.S. BUREAU OF THE CENSUS. *Statistical Abstract of the United States: 1965*, 86th ed. U.S. Government Printing Office, Washington, D.C.

2. EASTMAN, N. J., and HELLMAN, L. M. *William's Obstetrics*, 12th ed. Appleton-Century-Crofts, New York, 1961.

3. BUTLER, N. R., and BONHAM, D. G. *Perinatal Mortality: The First Report of the British Perinatal Mortality Survey*. E. and S. Livingstone Ltd., London, 1963.

4. U.S. DEPARTMENT OF HEALTH, EDUCATION, AND WELFARE, Public Health Service, National Center for Health Statistics. *Infant and Perinatal Mortality in the United States*. Series 3, No. 4. U.S. Government Printing Office, Washington, D.C., 1965.

5. AMERICAN PUBLIC HEALTH ASSOCIATION, COMMITTEE ON CHILD HEALTH. *Health Supervision of Young Children*. The Association, New York, 1955.

6. SIEGEL, EARL, and BRYSON, S. A redefinition of the role of the public health nurse in child health supervision. *Amer J Public Health*, **53**:1015–24, July 1963.

7. SCHIFFER, C. G., and HUNT, E. P. *Illness Among Children*. Children's Bureau Publication No. 405. U.S Department of Health, Education, and Welfare, Washington, D.C., 1963.

8. U.S. DEPARTMENT OF HEALTH, EDUCATION, AND WELFARE, Public Health Service, National Center for Health Statistics. *Vital Statistics of the United States.* Vol. 1. U.S. Government Printing Office, Washington, D.C., 1963.

9. PAKTER, J., ROSNER, H. J., JACOBZINER, H., and GREENSTEIN, F. Out of wedlock births in New York City: I. Sociological aspects. *Amer J Public Health,* 51:683–96, May 1961.

10. CLOSE, KATHRYN. Day care as a service for all who need it. *Children,* 12:157–60, July-August 1965.

11. AMERICAN PUBLIC HEALTH ASSOCIATION, COMMITTEE ON CHILD HEALTH. *Services for Handicapped Children.* The Association, New York, 1965.

12. ELIOT, MARTHA M. The Children's Bureau—fifty years of public responsibility for action in behalf of children. *Amer J Public Health,* 52:576–91, April 1962.

13. U.S. DEPARTMENT OF HEALTH, EDUCATION, AND WELFARE, Welfare Administration. *Crippled Children's Program Statistics, 1963.* Children's Bureau Statistical Series No. 80. U.S. Government Printing Office, Washington, D.C.

CHAPTER 12

HEALTH OF THE CHILD IN SCHOOL

Background and components of school health programs

Organization and administration of school health services

Characteristics and health problems of the school-age child

Elements of the school health program

Special considerations in the school health program

Summary

The health needs of the school-age child and how these needs are provided for within the school setting are discussed in this chapter. The first section briefly reviews the emergence of school health programs in the United States and enumerates the broad components of modern school health services. Patterns of administration of local school health programs, the organization of services within the school, and the contributions made by community, state, and national agencies and associations to the school health program are described in the second section of the chapter. The third section reviews some of the principal developmental characteristics of the school-age child and discusses numerous specific health problems that may be encountered in schoolchildren. The next section describes the various provisions of the school health program which are designed to promote the health and well-being of the child in school. Certain administrative considerations in the school health program are discussed briefly in the last section of the chapter.

BACKGROUND AND COMPONENTS OF SCHOOL HEALTH PROGRAMS

School health programs began in America concurrently with an awakening national concern for the health and welfare of children. The enactment of laws regulating child labor and making school attendance compulsory were early manifestations of this concern. With the enactment of compulsory education laws, new responsibility was imposed on local government as well as on parents. If a child is required to attend school, then government must provide the school, and, in addition, if there are any health hazards peculiar to school attendance, it becomes the responsibility of government to exert every reasonable effort to offset these hazards. It is in the discharge of this obligation that school health services were first developed. Gradually it became recognized that the school setting provides an opportunity to improve as well as protect the health of children.

The school health programs which began in the United States in the late nineteenth century were directed principally toward the control of communicable diseases and minor infections which were rampant in the school population. With improved methods of communicable disease control, this aspect, although still important, is not the major emphasis in the modern school health program. Contemporary school health programs have been broadened to include three primary components: medical, educational, and environmental.

The medical component of school health services involves the prevention of disease, the detection of physical or mental conditions which might handicap the schoolchild, and the provision of procedures for the correction of such defects. The educational aspect pertains to basic instruction in health for the child and to some extent for the school staff and the parents. The environmental component includes the provision and maintenance of sanitary, safe, and comfortable conditions in the school.

In the past, the greatest concentration of school health work has been with children in the first eight grades. The children in these grades are usually from 6 to 14 years of age and constitute approximately 65 per cent of the total school population. However, the age distribution is changing, and state and federal programs are providing for schooling for younger children, particularly those with working mothers or in one-parent families. There are increasing numbers of children in public and private schools, preschools, and nursery schools. Furthermore, with the increasing emphasis on scientific education and with a burgeoning younger population, an unprecedented number of young people are attending high schools, junior colleges, colleges, and universities. Table 12-1 illustrates the increase in

TABLE 12-1 School Enrollment, United States, Selected Years

	1930	1940	1950	1960	1962
			Number (in Thousands)		
Kindergarten	786	661	1,175	2,293	2,456
Grades 1 to 8	22,953	20,466	21,032	30,119	31,322
Grades 9 to 12	4,812	7,130	6,453	9,600	10,769
Higher education	1,101	1,494	2,659	3,216	3,726

Source: Adapted from U.S. Bureau of the Census. *Statistical Abstract of the United States, 1965,* p. 106.

all categories of school enrollment that has occurred during the period 1930 through 1962.

ORGANIZATION AND ADMINISTRATION OF SCHOOL HEALTH SERVICES

There are several elements in the organization and administration of school health programs. One element has to do with local agency jurisdiction, that is, which agency is responsible for school health services, whether one or more than one agency is involved, and how responsibility is divided if it is shared. Another element is the nature of the organization within the school itself. This includes the composition of the school health team, the roles performed by the different members of the team, and the physical setting provided for the school health workers, i.e., the school health office. Still other elements in the organization of school health programs include the kind and variety of community resources available and the programs and roles of state and national agencies.

Administration of Local School Health Programs

Throughout the United States, there is a wide variety of school health services ranging from comprehensive to minimal; in some communities there are no school health programs at all. There is also considerable variation from state to state and among communities with respect to the agency that is responsible for school health programs. Thus, school health services may be provided by a local, county, or state health department, or they may be provided by a department or board of education. In a number of instances, the services are administered jointly by the health department and the educational agency. Occasionally, still other kinds of administrative patterns occur, such as the provision of school health services by local medical groups.

Within the school system, patterns of administration and organization of health programs vary with the jurisdiction responsible for the program. In larger school systems, the health services may be a branch of a pupil personnel division, or they may constitute a special or auxiliary services division, usually the same division as for other pupil services such as child welfare and attendance, or vocational guidance and counseling services. Most health services are headed by a medical director, with supervisors representing the major disciplines serving as chiefs of their respective sections. Figure 12-1 illustrates, for one large metropolitan area, the organization of school health services within an auxiliary services division of the public school system.

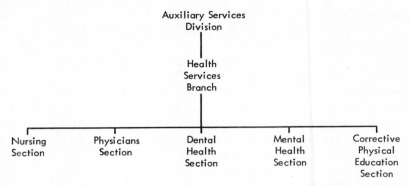

FIGURE 12-1. Organization of school health services, Los Angeles city school system.

Organization of School Health
Services Within the School

Composition and Roles of the School Health Team. In the more comprehensive school health programs, services are provided by a number of different persons representing various professional specialties. These include physicians, dentists, nurses, teachers, and, depending on the magnitude of the program, several other categories of specialists.

Physicians perform physical examinations of school pupils; almost all corrective work, however, is done in private offices, clinics, or hospitals. In large school systems that have numerous children with special problems (vision, hearing, heart, chest, neurologic, psychiatric, etc.), medical specialists are employed by the school district to render diagnostic services. These services are largely designed to assist in pupil placement in school and referral for prompt correction of remediable defects.

Dentists perform periodic dental examinations and participate in dental health education programs in the school. The school dentist may also do certain limited corrective work, although most dental corrections are done by private dentists and dental clinics.

Nurses assist the physicians in physical examinations of the children, make inspections of children referred by the teacher and arrange follow-up, and give first aid in minor injuries. The school nurse may assist the teachers in providing health instruction in the classroom and serve as a resource person. She may also visit parents in connection with health problems of their children, such as the need for correction of defects, and matters of personal hygiene, health habits, and school adjustment. She may arrange for treatment in free clinics for children whose parents are unable to pay for private care. Assisting parent-teacher groups in their health programs and helping to promote community understanding and participation in the school health program may also be important aspects of the work of the school nurse.

Teachers in many school systems provide formal health instruction as part of the regular classroom work and stimulate an interest in health among the children and their parents. In secondary schools, special health teachers conduct classes in personal hygiene, nutrition, and physical education.

Depending on the size of the health program, other specialists may participate in school health work, including audiometrists (who perform audiometric examinations at stated grades and on pupils especially referred because of suspected hearing problems), dental hygienists, clinical psychologists, psychiatric social workers, and others.

The physicians, nurses, and dentists may be employed either by the department of education or by the department of health. Special teachers in health and physical education are usually employed by the schools. When the health program is divided between the department of health and the department of education, the health department is responsible for the medical, dental, and nursing elements of the program, leaving the health instruction largely to the schools. When the entire health program is under the jurisdiction of the school system, these programs may be divided among different divisions; for example, there may be a health service in one division and a health education program in another division where the teaching staff has the major responsibility.

Since many children are congregated in the school setting, an excellent opportunity is afforded for the promotion of health through a variety of methods. Principals and teachers constituting one professional grouping and physicians, dentists, and other health workers making up another may interact with each other in a very meaningful way in accomplishing the goals of school health work. However, the activities may lose effectiveness if the health services are considered routine or inconsequential. In order for school health work to be of value, it must be relevant to pupil needs and to the school situation. Each contact with the physician, nurse, dentist, audiometrist, or other specialist should have meaning not only in terms of the child's physical state but also as an educational experience in which the pupil learns about health care and protection. As members of the team, teachers need to be informed about pupil health and ways in which the school can assist in health improvement.

In conducting a program, it is important to coordinate the school health activities with other health activities in the community in order to avoid duplication and waste of efforts. One of the major responsibilities of the school is discovering health problems that may interfere with the child's ability to benefit to the maximum from the educational experience; it is also a responsibility to see that these problems are corrected whenever possible. The case-finding activities of the school health worker gain in meaning when correction of defects is accomplished.

The School Health Office. The physical setting provided for the conduct of school health services is another aspect of the organization of the health program within the school. In city schools, a suite or room is set aside for the doctor or nurse. In rural schools, the principal's office or a classroom may be used for periodic physical examinations, examinations of especially referred pupils, special inspections, conferences with parents, and first aid given when necessary.

Whenever possible, a designated health office, properly equipped to perform the services needed, should be established in the school. Ideally, the health office should be situated adjacent to the school administrative offices in order to facilitate communication. In small schools, such a location allows easy access for the clerical staff, who handles most minor first aid for pupils with miscellaneous scratches and bruises. Larger school systems should provide a master plan for the health office unit which is adapted to the peculiar needs of the elementary school, the secondary school, or the college campus. Figure 12-2 shows a suggested floor plan for a health office unit in an elementary school.

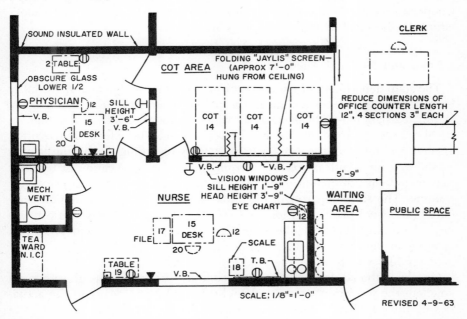

FIGURE 12-2. Elementary school health unit. (Source: Prepared by the Educational Housing Branch, School Planning Division, Los Angeles City Schools.)

The health office should be of adequate size to allow waiting area, nurse's room, physician's office, lavatory facilities, and a rest or isolation room. There should be sufficient space to provide 20 ft for vision testing with the Snellen chart, or 10 ft if a wall mirror is used. In large schools and colleges, there should be accommodations for one or more full-time physicians. A room for the physician for women and one for the physician for men may be advisable, as well as space for a secretary and adequate laboratory facilities.

Community Resources

Community interest and support are highly important for successful school health work. Community resources are used by the school health worker in follow-up activities required for the correction of remediable defects. The private physician, clinic, and parent-teacher association, as well as community service and church groups, are utilized to augment follow-up and corrective procedures.

Many communities have organized school health councils composed of representatives from official and voluntary agencies. School health representatives also work with civic and church representatives to coordinate school health activities. In large urban communities, the Welfare Planning Council has a school health committee. Local medical associations have school health committees, pediatric societies, or other relevant groups. Cooperation with these various organizations tends to maximize the school's efforts in the conduct of health programs.

State and National Agencies

The state department of education or instruction usually has responsibility for determining the curriculum in the public schools in the state. In many states, legislation has been enacted which requires health instruction on such subjects as accident and fire prevention and the effects of narcotics, alcohol, and tobacco; some states have statutes regarding teacher inspection of children for health problems.[1] Requirements for certification of teachers may include health qualifications and health education courses in preservice training. The state department of public health establishes sanitation standards for school plants and for food services. There should be close working relationships between the state departments of health and education in order to develop curriculum guides for health education and to coordinate services which affect the health of the schoolchild.

On the national level, numerous federally sponsored health programs augment the services offered in school health programs. Many of the activities of the Children's Bureau and the Public Health Service which were described in Chapter 11 in connection with young children also include the school-age child. The Office of Education (U.S. Department of Health, Education, and Welfare) is also concerned with the health of the schoolchild. The Consumer and Marketing Service of the U.S. Department of Agriculture administers the national school lunch program under authority of the National School Lunch Act of 1946, as well as the special milk program which was established under provisions of the Agricultural Act of 1954. In the national school lunch program, grants-in-aid to the states provide financial assistance to public and private schools, of high-school grade or under, operating nonprofit school lunch programs. The funds are provided to schools on the basis of their need for assistance and the number of meals served. Participating schools also receive foods bought specifically to help them meet meal standards and are eligible for foods acquired under price support and surplus removal programs of the U.S. Department of Agriculture. The special milk program is designed to increase the consumption of fluid milk by schoolchildren and, similar to the school lunch program, is available to nonprofit schools of high-school grade and under.

Many professional and voluntary organizations and associations are concerned with school health. The National Congress of Parents and Teachers is an important force in the promotion and support of health of the school-age child. The National Education Association and the American Medical Association have established a joint committee on school health policies and practices.[2] The American Public Health Association has a section on school health, with an annual meeting for the consideration of school health programs and problems. The activities of the American School Health Association, with more than 10,000 members, and the American College Health Association are devoted to the consideration and promotion of school health programs in the nation. The American Dental Association, the American Academy of Pediatrics, the American Nurses' Association, the American Psychiatric Association, and the American Orthopsychiatric Association are among the numerous other professional groups which have great interest in and concern for the school health program.

CHARACTERISTICS AND HEALTH PROBLEMS OF THE SCHOOL-AGE CHILD

Significant physical, mental, emotional, and social changes characterize the growth of the school-age child. Although certain norms may be used to describe the various stages of development, it should be kept in mind that deviation from the average does not necessarily constitute abnormality. Individual differences in the rates of growth must always be recognized. During childhood, growth rates also vary in the different body systems. For example, the child of six to ten years of age shows increasingly slow growth in height and increasing rapid gain in weight; this trend continues until the onset of puberty, when an accelerated gain in height and a still more accelerated gain in weight, normally occur. During this period, the child is exposed to common communicable diseases, malnutrition may be seen because of faulty or inadequate diet, and postural deviations may develop. During the adolescent period profound physical, emotional, mental, and social changes occur because of endocrine functioning, resulting in sexual growth and maturity. With growth, needs differ and the pattern of health care should be adjusted to meet the needs. The health program in the primary grades cannot be the same as that in a secondary school or college. Staff should be selected according to their ability and training to serve pupils at various school levels.

It is generally acknowledged that dental defects are the most common health problems found among school-age children. It has been estimated that dental caries are found in 50 to 70 per cent of all schoolchildren examined. Health problems of lesser frequency include defective vision, defective hearing, obesity, orthopedic and posture defects, diseases of the nose and throat, and nervous, emotional, and neurologic problems.

Teeth of the School-Age Child

Young children entering school at five years of age usually have 20 deciduous teeth. The first permanent tooth to erupt, i.e., the first molar, usually appears at six years of age. Frequently this permanent tooth is lost because of early neglect. Caries in the first permanent teeth is as important as in those that erupt at a later date. In certain endocrine states, the eruption of permanent teeth is delayed. However, there is a so-called normal schedule for the eruption of permanent teeth according to the age of the child.

Instruction in dental care is an important part of the school health program. However, cleanliness of the child's teeth depends largely on home training and example. Because of the high incidence of dental caries in the nation's children, efforts have been made to see that drinking water is appropriately fluoridated (1 ppm) in order to reduce the incidence of this health problem, and accordingly, many large cities in the United States have fluoridated their water. In many rural areas, the fluorine content of the water is sufficiently high that dental caries is greatly reduced in residents who use the water supply.

Some school systems have dentists or oral hygienists for examination of the teeth of pupils. Others rely on the inspections made by school physicians. Facilities for correction of dental defects found in schoolchildren are not adequate in comparison to need, which is one of the strong arguments in favor of fluoridating the water supply. It has been said that it would take all the dentists in California working full time for five years to fill the cavities that exist in the teeth of pupils currently enrolled in the Los Angeles city schools.

In the dental health education program, the teacher makes a valuable contribution to public health through efforts to stimulate pupil interest in mouth hygiene and in good dental care. This is accomplished in several ways: through instruction as to the structure, formation, and care of the teeth; through instruction about the relationship between diet and teeth; through attempting to see that each child is supplied with and properly uses a toothbrush; and through obtaining the interest and cooperation of parents.

Vision and the Eyes

It is recommended that for school testing of vision, the Snellen chart be used, either the regular letter chart or the illiterate E chart for pupils who do not know the alphabet. The chart has been precisely designed. Pupils able to read with ease on a well-lighted chart the line they normally should read at 20 ft distance from the chart are usually considered to have normal vision. Normal vision is described in terms of 20/20 vision. The numerator indicates the distance from the chart; the denominator indicates the line on the chart which normally should be read at that distance. The eyes are tested separately, with one covered by a card or occluder but not with the fingers because pressure against the eye may result in an incorrect reading if that eye is tested immediately. Children who have difficulty reading the "20/20 line" are asked to read the larger letters, and the findings are recorded as a fraction; the numerator representing the distance the child stood from the chart and the denominator representing the line read. Pupils who read below the 20/20 line (20/10, etc.) may be hyperopic and need further testing.

There are four kinds of visual defects which are commonly found among school-age children. *Myopia*, or nearsightedness, is the most frequent and tends to become more accentuated in older children. Handicapping myopia is readily discoverable with the routine vision tests used in schools. *Hyperopia* (hypermetropia), or farsightedness, decreases a little from about the ages of 8 to 25. The more severe grades of hyperopia are discoverable with vision tests in schools. *Astigmatism*, or blurring, may occur alone or with myopia or hyperopia. Vision may not be affected with slight astigmatism, but with a greater degree, there is diminution of acuity in both near and distant vision. Astigmatism is discernible through vision tests depending on the degree to which it impairs vision or causes symptoms. *Strabismus*, or squint, walleyes, or cross-eyes, is usually discovered by inspection rather than by testing the vision. Early detection and care may be important to prevent *amblyopia*, the loss of useful vision in an eye often because of disuse or suppression of vision in one eye to prevent double or blurred vision.

In addition to the defects which cause disturbance in vision, other conditions involving the eyes are encountered which are not primarily concerned with the function of sight. Thus, conjunctivitis is quite frequently seen in connection with colds, measles, and local infections. The condition known as "pinkeye" occurs among schoolchildren and is communicable. Diseases of the eyelids and evidence of injury are also encountered. These conditions may or may not affect vision, but sometimes require care or correction.

Hearing and the Ears

It is recommended that hearing be tested as early as possible in a child's school career and again in three or four years. Numerous children are referred to the school physician or nurse by the classroom teacher because of inattention and suspected hearing loss. However, hearing loss in many children is unrecognized until they are carefully examined by the physician, nurse, or audiometrist. Frequently children are considered to be slow learners when their basic problem is impairment of hearing. Testing at the secondary-school level gives a smaller but significant yield of hearing defects and should be done when feasible.

Hearing loss may be due to a conductive impairment, with the difficulty being in the outer or middle ear, or to nerve impairment, with involvement of the auditory nerve. Children who have congenital deafness with a large degree of permanent impairment should be given the advantages of early evaluation and appropriate training. When the cause of hearing impairment is due to infection, such as otitis media, medical care is important. Occasionally, impaired hearing may be due to wax in the external canal, which can be easily discerned by examination with an otoscope.

Many school physicians and nurses routinely do a screening test of hearing using the watch tick or spoken and whispered voice. Some states require that schoolchildren be tested with an audiometer. In California, testing of pupils' hearing is required, but use of an audiometer is optional, although recommended. In some school systems, children are given group screening tests utilizing various methods. When a hearing loss is recognized, careful follow-up should be done and adaptations made in the pupil's school program in order to assist him.

Tonsils and Adenoids

Although lymphoid tissues of the body are naturally of greater size during the early school years and tend to recede in size after 12 or 13 years of age, upper-respiratory-tract infections involving the nose and throat are still the most common cause of illness among children and youth. Reportedly, many respiratory-tract infections, now as always, involve tonsils and adenoids. However, with modern drugs and care the necessity for removal of tonsils and adenoids has been greatly reduced, and surgery is usually done only if other methods of treatment fail.

In more than 300,000 physical examinations done in the Los Angeles city schools in 1963–1964, approximately 5 per cent of the pupils were reported by school physicians as having greatly enlarged or diseased tonsils. These pupils were referred for further medical care and observation. The size of the tonsil alone is usually not the basis for referral, but rather a history of signs and symptoms of frequent recurring respiratory illness. Decisions for tonsillectomy should be based on factors directly related to the tonsils or closely related structures or general disturbance in which the tonsil becomes suspect, such as in rheumatic fever or other infections where a relationship may exist.

The adenoids, when enlarged, may almost fill the vault of the nasal pharynx, interfere with the flow of air through the nose, and obstruct the eustachian tubes causing mouth breathing and, in some instances, deafness.

Usually the voice has a nasal quality, and the child's facial expression is dull. Mouth breathing is present, especially during sleep. Surgical removal of the adenoids is indicated when these more serious symptoms persist. Usually the child's school performance improves when these conditions are corrected.

Posture and Skeletal or Orthopedic Defects

The way a pupil sits, stands, or walks may indicate many things, most important of which may be the way the individual esteems himself. The child who is filled with the joy of life will probably assume a very different attitude from the one who is depressed, unhappy, or indifferent. Chronic fatigue, malnutrition, improper clothing, or boredom may underlie poor posture. However, the school physician should also be constantly alert to the existence or development of orthopedic problems. It is estimated that there are about 400,000 children and youth in the United States who are handicapped more or less seriously by orthopedic conditions. Some of these defects are functional owing to faulty posture habits or improper body alignment or control. Some handicaps may result from muscle weakness, as frequently occurs following paralytic poliomyelitis. Some posture problems are congenital in origin, resulting from improper development of bones or joints. These defects may involve the spine, feet, or other bony structures. Still other handicaps are the result of infection, injury, amputation, or failure of growth. Some pupils show the effects of rickets due to faulty nutrition in infancy and early childhood. The severe orthopedic defects from tuberculosis of the bones and joints, osteomyelitis, and paralytic poliomyelitis are seen much less frequently than in former years, while congenital orthopedic defects and those due to accidents are more common.

In the ordinary school population, most orthopedic defects are functional in nature. Pupils can be assisted to improve posture and body alignment through well-directed physical education and corrective programs. Pupils with severe problems should be seen by orthopedic specialists to outline a school program with proper referral for early care when needed. Through special federal grants to states, most localities are able to arrange for expert care of children who are severely handicapped. With the great improvement of prosthetic devices, many children are able to attend school who formerly would have been excluded.

Heart Disease in Schoolchildren

Recent estimates indicate congenital heart abnormalities and rheumatic fever are the major causes of heart disease in the school pupil. The seriousness of the heart condition depends on the underlying pathology and whether it will respond to treatment. With the advent of the antibiotic drugs and the tremendous advances in cardiac surgery, many children who would have become cardiac cripples with a very short life expectancy are able to look forward to normal living.

Heart conditions can usually be classified as congenital, acquired (organic defects), or functional (no organic problem). *Congenital* heart lesions arise because of developmental defect. Important in the etiology are infections in the first trimester of intrauterine life. German measles is one of the important virus infections known to damage the embryonic heart structure and produce congenital lesions. Congenital lesions may be of numerous kinds, some complicated and difficult to correct; others may be amenable to correction, or relatively minor and producing few symptoms. Acquired heart disease in school-age children is usually associated with rheumatic fever, tonsillitis (as streptococcal sore throat), or one of the acute communicable diseases.

In the usual physical examination done at school, it may be difficult to distinguish between some of the functional, acquired, or congenital conditions. For this reason, examinations by heart specialists should be sought through private, school, or clinic diagnostic services. Because many children have heart murmurs which are functional in nature and disappear in later life, it is important that they be appropriately programmed in terms of regular school activity rather than treated as "heart problems." Limiting a pupil's physical activity unnecessarily deprives him of a very essential part of the normal childhood experience and should be done only after adequate examination has been made and type, degree, and length of limitation have been defined.

Nutrition

School statistics indicate that overweight is one of the more important problems among schoolchildren. However, malnutrition still is a frequent finding of concern to school health workers. The weighing and measuring of all pupils is an important part of the health evaluation, since growth is a significant index of health. Children in elementary schools should be weighed and measured annually, and the results entered on the child's health record. It must be borne in mind, however, that height-weight charts are based on the "average" child. Growth must be considered in terms of the individual pupil, giving consideration to his genetic endowment, family characteristics, body type, and phase of growth. The important fact is that a child is continuing to gain in weight and height, even though slowly, in a pattern "normal" for him.

Poor nutrition may be due to lack of adequate food intake, faulty choices in food, or chronic or acute infection or disease that interferes with normal nutrition. Malnutrition may range from mild to severe, and the problem may be exceedingly complex. Laboratory tests are valuable in ascertaining the nutritional status. In some examinations of very young children, tests are being provided in schools through federal programs, while for the older-age schoolchild such evaluations are usually done by referral to the family physician or to public or school clinics. Children suspected of having malnutrition should be referred for more definitive examination.

Part of the health education carried on in schools is instruction about adequate diet and food requirements. This instruction should be modified to incorporate food habits of differing ethnic groups and the foods available in the area. All individuals need not eat alike, but adequate and appropriate amounts of the four basic food groups are important, and these facts should be communicated as part of the school health instruction program.

Minor Infections and Infestations

In some areas where high levels of sanitation and body care exist, the incidence of the so-called nuisance diseases is greatly reduced. However, in other areas, this is not the case. Some of the more commonly encountered diseases of this kind are impetigo contagiosa, ringworm, pediculosis, and scabies.

Impetigo contagiosa is an infectious disease which spreads by direct contact. Although schools are restricted in their treatment activities, it may be necessary to recommend care in low socioeconomic areas where the disease is common. The usual treatment is a medication that can be supplied through the schools or obtained from a pharmacy without a physician's prescription, such as 5 per cent ammoniated mercury ointment, bacitracin, neopolycin, neosporin, or polysporin ointments to be applied after crusts are removed. If recovery is not prompt or if infection spreads, referral to a physician or clinic should be made.

Ringworm may involve the scalp (tinea capitis), the body (tinea corporis), or the feet (athlete's foot, or tinea pedis). Ringworm of the scalp is spread from person to person as well as from dogs, cats, and other animals; ringworm of the body or feet is spread by direct or indirect contact with the infected person. Since cases are sometimes resistant, treatment must be careful, complete, and continuing. This is especially true with ringworm of the scalp. Treatment depends on the type and severity of infection, and referral to a private physician or clinic is advisable.

Pediculosis (lice) usually is present on the hairy parts of the body and may be in the clothing. The infesting agent may be the head or body louse (*Pediculus humanus*) or the crab louse (*Phthirus pubis*). This infestation usually exists in the family and may spread in the classroom. The preferred method of treatment is 10 per cent DDT dusting powder for body and head lice; a 1 per cent benzene hexachloride ointment (Kwell) may be substituted, or one of the other commercial medications can be used for pediculosis of the hair and scalp, followed by a shampoo and careful removal of all nits with a fine-tooth steel comb.

Scabies spreads from child to child, and within the child's family. A 1 per cent benzene hexachloride ointment (Kwell) is usually applied to the whole body, with a cleansing bath and change of clothing. Personal cleanliness and thorough cleaning of all clothing and bedding after infestation is necessary to prevent reoccurrence.

The usual procedure for these various minor infestations and others is to permit children when under effective treatment to continue in school; otherwise they are excluded until free of infection. In areas of high incidence, a routine "morning inspection" of classes or of known contacts may be advisable. In rural areas where problems of infestation are particularly acute, it is frequently difficult for the nurse to get medical assistance, and she is often authorized to advise treatment previously outlined by the school physician or health officer. Whenever private or clinic medical care is available, pupils should be referred and every effort made to prevent the spread of these conditions to other children. When parents cannot afford even the simple materials necessary for treatment, medications may be supplied through funds made available by schools or welfare organizations. In some instances, parents do not see the importance of care and fail to give cooperation. They may themselves suffer from infection or infestation and thus serve as a source of reinfection to the pupil, or they may be indifferent to care. In certain instances it may be necessary to seek the assistance of child welfare personnel to reinforce the need for treatment.

Allergies

The term "allergy" is generally used to describe reactions resulting from antigen-antibody action within the individual in such a manner as to produce allergic symptoms manifest in the skin, respiratory system, gastrointestinal system, or in other ways. One of the most important of these allergic responses is anaphylactic shock. However, "hives," eczema, allergic rhinitis (hay fever), and asthma are the allergic conditions most commonly encountered in the school-age child. It is important that the school health worker have knowledge of the existence of allergic phenomena, particularly if emergency situations are likely to arise because of extreme sensitivity in a pupil. Certain environmental adjustments may be necessary for this child in the school situation; such highly allergic pupils should be under continued medical supervision.

Emotional Problems of Children

Most authorities agree that there is a rising incidence of nervous, emotional, mental, and social adjustment problems in the school-age child. The causes are likely to be multiple, complex, and frequently unknown, since there are many genetic, physical, and environmental influences that bear on the child's mental and emotional development. Some pupils come to school with a sturdier "psyche" than do others. The school experience may be very supportive and growth-producing; for some pupils, however, it may constitute, for numerous reasons, a time of crisis and distress.

Emotional disturbances may manifest themselves in a number of different ways. Poor achievement in a child who has normal or superior intelligence and no apparent physical problems or handicaps may be one manifestation. "Antisocial" behavior such as hostility, destructiveness, or cruelty may also signal emotional problems. Anxiety, nervousness, excessive efforts to gain approval, withdrawal, exhibitionism, or truancy may be among several other possible behavioral indicators of maladjustment. Many of the school dropouts among older children occur because of failure to adjust satisfactorily.

In a burgeoning population in a technologic era, there are increasing demands on people in every walk of life. This includes school-age children, on whom there are ever-increasing demands to excel. An appropriate amount of stimulation of the pupil to work for success may promote his mental health, but under pressures and a feeling of failure, there may be frustration, anxiety, apathy, and nonadjustment. School is the world of work for the child, just as industry, business, or a profession is the world of work for the adult. Inappropriate teacher or parental concern over a pupil's grades, "popularity," or athletic accomplishments may produce in him feelings of failure, fear, and worthlessness.

The importance of an emotionally stable and perceptive teacher, sensitive to the mood changes and emotional needs of pupils, cannot be overemphasized. Teachers sometimes need to be reassured that problems in school adjustment do not remain stationary; frequently with supportive help a child improves greatly with the passing of time. One of the most significant areas where the physician can help the schools is in relation to the emotional and social adjustment of the pupils. The school physician must recognize that the psychologic, emotional, and mental adjustment of pupils is an area in which he needs to be concerned and competent; as he recognizes the pupil's problem, he must be able to make recommendations for follow-up care. The school nurse, in turn, is important in seeing that follow-up activities are diligently pursued. Perhaps in no other area is the "team approach" more essential than in understanding and meeting the needs of the unadjusted pupil before crisis arises.

Some school districts maintain child guidance services, frequently supported by an auxiliary agency working in close cooperation with the school. An emotionally disturbed child with problems of school adjustment may be referred to this agency and a coordinated program of follow-up care established. If the pupil is mentally or emotionally ill and under private psychiatric care, a close cooperation with the school is necessary in order to effect optimal treatment. The return to school of a pupil after emotional or mental illness should be carefully handled. Here again, the school health worker assists the school and the pupil to effect a more comfortable adjustment by bridging outside and school care.

ELEMENTS OF THE SCHOOL HEALTH PROGRAM

The school health program serves many functions. Implicit in all its operation is the development of health awareness in the total school community, specifically as it relates to the needs of pupils and staff. A large portion of the school physician's time is spent in promoting this awareness through health examinations done at predetermined intervals and through health inspections. These examinations and inspections enable the physician to identify pupils who are in need of special school programs, remedial measures, and referral for care. Another valuable role the physician performs is that of consultant to the teachers or the administration about pupils who are having physical or emotional problems that interfere with pupil learning and frequently reduce effectiveness of the teacher's activities.

The Physical Examination of the Schoolchild

Early in the history of the school health movement, it was considered important that each pupil have a physical examination once a year, but experience has shown that careful examinations at wider time intervals are more meaningful. It is generally agreed that the best plan is a thorough health appraisal (consisting of a physical examination and history) made every four or five years during a pupil's school experience, with careful follow-up to see that defects are corrected. Decreasing the frequency with which all children are examined provides more time for the school physician to see pupils whose physical, emotional, or mental condition is regarded as unsatisfactory by the school nurse or teacher.

Examination services to pupils vary from school to school, but in general, *health appraisals* are recommended for kindergarten or first grade, fourth grade, seventh grade, tenth grade, and on admission to college. At any time during a pupil's school experience, however, *special referrals* for health examination may be made. The special referral is frequently the most important pupil examination. Usually, special referrals are made by a teacher or school administrator because of a pupil problem which may involve health. These referrals constitute a challenge to the school physician searching for reasons for pupil distress. *Health inspections* also are done and involve the examination of school pupils for participation in athletic teams, for driver instruction, for special school programs, or after illness or injury.

The physical examination done at school should be as thorough and complete as possible, using adequate time to elicit health history and to assess the child's physical and emotional status. Fifteen to twenty minutes should be allowed for the average examination. Careful recent medical histories and reports of teacher observation of abnormal symptoms in pupils may be significant clues to the school physician that further evaluations are necessary. Pupils showing any problems related to underlying illness or disease should be referred to their family physician or to a clinic or other medical facility where further study can be undertaken.

The findings of the physical examination should be reported to the child's parents or guardian, verbally or in writing. Pertinent information from the examination should be made available to teachers or concerned staff. Discussions about pupil health are frequently most successfully conducted in the "case conference" in which the principal, counselor, teacher, nurse, physician, and parent participate as appropriate. The problems of communication must always be recognized and surmounted, and in this respect the school physician, dentist, and nurse have great responsibility.

Inspection in Classes

For many years, a morning inspection of pupils by the teachers or nurse was recommended. However, in most situations where a well-organized school health program is in progress with staff alert to health problems, this routine is unnecessary. When a pupil in school has developed a major communicable disease, daily inspection of contacts during the incubation period for signs of illness is most important. This kind of inspection is usually done by the school nurse.

Health Records

Each pupil should have a health record on file containing identifying information, significant facts of the child's health history, findings of each physical examination, and an account of the health services provided (e.g., home visits, home notices, exclusions from school, communicable diseases, and correction of defects). The format of school health records varies, but they should be permanent, made of durable material, and large enough to accommodate entries for a period of several years. Figure 12-3 provides an example of a health record form that is in use currently in a large metropolitan school system.

The health record should be started when the child enters school and maintained throughout his school career. The record should accompany the pupil if he transfers from one school to another. Records should be filed so that they are available at all times for the reference and use of the school physician and nurse.

Referral for Treatment of Diseases and Correction of Physical Defects

There is an increasing tendency for the community to provide corrective services for children whose families are unable to pay for private medical care. Whenever a family cannot afford private medical care or does not have a family physician, the child should be referred to an appropriate

V _____ OT _____ P _____

SABIN 1 _____ 2 _____ 3 _____

POLIO SALK 1 _____ 2 _____ 3 _____

TRIVALENT 1 _____ 2 _____

Name: Last _____ First _____ Middle _____

Sex: M ☐ F ☐

LOS ANGELES CITY SCHOOLS
HEALTH RECORD

Residence	Phone	School	Date Arr.	Birth Date	Mo.	Day	Yr.
				Birthplace			
				Arrived in Calif.			
				Room Nos.			

PHYSICAL EXAMINATION

SYMBOLS

A — NEEDS ATTENTION GRADE URGENCY 1, 2, 3, OR 4

A — RECEIVED ATTENTION

F — FURTHER EXAM. NEEDED

O — OVER

Date of Examination	Name of Examiner	Grade	NUTRITION		EYES				EARS				NOSE & THROAT					TEETH					HEART			LUNGS	Orthopedic			Ner-vous System	Speech	Skin	Endo-crine	Misc.
			Hgt.	Wgt.	Vision R	Vision L	Path-ology R	Path-ology L	Hearing R	Hearing L	Path-ology R	Path-ology L	Ton-sils	Ade-noids	De-cay	Clean-ing	Gums	Ortho-dontia	Or-ganic	Func-tional						Pos-ture	Feet						

Rest: how long? _____

Assignment to Special Classes: _____

Corrective P.E. _____

Reg. Gym. _____

Driver Training _____

FORM 34-EH-5 50M 4-66 (STK. NO. 815301)   This card must be transferred with other record cards. Every child must have a health card or an "Excuse from Physical Examination."

390

PERSONAL HISTORY   Address

                              Date   Family Physician   Address
                                            Family Dentist

			IMMUNIZATIONS		FAMILY STATUS
Asthma	Tbc—Child	Dental Decay	Convulsions	Smallpox	Years	Father
Hayfever	Tbc—Family	Toothache	Fainting	Diph.		Mother
Eczema	Chickenpox	Freq. Colds	When?	Wh. Cough		Bros. Ages
Diabetes	Measles	Freq. Sore Throats	Nose Bleeds	Tetanus		
Heart Dis.	Ger. Measles	Freq. Coughs	Growing Pains	Polio:		Sis. Ages
Polio	Wh. Cough	Freq. Headaches	Operations			
Pneumonia	Mumps	Wears Glasses				
Rheum. Fever	Hernia	Tires Easily	Accidents			
Scarlet Fever	Eye Difficulty	Recent Bed Wtg.	Other Ser. Ill.			

Appetite   Milk Daily?   Food Allergies?

Breakfast   Bed Time   Rising Time

DENTAL RECORD				VISION SCREENING		PHYSICIAN'S, DENTIST'S, OR NURSE'S NOTES
Date Exam- ined	Name of Examiner	TEETH		Date	R L	Date

TEETH			
Decay	Clean-ing	Gums	Ortho-dontia

Audiometer   Date   Date   Date   Date   Date   Date   Mantoux   Date

R.

L.

FIGURE 12-3. School health record form.

clinic for medical service. More and more special facilities are being provided through federal programs to children of families with limited income.
In some areas parent-teacher associations provide a valuable diagnostic
and treatment service for pupils, expediting the correction of defects that
may interfere with school progress.

Prevention and Control of Communicable Disease

Immunization against those diseases for which an immunizing agent exists
is a first step in the prevention and control of communicable diseases in
schools. Recommended immunization schedules for infants and young children have been discussed in Chapter 11. If the child has been previously
immunized, boosters and revaccinations should be taken at specified intervals after he enters school. Immunization programs are conducted in some
schools as part of their health services, but where this is not done, the school
physician or nurse should, on a systematic basis, urge parents to have their
children vaccinated, revaccinated, or given boosters as needed.

Tuberculosis control is an important aspect of the school health program,
and tuberculin testing and x-ray programs are maintained in many school
districts for the prevention of tuberculosis among faculty and pupils. An
open case of tuberculosis discovered among teachers or pupils should serve
as an alert, and intensive case finding and follow-up procedures should be
inaugurated among contacts.

Since communicable diseases vary in severity and mode of transmission,
and since modifications are made in control measures from time to time, it
is important that school personnel be aware of the characteristics of communicable diseases and of the regulations regarding their control. Large
school districts may have a handbook of communicable diseases available
for use of administrative and school health personnel.[3] Local health departments have copies of the control regulations available that can be used in
schools, and these should be available in the school principal's office as well
as in the health office.

Although regulations and practices vary regarding the method of handling
a case of communicable disease, in general, a pupil suspected of being in
the early stages of such a disease is excluded from school immediately. If
he contracts the disease, he must remain out of school for a designated
period and be examined before readmission to school. For absence because
of a major communicable disease, a physician's certificate or health department permit may be required before a pupil is permitted to return to school.
Pupils known to have had recent exposure to a communicable disease are
either closely observed in school or temporarily excluded from school, as
required. The sibling of a pupil who contracts a major communicable disease generally may remain in school if he has been properly immunized
against the disease, is considered well and not a carrier, and if the patient
is isolated.

The question occasionally arises as to whether schools should be closed during an epidemic. Theoretically, if the school group is the focus, closure of the schools would separate those who are spreading the disease from those who are susceptible. Practically, however, when schools are closed pupils continue to intermingle with one another, generally in a less controlled manner. Most health authorities believe that regular attendance at school and daily inspection of pupils for signs of illness during an epidemic will do more to detect early cases and prevent the spread of the disease than closing schools.

Health Instruction

In addition to the learning experience implicit in pupil contacts with members of the health team, there is also much explicit teaching done as part of the school health program. The school physician, dentist, and nurse are appropriately regarded as resource personnel available to teachers to help them in their health instruction activities in the classroom. Health workers are frequently asked to give talks to pupil groups, and this is a valuable and important contribution particularly if part of an ongoing health instruction program. While the health worker does not usually assume the teacher's health instruction responsibilities on a regular basis, he may assist in developing audiovisual materials, radio and television programs, class presentations, and staff presentations of various kinds. It is worthwhile for the health worker to develop various communication skills in order that he may add to the effectiveness of the school health instruction program. The technique of arousing and sustaining the interest of children of various ages in developing optimal health attitudes and practices depends to a great extent on the workers' understanding of pupil growth and development.

More and more persons with formal training in health education are being used in schools as supervisors of health education or as teachers of health at the secondary and college level. However, in numerous instances, formal health classes are still taught by teachers of various backgrounds. Such teachers frequently need help with their health instruction program from the school health personnel. This contribution may be made individually, or through in-service training classes, workshops, lectures, curriculum committees, or demonstrations.

Physical Education

Although recess and physical education periods have traditionally been a part of the school day, in most areas an awakening interest in the individual's "physical fitness" has resulted generally in a stepping up of physical exercise and performance and endurance tests.

Physical education tends to relieve the tedium of the classroom and to reduce the fatigue incident to study, through properly placed rest and play periods. In the lower grades, these periods are quite frequent. In the upper grades, they occur less often and last longer. Usually, in the secondary schools the physical education program replaces the recess period. Pupils unable to participate in regular physical education are generally assigned on the physician's recommendation to modified physical education classes. When properly handled, physical education periods result in children being more alert and teachable, and they also provide an opportunity for the child to learn self-control, cooperation, and sportsmanship.

Provisions for the Handicapped Child

Separate classes which often have special equipment are provided for pupils with severe handicaps. Classes commonly provided are for the hard of hearing, the totally deaf, the blind and partially seeing, the crippled, the educationally handicapped, and the mentally retarded. Usually, these children are transported to school by bus, and especially trained instructors and appropriate medical services are provided. Frequently, the seriously handicapped pupils are assigned to special schools which are particularly designed and equipped for their care. These various kinds of special schools and classes are found in most of the major cities in the United States. Pupils with severe problems of adjustment, or teen-age pregnant girls, may be especially assigned until able to return to a regular classroom.

Emergency Care

Wherever there is a large congregation of people, accidents and injuries are likely to occur. Each year, there are many sudden illnesses, serious accidents, or deaths that occur in schools. Each year, somewhere in the United States, disaster strikes a school building and involves pupils. It is the responsibility of the administration and the school health staff to see that pupils are afforded maximum protection in the event of an emergency or crisis.

Every pupil on enrollment should file an "emergency card" giving the name, address, and telephone number of parents, nearest relative, and neighbor who might be reached in case there is an emergency at school. Similar information regarding the child's or family's physician should also be entered on the card.

Pupils at play receive minor cuts and bruises, most of which can be cared for in the principal's office by the school clerk. Any more serious injury is referred to the school nurse if she is present or can be called, and when a school physician is on the premises, he is always available to assist with major injuries. However, every school plant should have an established procedure in case of major emergency or disaster. Some school systems post an emergency information card in a conspicuous place in the principal's office, giving instructions for calling an ambulance, sending a patient to the receiving hospital, or notifying the police. It is important for staff to be aware of these procedures in the event the school physician or nurse is not available. School nurses provide a real service by offering courses in first aid so that all members of the school staff may be aware of accepted first-aid procedures. A first-aid kit should be well stocked and in a conspicuous place, and the nurse or someone whom she delegates should check the kits periodically to be sure they are in good order.

Health Supervision of School Personnel

Schools and universities in the United States are staffed with over 2 million teacher personnel and approximately 750,000 nonteaching personnel. Various methods of selection of teacher staff and other employees exist, differing widely in different areas. However, health standards for employment should be established and maintained in order to be certain that children are not unnecessarily exposed to employees suffering from tuberculosis or other communicable disease, nervous and emotional instability, or physical impairments that limit their competency and deprive pupils of an adequate school situation. Standards of appearance, vision, hearing, physical ability, and nervous and emotional stability should be considered as important requisites for employment. The healthy, adjusted teacher will undoubtedly bring more vigor and joy to the classroom than one who is physically or emotionally unfit.

SPECIAL CONSIDERATIONS IN THE
SCHOOL HEALTH PROGRAM

There are some differences of opinion regarding how the goals of school health programs can best be accomplished, one consideration being which of several possible administrative patterns, or jurisdictional arrangements, is preferable. There are both advantages and disadvantages if either the department (or board) of education or the department of health has *sole* responsibility for the administration of school health services. Even when the responsibility is *shared,* questions arise as to how the various components of school health service should be allocated between the two departments.

The jurisdictional arrangement which appears to some to be preferable places primary responsibility on the health department for planning and administering school health services, while the department of education is responsible for the approval of policies.[4] One advantage of this arrangement is that the health department remains the single agency responsible for all official community health programs, thus minimizing the possibility of fragmentation and duplication of services. Moreover, under this administrative pattern, the health department can endeavor to provide uniform services among all categories of schools—public, private, parochial, and special schools. Since the provision of health services is its customary activity, the health department may find it easier to develop a high-quality program and to attract better qualified personnel.

On the other hand, if the school system is responsible for the administration of school health services, there is the advantage that the services are an integral part of the educational program. Under this jurisdictional arrangement, school health workers are able to give their full attention to the conduct of the school health program and thus can engage in certain kinds of relevant activities that otherwise might not be possible. Within the school, this includes the design of special programs to meet the health needs of pupils with particular problems such as the physically handicapped, the emotionally disturbed, the teen-age pregnant girl, and others. Moreover, the school-based health worker frequently serves on policy-making committees, works closely with parent and pupil groups, participates in the development of the health curriculum, and is readily available as a resource person for the teaching and administrative staff. By maintaining a close working relationship with private physicians, the health department, and other health agencies, the school health worker can form a bridge between the school and the various health workers in the community.

Other administrative considerations in the school health program have to do with matters of policy, such as how much school health service should be provided for children whose families can afford private care, and how much should be provided for children from low-income families. In either case, certain problems arise from the fact that while the school health program offers preventive and some diagnostic and follow-up services, the child usually must go elsewhere for treatment regardless of his financial status. The principal problems in this arrangement pertain to where the child should go for such treatment, and how the goal of treating the "whole child" can be achieved when his care is divided among agencies.

There are also certain considerations regarding the optimal method of work for school health personnel, notably the physician and the nurse. Although the physician is able to perform many of his usual functions and some special ones in the school health program, his activities are limited largely to referral and follow-up of pupils with health problems. As a consequence, his customary role of providing treatment is markedly curtailed, which raises some question regarding whether his training and experience are being utilized sufficiently. With respect to the method of work of the nurse, some prefer that she be full time in the school program, while others consider that she can best carry out her responsibilities for the health of schoolchildren by functioning as a public health nurse in the community. Under the latter arrangement, she divides her time between the school, the health department clinic, and home visiting, thus serving not only the schoolchild but also his entire family. One work pattern of the nurse which appears to be emerging involves having public health nurses in elementary schools and full-time school nurses in secondary schools.[4] However, the pattern of having nurses assigned exclusively and full time to school health programs in both elementary and secondary schools is still considered to have numerous advantages.

SUMMARY

Interest in the health of the child in school emerged early in the twentieth century in the United States as part of an awakened concern about the health and welfare of children generally. Modern concepts of school health programs have broadened since those early days to include medical, educational, and environmental components.

Patterns of administration of school health services vary considerably throughout the United States, and these differences are reflected in the modes of organization of services within school systems. Within the school itself, the school health team ideally consists of physicians, dentists, nurses, teachers, and other specialists as needed; each professional specialty has a particular role which contributes to the goals of school health work. Most communities have several kinds of resources which serve as valuable assets to the school health program. Several official state and federal agencies as well as numerous professional associations and voluntary organizations support and promote school health work.

Growth of the school-age child is characterized by significant physical, mental, emotional, and social changes. However, the fact that there are considerable individual differences in growth rates is an important consideration in assessing a child's developmental status. Although schoolchildren constitute a relatively healthy segment of the population, certain health problems are likely to be encountered. Dental defects are the most common health problem found among children in school; some of the other problems which occur with lesser and varying frequency include defective vision, defective hearing, obesity and other nutritional disorders, orthopedic and posture defects, diseases of the nose and throat, heart disease, allergies, emotional disturbances, and minor infections and infestations.

Although the nature of school health programs varies widely, a comprehensive program provides numerous different elements of service. These elements include physical examinations at stated intervals; systematic maintenance of permanent, individual health records; referral procedures for the treatment of diseases and the correction of physical defects; prevention and control of communicable disease within the school; health instruction; physical education; provisions for the handicapped child; emergency care; and health supervision of school personnel.

There are several special administrative considerations in connection with the provision of school health programs and services. These considerations include the nature of local jurisdictional responsibility, certain matters of policy and practice, and methods of work of particular categories of school health personnel.

REFERENCES

1. NEMIR, ALMA. *The School Health Program.* W. B. Saunders Company, Philadelphia, 1965.
2. WILSON, CHARLES C., ed. *School Health Services,* 2nd ed. National Education Association and American Medical Association, Washington, D.C., 1964.

3. Los Angeles City Schools. *Communicable Diseases, Rules and Regulations.* School Publication No. 359, Los Angeles, 1966.

4. Harper, Paul A., and Stine, Oscar C. Health services for children. In: Sartwell, P. E., ed. *Maxcy-Rosenau Preventive Medicine and Public Health,* 9th ed. Appleton-Century-Crofts, New York, 1965.

ADDITIONAL READING

Randall, Harriett B. Mental health of teachers. *J Sch Health,* 34:411–14, November 1964.

School Nursing Committee, American School Health Association. The nurse in the school health program—guidelines for school nursing. *J Sch Health,* 37: entire issue, February 1967.

Sliepcevich, Elena M. *Summary Report of School Health Education Study* (sponsored by the Samuel Bronfman Foundation, New York). National Education Association, Washington, D.C., 1964.

Turner, C. E., Sellery, C. M., and Smith, S. L. *School Health and Health Education,* 5th ed. The C. V. Mosby Company, St. Louis, 1966.

CHAPTER 13

HEALTH EDUCATION

The background and processes of the health education component of health and medical services are discussed in this chapter. In the first section of the chapter, health education is defined, and its general nature and purpose are described. The second section reviews the role of behavior in health and disease and the factors which influence behavioral development, stability, and change. The place of health knowledge in health education, the analysis of the behavioral aspects of a health education problem, and considerations in the selection of methods to solve the problem are discussed in the next section. The fourth section reviews the elements and certain problems in evaluating the degree to which health education programs achieve their objectives. The last section of the chapter comments on a few special problems of contemporary health education programs in the United States.

THE NATURE AND PURPOSE OF HEALTH EDUCATION

Health education is that component of health and medical programs which consists of planned attempts to change individual, group, and community behavior (what people think, feel, and do), with the objective of helping achieve curative, rehabilitative, disease-preventive, and health-promotive ends. The health education process is complex, and to be effective it must go well beyond the methods conventionally used in education. However, all too frequently it is thought by lay persons and many health professionals alike that health education consists simply of instructing people about health matters, that its most appropriate place is in the schools where large numbers of children can be reached, and that it can be conducted by almost anyone who is able to communicate clearly and who has some knowledge of the nature of health and disease. Such conceptions for a long time have dimmed the understandi::g of the significance of health education and have masked the complexity of its nature and task.

Health education and psychotherapy may be said to have broadly similar functions in that both are directed toward influencing behavior. The distinction between them lies in the fact that psychotherapy is directed mainly toward the emotionally disturbed person whose behavior is not within the culturally defined normal limits for the community, whereas health education is concerned mainly with behavior which is, in itself, within normal limits. There is, of course, a considerable twilight area between normal and abnormal behavior, and there is also a basic continuity to all attempts to influence behavior of whatever kind.[1]

Education in the usual general sense is often regarded, particularly in the Western world, as good for its own sake and as an end in itself. *Health* education, however, must contribute to an outcome in which there is a behavior change associated with a demonstrably improved health status of the individual, group, and community. Thus, when selecting particular health education methods in preference to others, a primary consideration is the extent to which these seem likely to accomplish such an outcome. The one restriction is that the process, means, or methods should not violate the values of the community in which they are to be used. There is a relatively automatic safeguard in this connection, however, because methods that are incompatible with the values of the society are likely to fail, especially over the long run.

THE BASES OF HEALTH EDUCATION

An understanding of the nature of health education rests on a knowledge of the role of human behavior in the natural history of health and disease in the individual, the family and small group, and the community. The factors which influence behavioral development, stability, and change are also important considerations in health education.

The Role of Behavior in
Health and Disease

There are probably few if any diseases whose etiology is known or suspected, in which human behavior does not play a role, frequently a critical one. Perhaps the greatest achievement of medicine and public health, and more particularly of the laboratory, is the modern advance in knowledge of the communicable diseases. The major attention given to these diseases historically was a natural one in view of the direct responsibility they bore for high morbidity and mortality, especially among children. Most of the communicable diseases are now individually identifiable through clinical and laboratory procedures; for most, specific microorganisms have been identified as a causal agent whose life cycle, environmental sources, and mode of transmission have been determined; and perhaps greatest of all, for many, a specific immunization procedure has been developed. These striking successes, however, have encouraged a tendency to think of the microorganism as the sole, direct cause of its associated communicable disease. To this, epidemiology has applied the corrective of the host-agent-environment principle to show that the etiology of the communicable diseases is dependent on the states and relationships of all three.

With respect to the human host, it is readily apparent that no matter which communicable disease is examined, the behavior of the host is at least one important factor in causation. Thus, the physical proximity that people establish with one another; the dwellings they build; the way they dispose of their wastes; their use of animals for food, labor, or companionship; and their personal habits of hygiene all represent ways in which human behavior facilitates or obstructs the transmission of communicable diseases.

With the long-term chronic diseases, from what is now known of their etiology, human behavior is again centrally involved. The food people prefer and eat; what they drink; whether and to what extent they smoke; their daily cycles of rest, relaxation, exercise, and work; the way they relate with one another; and the way they rear their children are some of the many forms of behavior which have been implicated in the known or suspected etiology of the chronic diseases. Moreover, as society and human behavior change with man's restless activity, exploration, and enterprise, there is a constant creation of new problems or exacerbation of old ones, ranging from radioactivity, air pollution, and automobile accidents to changed emotional stresses, alcoholism, and drug addiction.

It would be somewhat misleading, therefore, to surmise that there is a special phenomenon of *"health* behavior," which suggests that some forms of behavior are peculiarly associated with disease-causative or health-promotive processes, while other forms of behavior are not. Rather, it would seem more reasonable to regard *all* behavior as being *health-related* in one way or another. Health-related behavior would also include some forms of behavior which could be described as *health-directed,* that is, instances where the individual or group acts with a clear awareness of the implications for health. Examples of such health-directed behavior are the ways people behave to relieve illness or to prevent it, the kind of help they seek, the use they make of available health and medical services, and the health programs which community groups might plan and implement. Individual or group decisions to give up smoking or to reduce weight for health reasons are clearly health-directed.

It should be kept in mind, however, that while human behavior plays an important role in the natural history of health and disease in the individual, much or even most of this behavior is not performed principally because of the individual's concern for his health. If it were possible directly to observe, in communities around the world, the total daily patterns of behavior and associated feelings and motivations, it would probably be found that specifically health-motivated and deliberately health-directed behavior has a relatively minor role. Getting on with others in order to have the emotional comfort of belonging, eating to satisfy hunger and for enjoyment, earning a living to be able to afford the necessities and possibly some of the luxuries of life, influencing children so that they will behave in culturally acceptable ways, and playing and physical activity for the fun of it would all perhaps more accurately reflect the real world of daily behavior.

In any event, if there is this intimate relationship between health and behavior, it seems clear that effective diagnostic, curative, rehabilitative, preventive, and health-promotive action leading to the control of both communicable and noncommunicable diseases is not possible without influencing human behavior in some way.[2, 3] This is true not only of the individual and the family in private life, but also of those leaders and power figures and organized groups who by their decisions and actions influence the state of health of their communities. From the remote African village with its chief and village council to the mayor and councilmen of a large American city, there are groups of power figures whose function is to influence, to control in varying degrees, and to exercise vigilance over the lives of others in manifold ways. To a differing extent in various communities, groups emerge to wrestle with problems not soluble by the action of individuals alone. Thus, the control of disease and the promotion of health depends on the degree to which it is possible to influence not only the personal, private behavior of the individual and family, but also the public decisions and actions of organized groups and community leaders.

Behavioral Development, Stability, and Change

If human behavior is important in public health and medical care and if affecting change in behavior is the basic task of health education, it is necessary to know more about behavior itself. This includes knowledge concerning the forms behavior takes in different individuals, groups, and communities; what factors make for stability in such forms of behavior; and how change in behavior occurs in natural, unplanned ways as against change brought about by deliberate planning.

No matter into which community an individual is born and in which he lives his life, maturation and learning during growth take place in a human relationship setting, surrounded by others who interact with him. In the first years, his parents or parent-substitutes take an active responsibility in rearing him in the ways of his community, and in differing degrees and at different stages, other members of his family and network of kin participate in the process. While each family, or child-rearing group, will have certain unique characteristics, at the same time it is in this immediate social life-space that the individual experiences and learns the customs of perception and thought, of feeling, and of outward behavior which are characteristic of his community as a whole. These customs will be based on universal human needs, but their form and expression are subject to great cultural variability, each community having a certain uniqueness in this respect.

In addition to being a member of his community as a whole, the individual is usually a member of a class within it. This class will have its own particular variations of customs which are characteristic of the total culture, and this membership of a class will also leave its mark on the individual. Children reared as members of a higher status or income class will, for example, have a different experience of growing up from those in a lower status or income class. Such socioeconomic class differences may be more marked in some communities than in others, and upward mobility from one class to another may be more restricted. Thus, the social distance, as it were, between a wealthy Ethiopian landowner and a tenant farmer on his land may be considerably greater than that between a New Jersey industrialist and a machinist in his factory.

During socialization, the complex belief, feeling, and behavior systems of the individual's community and social class become deeply embedded in his personality and in his view of the world. While socialization may be faster and exert more fundamental influence in the earlier years, the process of learning to live the life of one's group probably proceeds to some degree throughout life. However, regardless of the changes that the individual may exhibit from time to time, there remains a remarkable stability in the habit systems with which his earlier life experience endows him. This stability in individual behavior patterns is simply a reflection of a similar stability of the customs of his community as a whole.

The behavior or habits of the individual, and the customs of the community as a whole are not randomly assembled items. Rather, they form systems. A system consists of a set of elements which are related to one another in such a way that change in one or more elements will have associated change in other elements in the system. Thus, the habits of the individual are not free, discrete, independent elements, but rather tend to be linked with and dependent on one another. There is a certain internal consistency in the behavior of any single individual. In the same way, the customs of the community are closely related and interwoven with one another in the seamless fabric of culture.

Thus, the diurnal cycle of behavior in the individual may be seen as a stream of behavior rather than as a procession of discrete behaviors. The daily behavior of a Samoan fisherman and that of a Los Angeles office worker would each present a picture of a flow of action in which each episode was triggered by what preceded it. In the behavior of each, there would probably be a high degree of repetition from day to day with a generally predictable sequence as if the behavior had been carefully planned, scheduled, and practiced. Thus, the stability and the system properties of behavior are not only a function of one another and together make for a feeling of security, but also in these very characteristics represent a protection against change.

Since man is a social being, the individual and his group are inseparable. Isolated individuals are oddities in most communities and are frequently regarded as mentally ill. The behavior systems of individuals are largely the product of group pressures to conformity, are maintained by such group pressures, and are likely to be changed mainly (or often, only) through group influence and change. The rate and direction of change will vary from one community to another. It may take place more readily and rapidly in the vast migration and population area of southern California than in the more remote, isolated, homogeneous, and smaller population of the Yap Islands of Micronesia.

Moreover, in any human community there are individuals who exercise somewhat more influence than others both in maintaining the stability of customs and in inducing change. Of these, there are the more obvious, visible formal leaders who find their place in various organized community groups. Such leaders are usually clustered in the higher status classes in the community. By and large they recognize their own roles in this respect and are usually clearly seen by others as exercising such roles. Recent studies [4] have drawn attention to the fact that, in addition, there are to a great extent less visible, less formal leaders as well. Such opinion leaders, as they have been called, exercise a more informal, interpersonal influence within the families, small primary groups, and communication networks of which they are themselves members. The opinion leaders and their networks exist in all classes of a community and therefore have an important part to play in the acceptance or rejection of change through the whole range of social levels.

Thus, regardless of the forces making for perpetuation of habits and customs, there are also natural determinants of change. The use of the term *developing* countries is a recognition of their relatively rapid shedding of much of the conservatism and traditionalism that has characterized them for generations past. Contemporary history is replete with evidence of the pain and turmoil which often accompanies such change. As a single example, the rural-urban migration occurring today in those countries undergoing industrial revolutions is both a symptom and a determinant of change in the daily life behavior of millions of people.

All human communities are changing in different ways and at different rates. All people have felt needs not being met and are to some extent striving for something better from life. Not the least of these needs is greater freedom from the threat of disease and death.

THE HEALTH EDUCATION PROCESS

The Place of Health Knowledge in Health Education

The nature and task of health education gain greater meaning when viewed against the background of the role of behavior in health and of the natural, unplanned forces affecting both stability and change in behavior. Such a background helps to place the "educational" aspect of health education in proper perspective. Education is almost universally conceived to be an intellectual process or, more narrowly, the acquisition of knowledge. Education may be, and frequently is, expected to exert an influence on character and personality development. Nonetheless, at least in the Western world, within schools, colleges, and universities, the measure of achievement is essentially measurement of change in knowledge. There is, therefore, the tendency to transfer to health education the assumption that its functions are being fulfilled if it raises the level of general knowledge and information about health matters. Thus, its main task is often conceived to be the transmission of accurate health facts to the public at large.

Unfortunately, studies and experience both suggest that change in health-related behavior is only under special circumstances triggered by new knowledge alone. To dispense with knowledge altogether as a determinant of change would be patently absurd; clearly not only does knowledge contribute to the direction change may take, but perceptual and intellectual functions cannot be abruptly separated from the emotional and motivational.

It would appear, however, that human motivation, or what people feel they want, is one of the most important determinants of behavior change. To the extent that *new knowledge* provides a relatively simple, understandable, direct solution to a *felt need,* it is likely to be successful. Thus, polio may be felt as a threat which people want reduced and for which there is a highly effective and simple solution in the form of immunization. As a consequence, countries as widely differing as the United States and Israel can report outstanding success in having their respective populations seek immunization. On the other hand, cancer is at least equally threatening but, unlike polio, there is no single, simple, effective protective measure. In this case, the dissemination of knowledge about cancer may well produce defensive and rejecting reactions among the very segments of the population who need diagnosis and care the most. There are probably a great number of smokers in the Western countries today who know what is being said about the relationship between smoking and lung cancer, but this seems to have made little or no impact on the cigarette smoking habit, except perhaps among a few special groups such as physicians. They, incidentally, may be reacting as much to the pressures of their special image and role in the community as to the specific knowledge to which they have access.

The place of knowledge, per se, in bringing about behavior change is further illustrated by the similarities and differences between three problems in weight reduction and control presented, first, by obese middle-class American women; second, by normal or slightly overweight middle-class American women; and third, by obese Zulu women in South Africa. The content or knowledge component, nutritional in nature, for each of these three problems may well be the same in all essentials. There are, however, certain major differences between the problems from the standpoint of health education. Thus, the obese American women are outside the culturally acceptable limits in weight and appearance and may have marked emotional problems that require a psychotherapeutic component in the attempt to effect change. The second group is within the normal cultural limits for middle-class American women, has managed to maintain at least a near-normal weight even in the midst of an abundance of available weight-inducing foods, and therefore presents largely an informational task in the prevention of weight gain. The third group, consisting of obese African women, is within the normal cultural limits of that society, is actually regarded as somewhat more attractive than slimmer women, and therefore presents a task involving changes in the esthetic standards of the community as a whole.

Generally then, the nature and role of health education in its function of attempting to change health-related behavior are perhaps more evident in the work of behavioral scientists interested in change [5, 6] than in works concerned essentially with methods of communicating knowledge.[7] Clearly, however, the latter do have a place and this is largely a matter of emphasis.

Analysis of the Behavioral Aspects of a Health Education Problem

The effectiveness of any method used in the solution of a health education problem is dependent on an analysis of the nature of the behavioral aspects of the problem in the life of members of the target group and on the nature of the change to be brought about. This analysis prior to action would include at least three components.

The first component consists of identification of the target group whose health-related behavior is the objective of the change attempt. This might be the community as a whole or any category within it such as a specific socioeconomic class, a particular group such as industrial workers of a certain kind, an age or sex group such as the elderly or adolescent boys, and so on.

The second component of the analysis consists of an examination and assessment of the communication and influence networks of which the target group members are a part. This would include the more formal leaders as well as the opinion leaders who exert a special influence within these networks. Thus, obviously when dealing with young children as the target group, the adults, such as parents and teachers, who largely control or influence their lives are important and even indispensable in developing an effective program. On the other hand, with adolescent boys the role of adults in many societies may be relatively less significant, and the leadership within the ranks of the adolescent boys themselves would have to be identified.

The third component of the analysis concerns the nature of the behavior to be changed from the special point of view of its potentiality for change. Thus, the question has to be asked what the target group and relevant others know, believe, and feel about the problem, and what they may be doing about it.[8, 9] In this connection, the underlying consideration is whether a change in knowledge through the dissemination of information is likely to be effective, or whether there are deeper emotional and motivational obstacles and resistances to be overcome. Moreover, the practical feasibility of change also has to be considered. The proposed program, for example, may be demanding a radical change in the pattern of people's lives or the use of resources and facilities that simply are not available.

General Health Education Methods

There are numerous specific techniques which traditionally have been used in health education. These include the individual interview, group discussion, formal presentation to an audience, and the use of nonpersonal methods such as radio and television, films, posters, and pamphlets. However, the use of any of these techniques should always be based on an insight into the basic theory of how they work, and the kinds of target groups and tasks for which they may be most appropriate. There is little or no value to be derived from their routine or mechanical use.

In the health education process, there is a close relationship between the attempts to change behavior in the private life of the individual and the attempts, commonly known as community organization,[10] to develop organized groups of community members that will take public action for the health of the community as a whole or of particular groups within it. Thus, community organization involves the development of formal planning and implementation of health programs as a cooperative venture between agency and community, directed toward health education of the individual in his private life as well as the provision of conditions and services that make possible and facilitate behavior change in the individual. It may, for example, be not only the means whereby a building is provided in a suitable location for use as a clinic, but also the means for educating the target group to use it.

A recognition of the importance of health education in the control of disease and the promotion of health, and an awareness of the need for further development of health education theory and methods, have given rise to the development of a specific professional group known as health education specialists (called "health educators" in the United States). These personnel, qualified with a graduate degree in public health with concentration in health education, have the special responsibility for developing the health education component of services. A primary function of such specialists is to strengthen the health education role of other health personnel.

Thus, health education is also a function of all other health workers and of medical personnel who are in direct contact with the community. The physician in his consulting room giving guidance to the patient, the nurse in the maternal and child health program advising mothers on child care, the sanitarian persuading a restaurant owner to alter a practice in his kitchen are all attempting to influence health-related behavior. These personnel are, then, in one degree or another, health educators.

Selection of Appropriate
Health Education Methods

Current scientific knowledge is somewhat limited regarding the specific health education method which is appropriate for a given situation whose nature has been assessed through an analysis of the behavioral aspects of the problem to be solved. Studies and experience have to date, however, indicated certain possibly valid principles.

Nonpersonal and mass methods of communication may be quite appropriate where there is already a fairly strong felt need and where there is a relatively direct, effective line of action to accomplish the desired end. When these methods are considered appropriate in respect to any specific health problem, whatever media are to be used should be systematically pretested on a small sample of the target population. This makes possible some modification of the media if they appear unlikely to achieve their purpose. Sometimes pretesting may result in their rejection altogether. Thus, pretesting the responses of a sample of Zulu women to posters contrasting obese and slim women showed that the women rejected the message and favored the obese figure as a mark both of beauty and of affluence.

Interpersonal methods may be more appropriate wherever there is any kind of emotional resistance, where the message may be threatening, where there is no easy solution to a felt problem, or where there is no felt need. The relative power of interpersonal methods is perhaps best seen in small group techniques where, in group discussion and decision, use is made of group cohesiveness, of emotional support of the members for one another, and of relatively free self-expression to bring about change.[8] The special value of the interpersonal methods is that the individual or group target of the influence attempt is able to express reactions and feelings, thus enabling the educator and others to perform mutually interacting diagnostic and educative functions concurrently.

In any single health program, however, not one but a number of health education methods tends to be used. There is often, then, an intricate planning problem in the selection of methods in terms of their specific purposes, target groups, appropriate settings, various combinations, and possible sequence.

Whatever the specific methods being used, there is a basic consideration affecting them all. This is the degree to which they can contribute to the reduction of the sociocultural distance between the health professional and the community he is serving. In the first place, the health professional has health as his overriding concern and the conscious, central objective of his daily work. The health of any community is of fundamental importance. However, few if any of the communities, groups, or individuals with whom the health professional deals have health as the central, deliberate concern of their daily lives. This fact assumes added significance when it is combined with the general cultural and class distance that so frequently exists between professionals and the people they serve. Thus, for example, a Swedish physician in a WHO tuberculosis control program on his first assignment to an African country is likely to begin work with quite a considerable sociocultural gap between himself and the community. Similarly, a physician in private practice in his own country and working with fellow nationals but serving, say, mainly blue-collar workers and their families would have a somewhat narrower but no less real gap with which to contend owing to his higher socioeconomic status.

The health professional, therefore, has to learn to see the world through the eyes of the community. He needs to have an understanding of the community, its beliefs, felt needs, and aspirations, and of the place of the "problem" (which, incidentally, the community may not itself see as a problem) in the daily life of that community.[11]

Since this understanding is to be developed not for its own sake but in order to achieve some kind of prospective change, community organization is one important means for reducing the professional-lay distance beginning with the earliest stages of program development. Community organization involves working intimately with lay members of the community in defining and analyzing problems, in planning ways to deal with the problems, and in implementing the plans. Thus, it is important that those who do participate are at least partly drawn from the particular groups who are themselves most involved in the change. If membership of such organized groups consists predominantly or entirely of people drawn from classes or subcultures different from the target group, while they may provide power over certain resources, they may do little to reduce sociocultural distance and may even increase it. Thus, upper middle-class, Anglo-American "leadership" and community groups may have little influence among lower socioeconomic Mexican-Americans.

The various methods of bringing about change in health-related behavior require continuing study and research, both basic and applied, particularly by behavioral scientists. The methods also need experimental innovation and testing by practitioners in the field. The evaluation of the effectiveness of ongoing programs is one important source of knowledge about health education methods.

EVALUATION OF THE EFFECTIVENESS OF HEALTH EDUCATION

A perennial problem, and one which is gaining increasingly serious attention today both in the United States and in the rest of the world, is that of the evaluation of the health education component of health programs. Evaluation consists of all those procedures that provide an appraisal of the degree to which, and in what respects, the program or its health education component is achieving its stated objectives.[8, 9, 12] In this connection, it is important to have some knowledge of the change taking place independently of the program so that changes resulting predominantly from other factors are not attributed to the program itself.

Evaluation is often spoken of as if it were an independent form of appraisal not intrinsic to the program itself. In fact, the basic procedures involved in evaluation are basic and internal attributes of a sound program and are quite inseparable from it. Thus, in examining the nature and extent of the health education problem, part of the process is the establishing of quantitative base lines, or starting points. For example, one such base line might be the proportion of women of a certain age group in a specific community who made use of cervical cancer diagnosis facilities in a stated period of time. Base-line data give the program meaning and justification, indicate the extent of the task, and make possible the precise definition of an objective. However, they are also essential for proper evaluation since, unless change in the base line can be measured during progress of the program, there is no reliable way of telling whether and to what degree the program is effective in terms of the objective.

Evaluation is often desirably done not only in respect to the health education component as a whole, but also in respect to its constituent parts such as some of the specific methods being used. Thus, some methods may be included primarily to raise the level of public knowledge about a problem, others primarily to develop more favorable attitudes toward the particular agency concerned with the problem, and others to trigger action in those most personally affected by the problem. Measurement of the effectiveness of these methods in attaining their objectives is part of evaluation.

Since the objectives of health education are concerned with demonstrably health-related outcomes, the primary focus of health education evaluation should be on overt behavior change. However, evaluation may be, and perhaps too frequently is, concerned with the measurement of knowledge and of attitude change, both of which may be necessary precursors to changing overt behavior but which often are not. Thus, knowledge about and attitudes toward cigarette smoking are, in themselves, from the viewpoint of health and of health education less important than the act of smoking. Health education in this case would be concerned primarily with an actual reduction, say, of the smoking adoption rate by school-age children. This change in the smoking adoption rate may conceivably be brought about by means other than changing knowledge about and attitudes towards smoking —if, indeed, the latter can bring it about at all. It is conceivable that change in the smoking adoption rate of schoolchildren might be accomplished by increasing their supervised recreation and outdoor activity time. No doubt this would and could be accompanied by changes in knowledge and attitudes about smoking, but such changes may well be incidental to the development of more enjoyment and participation in outdoor games.

One basic problem of evaluation lies in the role of the practitioner, who, being far from disinterested in the success of his program and very much involved in its planning and operation, is attempting at the same time objectively to appraise its success. There may also be limitations on the evaluation methods which the practitioner can apply. The obligation of a service to do the best for the whole of the population for whose health it is responsible makes it difficult, for example, to apply experimental design in which control groups receive no such service or to resist modifying methods at the first indications they are ineffective and before the final data are collected.

SPECIAL PROBLEMS IN
HEALTH EDUCATION PROGRAMS

Health education deals with behavior variables that are far more elusive of identification and analysis than are physical and biologic variables. Furthermore, although its methods are generally accepted, they are not necessarily of proved effectiveness except in limited respects. For these and other reasons, patterns of health education tend to vary considerably according to the settings within which they are developed. Thus, there is quite a serious schism between the practice of health education in the community and the practice in school settings. Health education in the schools is generally considered to exercise its effect through the total experience of living and working in a healthful school environment, through the medium of school health services, and through classroom instruction.[13] Not unsurprisingly, however, it is the latter upon which reliance frequently is placed. When this occurs, school health education is simply conforming to the normal school reliance on classroom instruction that is used in teaching of mathematics, history, language, and other subjects. In marked contrast to the largely captive audience of the classroom is the vast noncaptive, target population of health education in community settings. Thus, the local public health department and the voluntary health agency, dealing with large populations and having disproportionately small staffs, rely heavily on mass media and community organization, coming face to face in their health education efforts with only comparatively small segments of the population. In further contrast is health education in medical care. Medical care works with comparatively much smaller populations of users, coping usually only with those with whom its physicians and nurses can come in face-to-face contact. Health education in medical care, therefore, is a function largely of the individual interview and of small, intimate groups of patients.

Another problem of serious importance in health education programs is the apparently inaccessible pockets of lower socioeconomic and subcultural groups, particularly in large urban areas. On the one hand, the curative needs of such groups may be quite considerable, but they may have access solely to overcrowded clinics whose personnel, if only through sheer work pressure, have a certain social and personal remoteness. On the other hand, the same groups also are often served by other health agencies, both official and voluntary, which are using, first, mass-media methods that are inadequately pretested for communicating with them and, second, community organization methods with participants who, in terms of cultural background and social class, are markedly different from the target group.

A further problem is related particularly to the fact, mentioned earlier, that the health, behavior, and way of life of a community are essentially a whole system of related parts and not a series of discrete, independent elements. Over against this unity and organization in the natural order of human life, agencies often appear to be a rather fragmentary array of more or less independent services. In many of the countries of Africa and Asia, personal health problems requiring the whole spectrum of curative, rehabilitative, preventive, and health-promotive action are handled by a single unit, the health center. The United States is in marked contrast, with an astonishing variety of specialized services as the rule rather than the exception. Thus, the individual and his family are called on to relate with a number of agencies and personnel, and the more serious the problems, the more numerous these tend to be. Health education is heavily dependent on a continuity and intimacy of relationship which is hardly possible under such circumstances. Furthermore, there are families in American cities who carry such heavy burdens of illness and allied problems that it would become almost a full-time occupation if they were to respond to all the exhortations of health education to use the vast number of different services which they appear to need.

SUMMARY

Health education is that function of health and allied services which seeks to bring about change in health-related behavior. Human behavior plays a critical role in the etiology of health and disease and in the means of achieving cure, rehabilitation, prevention, and health promotion. From the standpoint of health education, *all* behavior is considered to be *health-related* and includes some forms of behavior which are *health-directed*. In the life of the individual, however, behavior is motivated by many factors among which concern for his health is of relatively minor importance.

Behavior in the individual, in the family and other small groups, and in the community is in many respects stable and resistant to change, but there are also forces such as group and leader influences and unmet felt needs which contribute to change. Degrees of stability and change vary from one community to another. Health education is a form of planned intervention attempting to influence largely unplanned, natural processes in such a way as to bring about an improved health status.

In the health education process, the communication of health *knowledge*, although it clearly has a place, is frequently not sufficient in itself to bring about change in health-related behavior. Health education practice may utilize interpersonal methods, nonpersonal methods, or both in combination. Not only the health education specialist but also all other health workers and medical personnel function as health educators. In order to determine the health education method that is appropriate to solve a particular problem, it is necessary to make a careful analysis of the way of life, of the feelings and motivations, and of the beliefs and knowledge of those who are the target of health services. On the basis of such an analysis, health education methods can then be selected which will be most likely to accomplish whatever health objectives have been defined. A major determinant of the effectiveness of any health education method is the degree to which it can reduce the sociocultural distance between the health professional and the community he is serving.

Evaluation of health education programs is important in order to determine the degree to which stated objectives are being achieved. Evaluation includes the assembly of base-line data, the measurement of the effectiveness of specific methods once they are in operation, and the measurement of the amount of change in overt behavior that has occurred as the result of the health education program.

Some of the special problems in current health education programs in the United States include the wide variations in patterns of health education that occur depending on the settings in which they are developed; the inadequate provision of health education for lower socioeconomic and subcultural groups; and the difficulty of achieving continuity and intimacy of relationship in the health education process in view of the vast number of existing specialized, independent health services and agencies.

REFERENCES

1. MANN, JOHN. *Changing Human Behavior*. Charles Scribner's Sons, New York, 1965.

2. KING, STANLEY H. *Perceptions of Illness and Medical Practice*. Russell Sage Foundation, New York, 1962.

3. KNUTSON, ANDIE L. *The Individual, Society and Health Behavior*. Russell Sage Foundation, New York, 1965.

4. KATZ, ELIHU, and LAZARSFELD, PAUL F. *Personal Influence: The Part Played by People in the Flow of Mass Communication*. The Free Press, Glencoe, Illinois, 1955.

5. GOODENOUGH, WARD HUNT. *Cooperation in Change*. Russell Sage Foundation, New York, 1963.

6. LIPPITT, RONALD, WATSON, JEANNE, and WESTLEY, BRUCE. *The Dynamics of Planned Change*. Harcourt, Brace & World Inc., New York, 1958.

7. KLEINSCHMIDT, HARRY E., and ZIMAND, SAVEL. *Public Health Education— Its Tools and Procedures*. The Macmillan Company, New York, 1953.

8. SOPHE RESEARCH COMMITTEE. *Review of Research Related to Health Education*. Health Education Monographs, Supplement No. 1, New York, 1963.

9. VEENKER, C. HAROLD, ed. *Synthesis of Research in Selected Areas of Health Instruction*. School Health Education Research Monograph, Samuel Bronfman Foundation, New York, 1963.

10. ROSS, MURRAY G. *Community Organization: Theory and Principles*. Harper & Brothers, New York, 1955.

11. PAUL, BENJAMIN D. *Health, Culture and Community: Case Studies of Public Reactions to Health Programs*. Russell Sage Foundation, New York, 1955.

12. STUDIES AND RESEARCH IN HEALTH EDUCATION. *International Conference on Health and Health Education, Philadelphia, Pennsylvania, USA, June 30–July 7, 1962*. Published by International Journal of Health Education, Geneva.

13. JOINT WHO/UNESCO EXPERT COMMITTEE. *Teacher Preparation for Health Education*. World Health Organization Technical Report Series No. 193, Geneva, 1960.

SECTION IV

PUBLIC HEALTH CHALLENGES AND OPPORTUNITIES

CHAPTER 14

POPULATION, HEALTH, AND WELFARE

Excessive population growth, which is currently a matter of grave concern, and trends in solving the problems of overpopulation are discussed in this chapter. The first section of the chapter provides a brief account of the past growth of world population and some estimates of future growth based on current rates of increase. The next two sections review the principal factors which have influenced population increases and the numerous deleterious consequences of a too rapid rate of population growth. Indirect methods of controlling population increase are discussed briefly in the fourth section, and family planning—as probably the only method that can be effective in the long run—is described. The fifth section reviews the status of family-planning programs in the United States, including the role of government at various levels. The last section of the chapter describes the efforts being made by other nations to control population growth and provides examples of specific family-planning programs in several different countries.

THE THREAT OF OVERPOPULATION

The imbalance created by high birth rates and declining death rates and the social and economic consequences of this imbalance have become matters of worldwide concern.[1-3] Biologists, health experts, and biostatisticians have for several decades directed national and international attention to the implications and consequences of an accelerated rate of world population growth which ultimately may exceed the capacity to meet the needs for food, clothing, shelter, health care, education, and employment. To some extent, the impending population crisis can be alleviated by international planning efforts. Such planning would involve devising the means to expand agricultural production, to utilize and share available natural and man-made resources, and to improve education. However, it is becoming increasingly clear that such efforts must also be accompanied by specific measures to limit population growth, if the threats inherent in overpopulation are to be minimized.

Past and Future Growth of World Population

The world population doubled in about 1700 years from the beginning of the Christian era until the middle of the seventeenth century; it doubled again in about 200 years; doubled again in less than 100 years, and if the current rate of population increase were to remain constant, it would double every 35 years. This would result in a population of 6 billion by the year 2000 and about 24 billion by the year 2070. It was not until 1850 that the world population reached 1 billion, but it took only another 75 years for the second billion, and 35 additional years for the third billion. At the present rate, it will take only 15 years for the fourth billion and ten for the fifth billion. World population currently is increasing at the rate of about 2 per cent per year. If this rate of increase had existed since early Christian times, there would be about 20 million individuals in place of each person now alive, or 100 people to each square foot of space. If the present world population should continue to increase at its present rate of 2 per cent each year, within two centuries there will be more than 150 billion people.

The increase in world population is occurring because 130 million infants are born each year, whereas only 60 million people die annually, resulting in a net gain of 70 million. Such rapid population growth is undoubtedly out of proportion to present and prospective rates of increase in socio-economic development and the ability to advance human welfare. The long-term prognosis—according to the Committee on Science and Public Policy of the National Academy of Sciences—is that "either the birth rate of the world must come down or the death rate must go back up." [4]

Population Growth in
Various Parts of the World

The rate of population growth varies among regions of the world and among nations. One notable difference occurs between the more developed and the less developed areas of the world. This is illustrated by Table 14-1, which shows that the less developed areas already have almost three quarters of the world's population and among the highest rates of population

TABLE 14-1 Estimated Population in 1965, Annual Per Cent Increase, and Number of Years for Population Doubling, Major World Regions

	Estimated Population, 1965		Estimated Average Annual % Increase, 1960–1970	No of Yr for Population to Double at Indicated Rate
	Millions	Per Cent of World Total		
World total	3288	100.0		
Less developed areas	2383	72.5		
Latin America	245	7.5	2.9	24
Africa	308	9.4	2.4	29
South Africa	967	29.4	2.4	29
East Asia	863	26.2	1.7	41
More developed areas	905	27.5		
Europe	442	13.4	0.8	87
Soviet Union	233	7.1	1.7	41
Northern America	213	6.5	1.4	50
Oceania	17	0.5	1.6	43

Source: Adapted from Nortman, D. L. The Population Problem. National Educational Television, 1965.

increase. Thus, it is estimated that Latin America, Africa, and South Asia will double their populations in from 24 to 29 years and that East Asia will double its population in 41 years. Latin America is the fastest growing population region in the world, increasing at the rate of about 3 per cent per year, and the rate of increase is accelerating. The death rate dropped sharply following World War II, but the birth rates have remained high. Among the Asian nations, India and Japan provide a marked contrast. India, with a population of over 460 million, has more people than in North and South America combined and almost as many people as there are in Europe; [5] the population of India will be over 1200 million by the year 2000 if the present growth rate continues. Japan is unique among the Asian countries because it is the only nation of any size that is industrial, urban, and literate. Japan's birth and death rates are among the lowest in the world. Both rates have been declining since 1920, but the most significant change occurred during the ten years after World War II when there was a 50 per cent drop in the birth rate. The birth rate is now a little below long-term replacement of the population.

Among the more developed areas, Table 14-1 shows that the growth rate in Europe is the slowest of any region in the world, requiring about 87 years to double the population. Among European countries, the lowest rate of increase is in Luxembourg, Belgium, and Sweden, and the highest is in the Netherlands, Portugal, and Spain. Iceland has a very low death rate, a high birth rate, and hence the highest rate of natural increase. In contrast to Europe, the population growth rate in the Soviet Union, Oceania, and Northern America is more rapid, doubling in 41 to 50 years (Table 14-1).

The United States has undergone a steady increase in population since
the first census was taken in 1790. This is indicated by Table 14-2, which
also shows, however, that the percentage of increase has fluctuated widely.
The greatest increases occurred in the decades before the Civil War, after

TABLE 14-2   Population and Increase over Preceding Census,
United States, 1790–1960

	Number *	Per Cent Increase Over Preceding Census
1790	3,929,214	†
1800	5,308,483	35.1
1810	7,239,881	36.4
1820	9,638,453	33.1
1830	12,866,020	33.5
1840	17,069,453	32.7
1850	23,191,876	35.9
1860	31,443,321	35.6
1870	39,818,449	26.6
1880	50,155,783	26.0
1890	62,947,714	25.5
1900	75,944,575	20.7
1910	91,972,266	21.0
1920	105,710,620	14.9
1930	122,775,046	16.1
1940	131,669,275	7.2
1950	150,697,361	14.5
1960	178,464,236	18.4

Source: Adapted from U.S. Bureau of the Census. *Statistical Abstract of
the United States, 1965*, p. 5.
* Excludes Alaska and Hawaii.
† Not applicable.

which there was a decline, the percentage reaching an all-time low during
the depression years of the 1930's. The history of population growth in the
United States has been affected by several factors, including immigration,
which was stimulated by developments such as land expansion and the need
for labor manpower, and the birth rate, which has been subject to various
influences such as war and economic depression. Based on the increasing
growth rates of recent years, it is estimated that the population of the United
States will reach about 362 million by the year 2000.

INFLUENCES ON POPULATION INCREASES

The major influences on population increase are those that contribute
to increased longevity and a sustained high birth rate. A country with a
birth rate of 20 per 1000 population and a death rate of ten or less per 1000
population risks a doubling of its population in 40 to 50 years. Nations with

birth rates of 40 to 50 and death rates of 8.5 to 15 (per 1000 population) will have a much faster rate of population increase. Survival rates at birth, during the first year of life, and in early childhood have been spectacularly favorable in recent decades for most countries.

The first significant contribution to survival and longevity came through new knowledge of the causes of the epidemic diseases such as typhus, plague, yellow fever, dengue fever, and malaria. Discovery of the etiology and mode of transmission of these and other communicable diseases led to the development of effective control measures, including immunizations and vaccinations, and improved environmental sanitation practices such as the purification of public water supplies and the provision of waste disposal systems. The more developed nations first began to experience the benefits of these advances almost a century ago. Although the less developed countries began to share in the benefits only fairly recently, the period of time has been sufficiently long to effect a noticeable reduction in mortality rates even in those countries.

The increase in longevity accruing from the control of the communicable diseases has been augmented by several other medical advances and various social changes, at least in the more developed nations. Major discoveries in curative medicine, improved quality and greater availability of medical and nursing care, and expansion of medical care facilities and services have undoubtedly had an influence on survival rates. In addition to improved chances for surviving acute illnesses, the likelihood of surviving chronic and degenerative diseases has also become considerably greater. Improved nutrition, rising standards of living, and improved working conditions, supported by increased educational opportunities, are a few of several other kinds of factors that have probably helped to enhance life expectancy over the past several decades.

There are two significant results of increased survival and longevity, both of which affect population growth. One result is that more females survive into and through their childbearing period. Thus for a given generation of females, the possibility of having a maximum number of children is increased, and this possibility in turn is extended to their children and to their children's children, and so on. The second result is that an increasing number of people live into the period of old age, a possibility which will be further extended as the chronic and degenerative diseases are increasingly brought under control. Thus, the first phenomenon gives rise to a high birth rate, the second to a low death rate, and both together result in a rapid rate of growth for a given population.

CONSEQUENCES OF POPULATION INCREASE

There is grave concern about the possibility that the world's food-producing capacity may not be able to keep pace with the continued growth of the world population. For five years, the world's food supply has fallen short of population growth by at least 1 per cent a year and by 2 per cent in 1965. In addition, the food supply is not distributed evenly throughout the world. The distribution of arable land also is very uneven, and the supply of readily reclaimable land is becoming exhausted rapidly. Latin America can claim only 5 per cent of its area as arable, and India has very little additional land that can be brought into cultivation.[6] Widespread efforts to increase yields per acre on existing lands would encounter serious obstacles because many changes in agricultural techniques would have to be achieved, including the use of fertilizer in amounts that would exceed current world production.

In the less developed countries which have a predominantly agrarian economy, the struggle to obtain the bare necessities of life is particularly severe, and a rapidly growing population only presses harder against the relatively fixed resources of food and other production. A country with a high birth rate and a declining death rate has many dependents to provide for; for example, in the less developed areas, children under 15 years of age constitute between 35 per cent and 50 per cent of the population. Such an age imbalance presents not only a severe problem of support, but also an enormous burden of education in a nation which probably already has a low educational level and a high rate of illiteracy. Furthermore, until the educational deficit is overcome, these nations have little hope of obtaining the skilled manpower needed to achieve a more advanced economy. The average per capita income in less developed countries is estimated to be about $100 a year, and such marginal subsistence associated with high birth rates creates a trap from which neither families nor the nation can escape. When a rapidly expanding population is engaged largely in agriculture, the amount of cultivatable land that can provide employment becomes insufficient and there is not enough industry in urban areas to absorb the excess labor force. Thus in less developed areas, migration to urban centers often means only exchanging rural unemployment for urban unemployment.[6]

In the more developed nations, poverty and unemployment also present problems, but the most pressing, general consequences of excess population growth arise from large numbers of dependents and urban crowding, thus giving rise to environmental pollution, transportation congestion, and dwindling open space and recreational areas. The dependent population consists of first, a relatively large group of older persons steadily augmented by increasingly earlier retirement from the labor force and second, an even larger group of younger people that remains dependent longer as the period of education increases. As a consequence, people in the mid-age range support an increasing larger percentage of the population.

In the United States, the high birth rate that followed World War II will, alone, continue to have serious ramifications for many years to come.[7, 8] Thus, it is estimated that there will be an increase of about a million high school graduates a year and a tripling of college enrollments within 20 years. In the labor market, there will be a virtual avalanche of young persons seeking jobs at a time when automation is reducing employment opportunities. The result, it is expected, will be an increase by 1980 in the number of unemployed which, even at present rates, will be more than half as great as was experienced during the depression of the 1930's. Housing for about 800,000 new households each year will be required, with corresponding increases in the need for medical care provisions, environmental sanitation measures, transportation means, and recreational facilities. Thus, it is becoming increasingly clear that in a nation which is industrialized, urbanized, and becoming more automated, a too rapid population growth is a socioeconomic liability.

ALTERNATIVE METHODS OF POPULATION CONTROL

Indirect Methods of Controlling Population

In individual nations, population growth can be inhibited by certain economic factors. Thus, as population increases out of proportion to a country's gross national product, family limitation tends to occur, but only in the upper 10 to 30 per cent of the socioeconomic strata. There is also some evidence in Western Europe and in the United States of an inverse relationship between the labor force participation of married women and the size of their families. Economic depression serves to curtail population increase, but as indicated earlier in connection with trends in the United States, the decline is likely to be relatively temporary. The principal shortcoming of any of these economic factors as influences on population growth is that they are not likely to operate uniformly within a nation, among nations, or over long periods of time.

Social policies may be devised to limit population growth, such as the provision of incentives for later marriages and for smaller families. However, an attempt of this kind has been made only once in history, when a number of German states in the mid-nineteenth century restricted permission to marry to those couples who presumably would be able to support a family.[9] The social and political climate in most nations today are, of course, not favorable to such methods for controlling population growth.

Family Planning as a Method of Population Control

Family planning and family limitation programs constitute the most direct approach to the problem of overpopulation and, because they can be universally applied, are probably the only means which, in the long run, can be effective. The concept and methods of family planning are influenced by the social and cultural institutions of the various countries of the world. However, a growing appreciation of the small family and the practice of family limitation is found in both Western and Eastern countries, in industrial and agricultural societies, and among many social, economic, and religious groups.

In the ideal family-planning program, the children who are conceived and born are wanted, and the number of offspring are commensurate with family, community, and national resources, thus assuring a reasonable standard of living and the opportunity for personal development for all children. Furthermore, information on family planning is made available equally to all socioeconomic groups, and with a knowledge and understanding of the methods, the individual then has complete freedom to make a choice that is compatible with his cultural and religious background. Family-planning programs operate on a systematic, organized basis and include appropriate educational and medical services.

Family-planning methods and practices for the prevention of unwanted pregnancies have developed over the centuries and vary widely throughout the world. The oldest practices for family spacing are periodic or total abstinence and withdrawal, or coitus interruptus. One form of periodic abstinence is the *rhythm method,* which involves refraining from sexual intercourse while the woman is at highest risk of conception during ovulation. The principal problem in the rhythm method is that of establishing the true menstrual pattern and thus determining the exact period during which abstinence must be practiced (varying from 11 to 18 days). The failure rate of this method tends to be higher than with other methods. In addition to the rhythm method, there are other well-known techniques that are selectively used, such as various types of jellies, creams, foams, and douches; diaphragms; and, of course, condoms, which have been used for years in the Western world.

In recent years, oral contraceptives and various intrauterine devices have become popular and well-known. *Oral contraceptives* are synthetic progesteronelike steroid pills which prevent ovulation and permit the regular recurrence of uterine bleeding at about 28-day intervals.[10] This method affords a high degree of protection once it is regulated and carefully practiced. It is satisfactory for some population groups, but the costs and use requirements are beyond the reach of much of the world population. There are many *intrauterine devices* of various shapes, generally made of flexible plastic material. These plastic rings, coils, or other shapes are inserted through the cervical canal and return to their original form in the uterus. This method of contraception is believed to be both safe and very effective, requiring little action by the individual once the device is implanted. It has a low cost, is protective over a long period of time, requires only the decision to use it, and probably is the most effective contraception for the less educated, less motivated, and less self-controlled.

There is evidence that *sterilization* is being used by an increasing percentage of selected population groups in the United States, Japan, and India. This method of birth control requires a safe, simple surgical technique in either the male or female. The vasectomy for sterilization of the male is the surgical removal of a portion of the vas deferens, which is the excretory duct of the testicle. Female sterilization is also a safe procedure requiring a small abdominal incision to tie and cut the fallopian tubes, which prevents the ovum, or female egg, from reaching the uterus and being united with the male sperm. Both male and female sterilization is popular in Japan and India, and female sterilization is popular in Puerto Rico. The advantage of this method is the degree of permanency and the freedom from the need for continuous application that characterizes other methods of contraception. Owing to the permanency, use of this method is often delayed until the family has "enough" children (an average of about four). Thus, this procedure tends to be used by older age groups. There is rarely any psychologic or related physiologic reaction following the sterilization and none in cases adequately evaluated and selected beforehand.

Induced abortion has been and is being used as a means of birth control, but because of potential dangers to the woman's health, it is no substitute for a national policy supporting and promoting natural and other more acceptable methods of family planning. The rate of abortions and the death rates due to illegal or spurious abortions will continue in many groups until there is universal opportunity for family-planning information and services. However, circumstances such as rape, risk to the life of the mother, or risk of producing a malformed infant will continue to require laws which will permit controlled legal abortion unrelated to birth control.

There are arguments, supported somewhat by European (particularly Scandinavian) and American experience in the past, that population groups with higher standards of living and increased education will practice family planning, utilizing the methods that are available and acceptable. While improved socioeconomic conditions may have a favorable influence in reducing population increase, the goal of achieving population balance demands realistic world programs of control through voluntary individual family planning, irrespective of economic considerations. In general, for programs for voluntary control of family size to be effective, there needs to be both a high degree of individual motivation *and* availability and knowledge of the utility of birth control procedures.

Research will undoubtedly in the long run lead the way to the most efficient, practical, and acceptable methods of birth control. Immunologists may some day develop a vaccine for the female against the spermatozoa or against the development of placental tissues. A vaccine for males may be discovered some day which would prevent the development of active sperm mobility or of sperm ability to fertilize the ovum. Vaccination is a procedure well accepted and would enhance fertility control. In the meantime, it will be necessary to continue to incorporate already available family-planning methods into regular health and medical care practice as an essential part of comprehensive health care.

FAMILY PLANNING IN THE UNITED STATES

The American public, the various levels of government, and professional and religious groups have been reluctant to recognize the potential effects of excessive population increases on future health and welfare. This has resulted in a lag in generating broad and systematic programs in family planning in the United States. The higher socioeconomic groups of the population have been able to some extent to obtain advice and assistance through private medical care, but because of past religious and political fears, the poor, who rely on public tax-supported programs for much of their medical care, have been denied family-planning services.[11]

In spite of general apathy and resistance, efforts have been made during the last several decades to promote and provide programs in family planning. A number of local health departments for many years "bootlegged" family planning and counseling into their maternal and child health programs. The Population Council and the Planned Parenthood–World Population organization—the latter founded by Margaret Sanger 50 years ago—promoted family-planning clinics, public education, and demonstrations. Policies and positions in support of family planning were developed by many state health and welfare agencies, the World Health Organization, the United Nations, the National Academy of Sciences, and several professional groups (e.g., the American Public Health Association, the American Social Welfare Association, and the American Medical Association).

More recently, attitudes have begun to change, so that a large majority of the public now expresses approval of making birth control information available to everyone who wants it. There is a growing recognition of the desirability of family planning as a means of permitting the American woman to make an independent contribution to society. Family planning allows her to be both a mother and a participant in the labor force if she wishes, to protect her own health and that of her children, and to assist in the maintenance of a more economically secure family unit.

Interests of the United States
Government in Family Planning

There is increasing involvement of various agencies of the federal government in family-planning services stimulated by both the executive and the legislative branches. In 1966, President Lyndon B. Johnson in his special message to Congress stated that, "We have a growing concern to foster the integrity of the family and the opportunity for each child. It is essential that all families have access to information and services that will allow freedom to choose the number and spacing of the children within the dictates of individual conscience."

The national government's role in family-planning programs is indicated

TABLE 14-3 Federal Financial Support for Family Planning, by Fiscal Years

	1965	1966	1967
		(in Thousands)	
Department of Health, Education, and Welfare	*	$ 8,956	$13,406
Office of Economic Opportunity	$ 437	1,963	3,000
National Science Foundation †	347	167	—
Department of the Interior	2	43	52
Department of State	247	333	398
Agency for International Development	1,328	3,240	8,425
Total	2,361	14,702	25,281

Source: The Population Crisis Committee. *Population Crisis.* The Committee, Washington, D.C., January–February 1967.
* Not available.
† Selected biology projects.

by Table 14-3, which shows the principal participating agencies and the increasing magnitude of federal financial support, totaling $42.3 million for the three-year period of 1965 through 1967. Although the figures are estimates, they include readily identifiable family-planning activities in the fields of information, counseling, services, training, research, and demonstration. Leadership at the federal level, it is anticipated, will help to stimulate increasing services by state and local agencies, hospitals, voluntary clinics, and private physicians.[12] The recent initiation of a program to assist communities and educational institutions in the provision of family-life education and sex education indicates that new federal policies are emerging.

The U.S. Department of Health, Education, and Welfare supports family planning through programs in the Public Health Service, the Food and Drug Administration, and the Welfare Administration. The *Food and Drug Administration* assesses oral contraceptives and intrauterine devices. The *Public Health Service* supports some family planning activities as part of grant-in-aid programs for state and local direct health services, training of personnel, and demonstration projects. Family-planning information and services are incorporated in the medical care programs provided for personnel of the uniformed services and their dependents, for American Indians, and for Alaska natives. Research related to family planning is supported by the National Institute of Child Health and Human Development, including studies in the biologic and behavioral process of reproduction, the determinants of population growth rates and family size, and new techniques of family planning. The Public Health Service also supports a variety of training programs directly or indirectly related to family planning.

Activities of the *Welfare Administration* that are related to family planning include an extensive program supported by the Children's Bureau, which provides family-planning assistance as part of comprehensive maternity care for low-income women. This program involves over 50 projects in 30 states, the District of Columbia, and Puerto Rico; the program also supports research and training activities in family planning. The Administration's public assistance medical care program under the Social Security Act—which, it will be recalled, was described in Chapter 5—may include expenditures for family-planning clinic services, and such provisions also are part of the new Medicaid program (Title XIX of the Social Security Act). Under this program, California, for example, has included family planning as a part of the medical services for indigent women, and private physicians, hospitals, and private agencies are eligible for reimbursement for the family-planning services they provide.

The Office of Economic Opportunity, through its Community Action Program Division, has stimulated and supported direct family-planning services for low-income women. This program ultimately may be especially effective because the clinics are, by design, situated in locations that are convenient for the women they intend to serve. The clinics also utilize aides who are recruited from the local neighborhoods.

In addition to these various agency programs, further evidence of the interest of the federal government in family planning is indicated by the fact that the United States Congress is giving increasing attention to the problem of population growth and limitation of family size.[12] Legislation has been proposed which would provide for an office of population affairs and a new post of Assistant Secretary in the Department of Health, Education, and Welfare. The new office would develop and coordinate all programs and activities in the field of family planning in the United States. Legislation has also been proposed to authorize the Secretary of the Department of Health, Education, and Welfare to make grants to state and local public agencies and to private organizations for the support of comprehensive family-planning programs.

The States and Communities in Family Planning

Thirty-two state health departments and the District of Columbia and an estimated 20 per cent of local health departments have some kind of official family-planning programs. Both the need and the potential for continued development of family-planning services have been well documented.[12] The women presently denied access to these services can be identified, and in general, it is known how to design programs with respect to optimum location, auspices, budgeting, and staffing. Adequate technology exists and further improvements will be forthcoming. Costs are modest compared to other social and medical programs, and long-run results are likely to be significant if relevant professions, public agencies, and hospitals implement and broaden existing programs.

The physician in private practice has an important role in promoting family planning. The advantages of planning and spacing pregnancies can be discussed with pregnant women before and after delivery. While nursing and social welfare personnel may indoctrinate, attempt to educate and influence, and refer women for family-planning services, it is the medical profession that is expected to respond in a positive, realistic way. Physicians need to stimulate the interest of patients in family planning, and they should advise the use of whatever contraceptive method is consistent with the cultural and economic background of the patient.

The cooperative efforts of the health science professions, official health agencies, and voluntary organizations can create the environment for effective programs of family-planning services in the community. Various programs are emerging, including public education, in-service training of personnel, demonstration service centers, and systems of referral and follow-up. For example, Colorado has involved a broad range of community resources in a series of family-planning clinics.[13] Some of the clinics are staffed entirely by the public health department; others are staffed by public health nurses and by volunteer physicians; and still other clinics, which are held in various public buildings, are staffed entirely by volunteers. Some degree of case finding and follow-up activity occurs in each of the arrangements. Many other states and communities have demonstrated that effective family-planning services can be developed through the resources of local health and welfare agencies, hospitals and outpatient clinics, and the medical profession.

Future Needs in Family Planning

Research is urgently needed to develop additional effective, safe, and acceptable methods of family planning. The National Advisory Child Health and Human Development Council has stressed the need for research on population dynamics, fertility, and sterility.[14] In addition, further development of specific contraceptive techniques is required through research, such as vaccines that would be relatively long lasting, a type of sterilization that would be reversible, pills that could be taken less frequently than is now necessary, or injections that could be given once a month or less often.

There is a great need for more complete awareness and understanding of the stresses that future generations will experience, if excessive population increase is allowed to continue. It is difficult for one generation to be concerned with the health and welfare of future generations, and usually only a relatively small minority of persons express such concern at any particular time. Furthermore, efforts to reduce the threat of overpopulation have been deterred by small, but powerful, organized groups whose influence has been out of proportion to their representation in the population, and whose views have been in conflict with public aspirations. In order to overcome these obstacles, the support of political statesmen, theologic leaders, and socially conscious economists and industrialists is essential.

Wholehearted support and concerted action on the part of state and local governing bodies is also required in order to achieve the goal of a population of optimum size.

Educational systems should make special efforts to foster and encourage the inclusion of family planning into existing courses and in the development of new courses. Special attention should be directed to the training programs for the professions of medicine, law, theology, teaching, nursing, social work, health education, and related groups. Such programs should include the study of the problems of excessive population increase and unwanted children and the methods of alleviating such problems.

FAMILY PLANNING IN OTHER COUNTRIES

A vast complex of cultural, socioeconomic, and political factors influence population growth in a particular nation. Furthermore, these factors differ from one country to another and play an important role in determining the success or failure of particular population control measures. During the past decade, an increasing number of nations that are particularly hard pressed by overpopulation began to deal with these complicated issues. In this relatively short period, a number of governments have reached or are working toward a national policy on population. In 1962, when the United Nations was formulating a policy on technical aid in the field of fertility regulation, virtually all the Asian and Arab nations voted in favor of the proposal; opposition came largely from the European countries, which, as indicated earlier, already have low birth rates. Thus, the present trend among developing nations to effect control of their population growth is motivated by forces within these nations, rather than being due to the imposition by Western countries of the kind of behavior which has helped to achieve their own favorable population balance.[15]

A number of international organizations offer support and assistance to the countries throughout the world that are trying to cope with a too rapidly growing population. During the 1965 World Health Assembly, the member nations of the World Health Organization unanimously approved a policy supporting research and technical aid in the field of human reproduction and fertility control. This will make available to governments, on request, a vast range of reference and expert advisory services. It will be recalled from Table 14-3, shown earlier in this chapter, that the Agency for International Development is the second largest recipient of United States government financial support for family-planning programs. The Agency provides needed technical and advisory help to more than 20 nations for population programs, training, and research. It also encourages developing countries that need aid for family and population planning activities to request whatever assistance is required.[16] Among the private and voluntary organizations that conduct valuable international programs in population control are the International Planned Parenthood Federation, the Population

Council, the Ford Foundation, the Pathfinder Fund, and the Rockefeller Foundation.

India initiated a national family-planning program in 1952 that was in effective operation by about 1956. In succeeding years increasingly large sums of money have been allocated for the program. As a result, more than 8000 rural and urban family-planning centers have been opened, and demonstration projects have been undertaken in a number of areas. There are educational programs directed to the public, for the training of personnel, and for the orientation of village leaders. Sterilization efforts were expanded in a few states, and sale of contraceptives has increased markedly in recent years. Although India has far to go in achieving an optimal rate of population increase, there are indications that at least in cities such as Bombay, the birth rate is declining.

Pakistan (with a large population) and *South Korea* (with a much smaller population) also have official national programs in family planning. In Pakistan, family-planning services have been added to 1600 medical units throughout the country, and there are also short training courses for medical and paramedical personnel. A National Research Institute for Family Planning has been established, and public education programs are being offered.[15] In South Korea, two or three full-time family-planning workers are employed in each of the country's 189 health centers, and 1400 assistant workers serve smaller areas. In addition, there are more than 1100 clinics which provide intrauterine devices and 700 vasectomy clinics. In 1966, there were nine family-planning teams working in the provinces as mobile units.

Taiwan has had a Family Planning Association for at least a decade, and an islandwide program in family planning has been in effect since 1965. The program is financed by the Population Council and the Joint Commission for Rural Reconstruction, a semiautonomous agency in Taiwan. Intrauterine devices are manufactured in Taiwan, and recently about 10,000 insertions have been performed each month. The Taiwan Population Studies Center, which was established in 1961, is responsible for evaluating the family-planning program. As part of a recently approved, long-range manpower development resources plan, the government has advocated a family-planning program to reduce the rate of population growth to 2 per cent per year.

The Philippines now has a nationwide family-planning program which, although it is not sponsored by the government, has significant governmental, medical, and church backing. The Family Planning Association, created in 1965, operates nine clinics in five different cities. Three of the health centers in Manila offer family-planning services, and there is a training project open to the staff of the city's 40 health centers. Oral contraceptive programs are being conducted in ten barrios.

Japan, as indicated earlier, has already been successful in planning and effecting a balance between population growth and resources. As the result of markedly increased rates of abortions occurring in the 1940's, the Eugenic

Protection Law permitting induced abortions was passed in 1948 and followed by various liberalizing amendments. The original intent of the law was to protect the health of the Japanese women rather than to control population. The Japanese people see no ethical or religious objection to abortion, and the general consensus is that abortion was an important or even principal factor in the decline in births in the postwar period. However, it was recognized that this practice was not a substitute for successful family planning and the use of contraceptive methods. As a consequence, Japan was one of the first nations in the world to undertake experimental and pilot projects in family planning. Japan's success in population control is attributed to abundant medical personnel and health centers, to adequate supplies and facilities, and to the high literacy and motivational levels of the people.[5]

In addition to South Asia and the Far East, there is also growing awareness of the problems of population pressure in other parts of the world. In the Near East, *Turkey* in 1964 repealed the strict antibirth control legislation which had been enacted during the 1920's and since then has initiated an extensive national family-planning program. *Iran* now includes family planning as an official part of the government's maternal and child health services, and in *Jordan,* the government has licensed the Jordan Family Planning Association to conduct clinics which are now in operation in several principal cities. The *United Arab Republic* has created a strong organizational framework directly under the Prime Minister which promotes national family planning. In 1965, the National Assembly resolved that contraceptives should be manufactured within the country and made available free of charge and that a campaign to educate the people in the importance of birth control should be started and should include the information that Islam presents no moral or theologic barriers to family planning.

In Africa, there is currently a rapid increase in the number of countries with voluntary family-planning associations and/or official family- and population-planning policies and activites. In *Tunisia,* legal restrictions against family planning were repealed in 1961, and an experimental program began in 1963. Fifty-nine hospitals and health centers are now providing intrauterine devices. *Nigeria* began organized family-planning work in 1958, and the Family Planning Council of Nigeria was set up as a national organization in 1964. Several family-planning clinics have been established, and a pilot project in the use of intrauterine devices is under way in Western Nigeria.

In Latin America, interest in family planning is now apparent in many countries, mainly in recognition of its importance for improving maternal and child health and because of growing concern over a sharply increased incidence of abortion. At least six Latin American countries now have national family-planning programs, and many others have substantial non-official family-planning organizations and activities. *Chile* has the most advanced program in Latin America, with family-planning clinics in government hospitals and health centers which serve over 150,000 women each year. In *Uruguay*, there is a family-planning clinic at a hospital in Monte-video, a research program is being conducted, and a variety of community projects are under way in family planning and sex education. In *Venezuela*, the Ministry of Health has established a Population Division, and the principal maternity hospital in Caracas has conducted a family-planning program since 1963.

These examples provide an indication of the kinds of attempts that are being made throughout the world to control excessive population growth. Numerous other nations have population control programs of various sorts, but a large number of countries have no program at all, even though they are also experiencing rapid growth rates.[16] Existing family-planning pro-grams in developing countries vary widely in scope, and most still are not adequate to meet the needs. A number of the more comprehensive programs are so new that it is not yet possible to assess their effectiveness. Some pro-grams operate under a handicap because they lack government sponsorship, even though they may have official approval. Thus, the problems of popula-tion control for the world as a whole are far from solved. Nevertheless, the serious efforts that are currently being made provide striking evidence of the fact that nations are no longer willing to endure the hardships and deprivations associated with uncontrolled population growth.

SUMMARY

The rapid growth of the world's population threatens to exceed the capacity to meet even the essential needs of daily living. Estimates of the magnitude of the population in future years, based on current rates of increase, indicate that measures to limit excessive growth are urgently needed. Although in Europe it will take almost a century for the population to double at its present rate of growth, in Latin America, Africa, and South Asia it will take only about a quarter of a century. Other major areas of the world range between these two extremes.

A rapid rate of population growth results when there is a high birth rate and a low death rate. Both rates are due to increased survival and longevity, which in turn are the result of several influences, including the control of communicable diseases, other medical advances in the control of acute and chronic illnesses, improved nutrition, and rising standards of living. As a consequence, females are now more likely to survive into and through their childbearing period, and an increasing number of people live into old age.

Unless excessive population growth is controlled, there is considerable doubt about the world's capacity to produce sufficient food. This is by no means the only cause for concern, however. In developing countries, there is not only a struggle for the bare necessities of life, but also a heavy burden of dependents, a low per capita income, a high rate of general unemployment, and many other deleterious social and economic consequences. In more developed nations, the most pressing problems resulting from excess population growth are large num-bers of dependents and urban crowding, which give rise to several other un-favorable circumstances.

There is some evidence that certain social and economic factors can inhibit population growth in a particular nation, but it would appear that these cannot be relied upon to alleviate the present threat. Family-planning and family limitation programs are probably the only measures which can be effective in the long run. Such programs help to ensure that only wanted children are born and that once born they can be provided for adequately.

In addition to several traditional techniques of family planning, two more recently developed methods are oral contraceptives and intrauterine devices. There is also evidence that sterilization of either the male or female is being used increasingly in various parts of the world as a method of birth control.

In the United States, long-standing resistance to family-planning programs gradually is being overcome, and recognition of the need for and desirability of such programs is increasing. There has been greater involvement of the federal government recently in the provision of family-planning services through the programs of several official agencies, and various legislative measures are under consideration by the United States Congress which would further strengthen the government's role in the field of family planning. A considerable number of state health departments, but far fewer local health departments, presently have official family-planning programs. Future needs in the United States include further research to develop additional methods of family planning, greater public understanding of the consequences of uncontrolled population growth, increased support of family-planning programs by influential groups and by governing bodies, and more education of professional groups in the need for and methods of family planning.

Factors that account for population growth, and solutions to the problems of excessive growth, are highly complex matters. Developing nations in particular are hard pressed by the magnitude of the problem and the complexities of the issues. Nevertheless, a number of nations have established national policies on population which are reflected in government-sponsored family-planning programs, and some other countries have begun to develop such programs on an official or unofficial basis. Many of the nations are being aided in their efforts by the resources of several international organizations. In general, trends in the direction of family planning are promising, although the problems of overpopulation in the world as a whole are still far from solved.

REFERENCES

1. BERELSON, B., ANDERSON, R. K., HARKAVY, O., MAIER, J., MAULDIN, W. P., and SEGAL, S. J., eds. *Family Planning and Population Programs: A Review of World Developments.* University of Chicago Press, Chicago, 1966.

2. SHEPS, M. C., and RIDLEY, J. C., eds. *Public Health and Population Change: Current Research Issues.* University of Pittsburgh Press, Pittsburgh, 1965.

3. MURAMATSU, M., and HARPER, P. A., eds. *Population Dynamics.* The Johns Hopkins Press, Baltimore, 1965.

4. NATIONAL ACADEMY OF SCIENCES-NATIONAL RESEARCH COUNCIL. *The Growth of World Population.* Publication 1091. National Research Council, Washington, D.C., 1963.

5. NORTMAN, D. L. *The Population Problem.* National Educational Television, New York, 1965.

6. MERRILL, MALCOLM H. An expanding populace in a contracting world. *JAMA*, **197**:114–19, August 1966.

7. BOGUE, DONALD J. Population growth in the United States. In: Hauser, P. M., ed. *The Population Dilemma*. Prentice-Hall, Englewood Cliffs, New Jersey, 1963.

8. CORSA, LESLIE, JR. Recent developments in public health family planning programs in the United States. In: Muramatsu, M., and Harper, P. A., eds. *Population Dynamics*. The Johns Hopkins Press, Baltimore, 1965.

9. GLASS, D. V. Population growth and population policy. In: Sheps, M. C., and Ridley, J. C., eds. *Public Health and Population Change: Current Research Issues*. University of Pittsburgh Press, Pittsburgh, 1965.

10. TAYLOR, HOWARD C. Evaluation of recent developments in contraceptive technology. *Amer J Public Health*, **56**:74–79, January 1966 (Supplement, Part II).

11. CORSA, LESLIE, JR. Family planning programs in the United States: introduction. *Amer J Public Health*, **56**:1–5, January 1966 (Supplement, Part II).

12. PERKINS, G. W., and RADEL, D. *Current Status of Family Planning Programs in the United States*. Planned Parenthood-World Population, New York, 1966.

13. TEPPER, SHERI E. A "package" plan for extension of birth control services. *Amer J Public Health*, **56**:22–28, January 1966 (Supplement, Part II).

14. U.S. DEPARTMENT OF HEALTH, EDUCATION, AND WELFARE, Public Health Service, National Institute of Child Health and Human Development. *The Recommendations of the National Advisory Child Health and Human Development Council on Research on Fertility, Sterility, and Population Dynamics*. U.S. Government Printing Office, Washington, D.C., 1966.

15. NOTESTEIN, FRANK W. Population growth—a challenge to public health. *Amer J Public Health*, **56**:80–84, January 1966 (Supplement, Part II).

16. AGENCY FOR INTERNATIONAL DEVELOPMENT, Office of Technical Cooperation and Research Health Service, Population Branch. *Assistance for Family Planning Programs in Developing Countries*. The Agency, Washington, D.C., 1967.

CHAPTER 15

PROFESSIONAL SERVICES AND CAREERS IN COMMUNITY HEALTH

Status of manpower in the health services

Medical and other professional practitioners

Nursing and related services

Laboratory services

Pharmacologic services

Nutritional and dietetic services

Special therapeutic services

Social work in the health services

Environmental health specialties

Training opportunities in public health

The many health fields which exist today, and the numerous expanding opportunities that these fields offer for professional careers and occupations in the health services, are described in this chapter. The first section of the chapter reviews the growth and current status of health professions and occupations in the United States and the contemporary concerns regarding manpower shortages in the health fields. In the next several sections of the chapter, the nature of the services provided and characteristics of the principal professions and/or occupations are described briefly for each of a number of selected health fields. The fields include medicine, dentistry, visual services and eye care, veterinary medicine, and nursing and related services. Other fields discussed are laboratory services, pharmacologic services, and nutritional and dietetic services. Several special therapeutic services—i.e., physical therapy, occupational therapy, and others—are also described, as well as social work in the health services and various environmental health specialties. The last section of the chapter discusses the training programs for professional careers in public health that are provided by schools of public health in the United States.

STATUS OF MANPOWER IN THE HEALTH SERVICES

The complex network of community health agencies engaged in the provision of health programs and services requires many different kinds of professional and technical personnel, as well as administrative and supportive staff. In the United States, as health services have expanded to meet the needs of the population, the number of health workers has, of course, also grown. Among a total of 71 industries in 1960, the health services ranked third in the number of civilian labor force employees, exceeded only by agriculture and construction.[1] In the decade between 1950 and 1960, workers in the health services industry increased 54 per cent, from about 1.7 million to 2.6 million. Among the nine largest industries, only government educational services had a larger gain, and among all 71 industries, only seven exceeded the relative growth of the health services.

The rate of growth of specific health professions and occupations varied in the period of 1950 to 1960. Manpower in the medical and dental fields each increased about one third in number, and nursing increased almost one half. Personnel in environmental health occupations almost doubled, and scientists engaged in health research (excluding physicians, dentists, and veterinarians) increased fourfold.[1] The picture is less favorable, however, when viewed in relation to the population growth of the United States. Thus, for example, Table 15-1 shows that over a 15-year period from 1950 to 1965, the increase in the number of physicians and dentists barely kept pace with increases in the population. Only the nursing profession gained personnel at a more rapid rate than the population grew (Table 15-1), but the effective increase has not been as great as it might appear since some of the added number worked only part time.

TABLE 15-1   Physicians, Dentists, and Professional Nurses in Relation to Population, United States, Selected Years

	Number per 100,000 Population		
	Physicians *	Dentists	Professional Nurses
1950	149	57.2	249
1955	150	57.2	251 †
1960	148	56.4	282
1965	153	56.2	306 ‡

Source: Adapted from U.S. Department of Health, Education, and Welfare, Public Health Service, National Center for Health Statistics. *Health Resources Statistics—Health Manpower, 1965,* pp. 46, 100, 111.
* Includes doctors of medicine and doctors of osteopathy.
† Data are for 1954.
‡ Data are for 1964.

In 1965 in the United States, about 3 million persons were employed in more than 30 different health fields, and in from 200 to 300 occupations within those fields. These numbers include only persons who have had special education or training for work in a health setting; excluded are many other persons who perform the business, clerical, and maintenance services essential to the operation of health facilities and agencies, but whose occupations are not unique to the health field. Table 15-2 shows the principal health fields arrayed in descending order of the estimated number of

TABLE 15-2   Health Fields and Estimated Numbers of Persons Employed, United States, 1965

Estimated Persons Employed	Health Fields (and Typical Occupations)
1,409,000	Nursing and related services
	(Professional nurses; practical nurses; aides, orderlies, attendants; home health aides, homemakers)
305,100	Medicine and osteopathy *
	(Physicians: doctors of medicine and doctors of osteopathy)
230,900	Dentistry and allied services *
	(Dentists; dental hygienists, assistants, and laboratory technicians)
150,000–250,000	Secretarial and office services
	(Medical, dental, and optometrists' assistants, secretaries, and receptionists)
118,000	Pharmacy †
	(Pharmacists, pharmacy helpers)
85,000–95,000	Clinical laboratory services
	(Clinical chemists, microbiologists, and other biologic scientists; clinical laboratory technologists, technicians, and assistants)
70,000	Radiologic technology
	(Radiologic technologists, or medical x-ray technologists or technicians)
44,200	Basic sciences in the health field
	(Microbiologists, geneticists, physiologists, parasitologists, biochemists, biophysicists, biomathematicians, etc., engaged in medical research)
40,400	Visual services and eye care
	(Optometrists; opticians and optical technicians; orthoptists)
37,000	Medical records
	(Medical record librarians, technicians)
31,500–37,000	Administration of health services ‡
	(Public health, hospital, nursing home, voluntary health agency administrators; administrative officers, assistants; program analysts; program and field representatives)
32,500–35,000	Environmental health †
	(Sanitarians and sanitarian technicians; environmental health engineers, scientists, specialists, technicians; engineering aides)
30,000	Nutritional and dietetics services §
	(Nutritionists, dietitians, other food service staff)
23,700	Veterinary medicine *
	(Veterinarians)
17,500	Social work †
	(Medical, psychiatric social workers)
16,700	Health education
	(Public health educators; school health educators, coordinators)

TABLE 15-2 (continued)

Estimated Persons Employed	Health Fields (and Typical Occupations)
16,500	Food and drug protective services (Food technologists, government food and drug inspectors and analysts)
14,000	Speech pathology and audiology (Speech pathologists; audiologists)
12,000	Physical therapy † (Physical therapists, physical therapy aides)
9,000	Psychology (Clinical, counseling, social, measurement psychologists)
8,000	Library services in the health field ¶ (Medical librarians, patients' or hospital librarians)
7,600	Podiatry (Podiatrists)
7,500	Biomedical engineering (Biomedical or medical engineers and biomedical engineering technicians engaged in inventing, adapting, and maintaining medical devices and instruments)
6,200	Miscellaneous hospital services # (Inhalation therapists; electrocardiograph, electroencephalograph technicians; surgical, obstetric, and pediatric aides)
6,000	Occupational therapy † (Occupational therapists, occupational therapy assistants)
5,300–5,900	Specialized rehabilitation services (Corrective, educational, manual arts, music, recreational therapists; homemaking rehabilitation consultants)
5,000	Health information and communication (Science writers and health information specialists; technical writers; illustrators, poster and display artists, and draftsmen; medical illustrators)
4,200	Vocational rehabilitation counseling (Rehabilitation counselors)
3,300	Orthopedic and prosthetic appliance making (Prosthetists, orthotists)
1,400–2,400	Health and vital statistics ** (Health statisticians or biostatisticians, statistical clerks, vital record registrars, health demographers)
600–800	Anthropology and sociology (Physical and cultural anthropologists; sociologists and medical sociologists)
500	Economic research in the health field (Health economists engaged in research and analytic studies)
300	Automatic data processing †† (Systems analysts, programers, computer operators)

Source: Adapted from U.S. Department of Health, Education, and Welfare, Public Health Service, National Center for Health Statistics. *Health Resources Statistics—Health Manpower, 1965,* p. 177 and individual chapters.

* Estimate includes total personnel (active and inactive) for physicians, dentists, and veterinarians.

† Estimates not available for aides and technicians.

‡ Excludes business, clerical, and maintenance workers.

§ Estimates not available for food service supervisors and clerical and other workers.

¶ Estimate includes technical and clerical workers in medical libraries; estimate not available for patients' librarians.

\# Estimates not available for electrocardiograph technicians and hospital aides.

** Estimate not available for statistical clerks.

†† Estimates not available for programers, operators, and electronic technicians.

persons employed and indicates one or more typical occupations within each field. There were 1.4 million persons employed in the field of nursing and related services in 1965, followed by medicine and osteopathy with 305,000, and dentistry and allied services with almost 231,000. The large number of remaining health fields ranged in magnitude from more than 100,000 persons to several hundred (Table 15-2).

Health workers are employed in many different kinds of settings, from private offices to large and complex health organizations where numerous occupations are represented. Hospitals are an example of the latter, and nationally, they employ the largest number of health personnel. State and local health departments in 1964 employed a total of about 71,000 persons in a diversity of occupations. These occupations and the numbers of full-time state and local health department employees are shown in Table 15-3. Other settings in which health personnel are employed include many vol-

TABLE 15-3　Occupation of Full-Time Employees of State Health Departments and Local Health Units: January 1, 1964 and 1965

	State Health Department Employees		Local Health Unit Employees,
	1965	1964	1964 *
All Occupations	22,697	19,009	51,632
Physicians	708	609	1,668
Public health nurses	1,571	869	16,058
Clinic nurses	95	61	841
Dentists	166	164	402
Dental hygienists	66	58	496
Engineers	996	830	464
Sanitarians	1,072	688	7,508
Other sanitation personnel	544	350	2,188
Laboratory personnel	2,285	2,158	1,546
Health educators	286	233	361
Nutritionists	187	146	177
Social workers	291	230	688
Psychologists	66	69	156
Analysts and statisticians	544	387	250
Veterinarians	62	51	209
Public health investigators	403	337	543
X-ray technicians	197	222	380
Physical therapists	127	82	249
Administrative management	1,443	1,128	795
Clerical	8,776	7,733	11,634
Maintenance and service	2,101	1,677	3,143
Other personnel †	711	927 ‡	1,876

Source: U.S. Department of Health, Education, and Welfare, Public Health Service, National Center for Health Statistics. *Health Resources Statistics—Health Manpower, 1965,* p. 14.

* 1965 data not available.

† Includes some personnel in special programs, such as air pollution, water pollution, radiologic health, industrial hygiene, alcoholism, and community health.

‡ Includes attorneys, consultants, program representatives, and others who work with administrative management and were included in that group in 1965.

untary health agencies, as well as school systems, clinics, and laboratories. Business and industry also employ health workers in the conduct of occupational health programs and services.

In spite of increases in the number of health personnel in recent years, the manpower shortage remains one of the most serious problems confronting community health programs today. It will be recalled that reference has been made to this problem in preceding chapters, and it has been the subject of extensive analysis by government officials and members of the health professions who are continuously seeking ways to overcome the manpower deficit.[1-4] The need for additional health personnel is not only immediate but it is also expected to remain a consistent future concern. It has been estimated that an increase of a million individuals, above present totals, will be needed in all health occupations together in order to meet national requirements for health manpower through 1975.[5]

In the field of nursing, a 25 per cent increase over the present supply of professional nurses is expected by the 1970's, but this will still fall far short of meeting the full need.[6] Even in 1965–1966, there were budgeted vacancies for at least 75,000 registered nurses and 25,000 licensed practical nurses.[7] In dentistry, the backlog of unmet dental needs grows larger every year in spite of steady advances in dental science, services, and education. The number of practicing dentists is expected to increase 17 per cent over present numbers by 1975—but the population of the United States will have increased by an estimated 23 per cent.[6] Although the gap between supply and demand is larger in nursing and dentistry than in some other health fields, there are needs for increasing numbers of personnel in many other health occupations as well. For example, many more physicians will be needed merely to maintain the current physician-population ratio. In pharmacy, about 45 per cent of the nation's hospitals do not have a pharmacist on their staff even though the number of full- and part-time hospital pharmacists doubled in the period 1947 through 1962.[7] It has been estimated that the number of medical technologists in hospitals should be doubled in order to keep pace with the steadily increasing quantity and complexity of laboratory procedures.[7] Parallel instances of increasing manpower needs are to be found in almost any of the several hundred health occupations.

Thus, the health services offer countless future opportunities for careers in a wide diversity of fields, occupations, and settings—careers that can be both challenging and satisfying. The "knowledge explosion" has revolutionized the health fields, and many more skilled persons will continue to be required to develop and apply modern medical science and technology. Progress in the health sciences not only creates new health careers but also increases the number of people needed in those already well established.[6] For example, aerospace medicine, as a key element in the development of manned space flight, is a new frontier in the field of medicine. Not only are physicians engaged in the advancement of aerospace medicine but many other kinds of health personnel are also contributing, including veterinarians, who are closely involved in the research and medical care aspects of animals in space flight programs. In addition to scientific advances, another factor contributing to expansion of the health fields is the growth of the population, which is of particular significance since the relative rate of growth is highest among children and older people where health needs are greatest. A further factor is the increasing public demand for attaining and maintaining ample and high-quality health services; this demand continuously requires more, and well-trained, workers.

MEDICAL AND OTHER
PROFESSIONAL PRACTITIONERS *

There are several health services in which professional practitioners are required to have advanced training at the doctoral level or beyond. This includes general practitioners and the many specialists in the field of medicine, as well as dentists, optometrists, and veterinarians in their respective fields. These practitioners share a common concern for the promotion of general health, and various aspects of their fields are particularly relevant to public health practice.

Medicine

In the United States and outlying areas at the close of 1965, there were 292,088 physicians who held the degree of Doctor of Medicine (M.D.) and 13,027 who held the degree of Doctor of Osteopathy (D.O.).[3] Physicians are in private practice and in group practice, as described in Chapter 5, as well as in hospital service, teaching, public health and preventive medicine, research, and other forms of practice. Currently, fewer than two out of three physicians are in private practice, and the proportion has been declining over the years.

The growing number of specialists in the medical profession (also referred to in Chap. 5) has resulted in an outnumbering of general practitioners by about two to one among the active doctors of medicine. In addition to general practice, the profession recognizes almost 30 specialties which may be grouped into four major categories: medical specialties (e.g., cardiovascular disease, internal medicine, pediatrics); surgical specialties (e.g., general surgery, orthopedic surgery, obstetrics and gynecology, ophthalmology, urology); psychiatry and neurology; and other specialties such as administrative medicine, pathology, radiology, occupational medicine, physical medicine and rehabilitation, general preventive medicine, and public health.

* Information contained in the next eight sections of this chapter (pp. 442–57) is based to a large extent on *Health Resources Statistics—Health Manpower, 1965* (U.S. Department of Health, Education, and Welfare, National Center for Health Statistics) and *Health Careers Guidebook* (U.S. Department of Labor, Bureau of Employment Security).

Training as a physician takes at least eight years after graduation from high school and may extend from 10 to 15 years. A license to practice is required in all states and the District of Columbia. To qualify for a license, a candidate must have been graduated from an approved school, pass a licensing examination, and—in more than half the states—serve a one-year hospital internship. There are 84 medical schools and five osteopathic colleges in the United States which award M.D. and D.O. degrees, respectively, to those completing a required four-year course.

Physicians with a specialty in public health are certified by the American Board of Preventive Medicine. In addition to a medical degree and training as a general practitioner or a specialist, the career public health physician usually has a graduate degree in public health. Such physicians are employed by federal, state, and local health departments and by voluntary health agencies. Their activities range from clinical practice to consultative and administrative positions. They work closely with other public health personnel, such as nurses, sanitarians, health educators, and social workers. Many public health physicians specialize in particular areas, including maternal and child health, chronic disease, communicable disease, mental health, alcoholism, and others.

Dentistry

The Dental Profession. Almost all dentists provide care to patients, primarily in private dental offices, but also in public and private clinics and hospitals, military installations, and other institutions. Some dentists, however, are engaged in nonclinical activities, such as teaching, research, or administration of dental programs; the settings in which these dentists work include dental schools, public health departments, dental societies, and various other public and private organizations.

In mid-1965, there were approximately 109,300 dentists, including 102,175 nonfederal dentists located in the 50 states and the District of Columbia (about 86,320 of these were professionally active) and 7125 federal dentists in the Armed Forces, Public Health Service, and Veterans Administration. Although most dentists are general practitioners, there were almost 6500 specialists in 1965, the number having more than doubled since 1955. There are eight recognized areas of dental specialization, but over one half of the specialists engage exclusively in orthodontia (straightening of teeth), and about one quarter limit their practice to oral surgery. To be recognized as a specialist, a dentist needs at least two years of advanced study and several years of experience in his specialty.

All dentists must be graduates of an accredited dental school and must obtain a license before practicing dentistry. Dental schools in the United States (of which there were 49 in 1965, including one in Puerto Rico) offer a four-year course leading to a degree of Doctor of Dental Surgery (D.D.S.) or Doctor of Dental Medicine (D.M.D.). No distinction is made between these degrees by the profession or licensing agencies. To qualify for licensure in a state, the dental school graduate must pass both a written and a clinical examination.

Dental Diseases. There are several major kinds of dental diseases which are of particular concern to dental practitioners. *Dental caries* (tooth decay) is the most common disease in the United States, afflicting over 95 per cent of the population. *Periodontal disease* (pyorrhea or diseased gums) affects the bony and soft-tissue support of the teeth. If untreated in adults, it is progressive and terminates with the loss of teeth. After age 35, periodontal disease is the single most important cause of tooth loss. *Malocclusion* (crooked teeth) occurs when teeth or jaws are not in normal alignment with each other. Although such orthodontic deformities are common, a majority of the cases do not constitute a serious health hazard to the individual; however, in the more extreme cases, severe psychologic and physiologic handicapping can result. *Cleft palate and cleft lip* are more serious deformities which originate as birth defects in one out of every 700 or 800 live births and represent 13 per cent of all birth anomalies. Treatment of oral clefts is an extremely complicated and frequently prolonged procedure, requiring the combined efforts of surgeons, orthodontists, prosthodontists, speech therapists, and psychologists. *Cancer of the mouth* accounts for an estimated 3 to 4 per cent of all cancers, and there are over 4000 deaths each year from oral carcinoma. Early detection and prompt treatment can reduce mortality by as much as 89 per cent for lip cancer, but by only 30 per cent for cancer of the tongue.

Treatment and Prevention of Dental Diseases. Early diagnosis and treatment of dental diseases are necessary to ensure the proper chewing of food and to maintain normal speech and facial appearance as well as general health. Modern dentistry also places great emphasis on the prevention of dental disease. Prevention includes such measures as the fluoridation of community water supplies, topical applications of fluoride solutions to the natural teeth, the addition of fluorides (tablets or drops) to the diet, and the reduction of fermentable carbohydrates in the diet. Dental health educational programs stress the importance of proper diet, correct oral hygiene practices, and regular dental examinations. Dental research, both basic and applied, is contributing increasingly to advances in the treatment and prevention of dental disease. At present, dental research is reaching out in its investigations into many fields of biology and into many areas of the physical sciences, biochemistry, physiology, and radiobiology.

Dental Public Health. One of the newest specialties in the field of dentistry is dental public health. Dental public health programs, provided through state and local health departments and several federal agencies, place major emphasis on promoting the preventive aspects of dental care and on the education of the public to the importance of dental health. The public health dentist assesses the dental health needs of a community, and assists in the planning and development of programs of education, prevention, and care on a communitywide basis.

Direct services on the *local* level are primarily for the treatment of indigent children. A few large cities have fairly extensive programs, employing dentists in local clinics. Dental public health programs on the *state* level provide dental consultation and technical assistance to other departments within the state government and to local communities. Such programs also offer diagnostic laboratory services to practicing dentists; conduct screening examinations, postgraduate training, research, and demonstration projects; and provide dental treatment for patients in state institutions. In some states, direct services are made available to indigents and to persons in isolated areas by dentists and dental hygienists employed by the state. More often, the department of public welfare administers the dental program for eligible beneficiaries who receive authorized treatment from private practitioners.

On the *national* level, the Public Health Service provides consultation, technical assistance, and funds for research and demonstration projects. Public Health Service dentists provide direct care for Service personnel and for the special population groups for which the Service is responsible. The National Institute of Dental Research of the National Institutes of Health carries on research in the basic sciences of dentistry and the epidemiology of dental diseases. It also provides training and research grants to schools and individuals engaged in dental public health education and research. The Children's Bureau provides grants-in-aid to state and local governmental programs to promote maternal and child dental health. In addition, the Crippled Children's Program, federally supported through state agencies, has been most successful in the correction of many oral defects. The Armed Forces and the Veterans Administration employ dentists who render direct care to military personnel and in Veterans Administration hospitals, respectively.[8]

Allied Occupational Groups in Dentistry. There are three principal allied occupational groups in dentistry: dental assistants, dental hygienists, and dental laboratory technicians. *Dental assistants,* who numbered about 91,000 in 1965, assist the dentist at the chairside by preparing the patient for treatment, keeping the operating field clear, mixing filling materials, passing instruments, etc. Other duties involve exposing and processing x-rays, sterilizing instruments, assisting with laboratory work, ordering supplies, and handling the office records and accounts. More than 85 per cent of the dentists in private practice now employ one or more dental assistants. Traditionally, dental assistants have been trained on the job by their dentist employers. However, the number of institutions offering accredited training programs for assistants increased from 26 to 64 within the four-year period of 1961–1965.[3]

Dental hygienists are the only dental auxiliaries who provide service directly to the patient and who, like the dentist, are required in each state to obtain a license to practice. The hygienist, working under the direction of the dentist, performs prophylaxes (scaling and polishing of the teeth), exposes and processes dental x-ray films, applies fluoride solution to the teeth of children, instructs individual patients in toothbrushing techniques and proper diet as related to teeth, etc. In 1965, an estimated 15,100 dental hygienists were in practice, but there are still only 16 active hygienists per 100 practicing dentists and a number of these are employed part time.[3] The number of schools offering training in the dental hygiene program has increased significantly in recent years, from 37 in 1960 to 56 in 1965.

The *dental laboratory technician* is a highly skilled craftsman who performs many tasks involved in the construction of complete and partial dentures, fixed bridgework, crowns, and other similar dental restorations and appliances. The technician does not have direct contact with the patient but performs his work in accordance with instructions received from the dentist. There were an estimated 25,500 technicians in 1965, approximately 20,200 of whom worked in commercial dental laboratories; the remainder were employed by dentists in private practice.[3]

Visual Services and Eye Care

The responsibility for visual services and eye care is divided among three categories of health personnel: ophthalmologists, optometrists, and opticians. *Ophthalmologists*, constituting one of the surgical specialties mentioned earlier in this section, are physicians who specialize in the medical and surgical care of the eyes and who may prescribe drugs or other treatment as well as lenses.

Optometrists specialize in vision analysis by examining the eyes, and they prescribe lenses and other vision aids, visual training and orthoptics, or other forms of treatment. They do not treat eye diseases or perform surgery. There are about 17,000 active optometrists in the United States, the number having been relatively constant for many years. Nearly three quarters are in private practice, either solo or group practice. All states and the District of Columbia require a license for the practice of optometry. To qualify for a license, the applicant must be a graduate of an accredited school of optometry and pass a state board examination. In 1965, there were ten accredited colleges of optometry in the United States, requiring a six-year curriculum leading to the degree of Doctor of Optometry (O.D.).

Opticians fit and adjust eyeglasses according to prescriptions written by ophthalmologists or optometrists; they do not examine eyes or prescribe treatment. The actual grinding and polishing of lenses and assembly in a frame are done by an *optical technician*, who is also known as an optical laboratory mechanic, lens grinder, or polisher. The dispensing optician then fits and adjusts the eyeglasses to the individual's requirements. There were an estimated 23,000 opticians and optical technicians employed in the United States in 1965. Opticians are required to be licensed in 17 states; some of these states also require licenses for optical technicians in retail optical shops or for the retail optical establishment itself.

The public health aspects of visual problems and eye care are becoming increasingly recognized. There is a growing awareness of the importance of community-based planning and development of programs for the diagnosis and treatment of eye disorders so that all segments of the population who need eye care services will receive them. Public education regarding eye care and the desirability of early diagnosis and optimum treatment to forestall visual impairment is an important part of such programs. Glaucoma, which is a major eye disorder, is a particularly important public health problem because the blindness to which it may otherwise lead is preventable if the disease is discovered in its early stages. Similarly, cataracts are the most common present cause of blindness in the United States, but the onset of blindness can be prevented by early detection and restoration of sight through surgery. Early detection of these and other eye conditions depends on the provision of broad programs for examining apparently healthy eyes —by specialists in their own offices and by comprehensive screening and testing programs.

Veterinary Medicine

The Veterinary Profession. Veterinary medicine deals with the prevention and treatment of disease and injury in animals. Veterinarians, in addition to providing treatment, also give advice regarding the care and breeding of animals and help prevent the outbreak and spread of disease among them, by physical examinations, tests, and vaccinations. One of the newest developments in the health field is the veterinarian's role in disease prevention among human beings by protecting them from the various diseases that can spread from animals to man, including tuberculosis, rabies, brucellosis, and salmonellosis.

The number of veterinarians in the United States increased from 15,800 in 1950 to 23,700 by the end of 1964.[3] All states and the District of Columbia require that veterinarians have a license to practice. To obtain a license, an applicant must be a graduate of an approved veterinary school and pass a state board examination. A few states also require some practical experience under the supervision of a licensed veterinarian. Graduates of a veterinary school earn the degree of Doctor of Veterinary Medicine (D.V.M.), which requires a minimum of six years beyond high school. In 1965, there were 18 approved schools of veterinary medicine in the United States.

More than half of the veterinarians go into private practice, and most handle all kinds of domestic animals. An additional number work directly in regulatory and public health aspects of veterinary medicine for federal, state, or local governments or are engaged in teaching, research, and other types of practice. For positions in public health, research, or teaching, the master's or doctoral degree in a field such as pathology, epidemiology, public health, or bacteriology may be required, in addition to the D.V.M. degree.

Veterinary Public Health. Veterinary public health is a specialty within the broad field of veterinary medicine. Veterinarians in public health conduct research, develop diagnostic and laboratory methods, provide special training and advisory services, and conduct epidemiologic investigations and preventive medical programs concerned with diseases transmissible from animals to man.

More than 11 per cent of all veterinarians work for the federal government, state or local agencies, and international groups.[6] For example, the Agricultural Research Service of the U.S. Department of Agriculture has a full-time staff of veterinarians to inspect meat in packing plants and to work throughout the country on the control and eradication of animal diseases. Other veterinarians in this Department supervise stockyards, inspect poultry, and enforce quarantine regulations and the various rules about the importing and exporting of animals and animal products; in addition, they conduct research and supervise the licensing of firms manufacturing serums and vaccines for animals. The Food and Drug Administration also employs veterinarians.

A veterinary public health section has been organized in the Public Health Service to develop programs for controlling animal diseases that affect public health, to help the states establish veterinary public health programs, and to serve as consultants in other Public Health Service activities. This nationwide service provides a broad base for tackling widespread problems and has proved effective in reducing the spread of many diseases from area to area. Other goals of veterinary medicine within the Public Health Service are to collect and evaluate statistical data on human illnesses caused by animals, to study the effects of air pollution on animals, and to conduct basic research on chronic and communicable diseases.

Veterinarians employed by state and local health departments cooperate with private practitioners and federal field workers to control disease among animals and also to protect human health. Some counties and many cities employ veterinarians to see that meats and dairy products are wholesome and are sold in clean surroundings. In other instances, veterinarians supervise the production of biologicals—serums, antitoxins, and the like—used in the prevention and treatment of disease in human beings.

Internationally, veterinarians are on the central and regional staffs of the World Health Organization and the Food and Agriculture Organization of the United Nations. During the years following World War II, veterinarians worked with the United Nations Relief and Rehabilitation Administration to help war-torn countries build up their supply of food animals. Currently, they are working with the Foreign Operations Administration to provide economic and technical aid to less developed countries.

NURSING AND RELATED SERVICES

Professional nurses, of course, constitute the key group of personnel in the field of nursing services. They may be supplemented by, and often supervise, several other types of nursing personnel, including practical nurses, aides, orderlies, attendants, and ward clerks. Two relatively new categories of workers in the nursing services consist of home health aides and homemakers.

Professional Nurses

Professional nurses, who are also known as registered nurses (R.N.'s) or graduate nurses, are responsible for the nature and quality of all nursing care that patients receive. They carry out the physicians' instructions and supervise practical nurses and nonprofessional personnel who perform routine care and treatment of patients. There were about 582,000 professional nurses in practice in the United States at the beginning of 1964, and they were employed in a variety of settings.[3] About two thirds (67 per cent) worked in hospitals, nursing homes, and related institutions, and 11 per cent were self-employed private-duty nurses. An additional 10 per cent were public health, school, or occupational health nurses. The remainder worked in offices or were engaged in nursing education or other areas of practice.

There are a number of clinical specialties in the nursing profession. For example, pediatric nurses specialize in caring for children; obstetric nurses care for mothers and new babies; and medical-surgical nurses care for patients before, during, and after surgery and in most types of illness. Other nursing specialties include the care of patients with particular diseases, such as cardiovascular illnesses, cancer, and pulmonary ailments. Positions in these and other specialties require experience and additional courses of study beyond the basic preparation, usually at the master's or doctoral level.

A license is required to practice professional nursing in all states and the District of Columbia. For licensure as a registered nurse, an applicant must have graduated from a school approved by the state board of nursing and pass a state board examination. In 1965, there were 1191 schools of nursing in the United States (including Puerto Rico) which offered one of three possible training programs: a program leading to an associate degree (usually a two-year course), to a diploma (usually three years), or to a bachelor's degree (usually four years, but sometimes five).[3]

Practical Nurses

Practical nurses, known also as vocational nurses, give bedside nursing care to patients who are not acutely ill and assist the professional nurse with patients who are more seriously ill. They must be licensed to practice as L.P.N.'s (or as L.V.N.'s in California and Texas). There were about 282,000 practical nurses employed in the United States in 1966.[3] The majority work in hospitals, clinics, homes for the aged, and nursing homes. Many others are employed in private homes, and some work in doctor's offices, schools, and public health agencies. Training as a practical nurse usually requires 12 to 18 months and may be obtained in trade, technical, or vocational schools operated by public-school systems or in private schools controlled by hospitals, health agencies, or colleges. In 1964, there were 913 approved programs of practical nursing education offered in the United States and outlying areas.

Related Nursing Services

There are several kinds of workers who provide auxiliary nursing services in hospitals, clinics, and nursing homes. *Nursing aides,* who are usually women, assist professional and practical nurses by performing less skilled tasks in the care of patients. *Orderlies* and *attendants,* who are usually men, perform routine duties in caring for male patients and certain heavy duties in the care of the physically ill, mentally ill, and mentally retarded. There were an estimated 500,000 of these auxiliary workers in the United States in 1965.[3] Such occupations are not licensed (except for psychiatric aides, who are licensed in Arkansas, California, and Michigan), but hospitals generally have their own standards of service and their own training programs. *Ward clerks,* sometimes also known as floor clerks or ward or unit secretaries, act as receptionists and relieve the nurse of much of the paperwork in the patient-care units of an institution. They receive on-the-job training for duties such as preparing patients' charts, distributing the records needed by physicians on their rounds, and similar clerical tasks.

Workers who provide auxiliary nursing services in the home rather than in an institutional setting are *home health aides* (also known as home aides or visiting health aides) and *homemakers.* In general, the duties of the home health aide include a large element of personal care for persons who are ill or disabled, while those of the homemaker are more likely to be associated with various problems of household management that have arisen because of illness or disability in a family. Home health aide–homemaker services are organized and administered under various auspices, including more than 500 public or voluntary agencies which provide such programs. The number of home health aides and homemakers was estimated to be in excess of 6000 in 1965 in the United States.[3] Such workers receive on-the-job training and work under professional supervision.

Public Health Nursing

Public health nursing is a specialty within both professional nursing and the broad area of organized public health practice. It is responsible for the provision of nursing service on a family-centered basis in the home and for individuals and groups at work, at school, and in public health centers. The public health nurse works to prevent disease and promote health through case finding, by encouraging individuals to seek medical care, and by providing facts about health to the individual, the family, and the community.

Local health departments constitute the typical settings in which public health nurses are employed. Public health nurses also work in voluntary agencies, notably visiting nurse associations. In addition, school nurses and occupational health, or industrial, nurses are often considered a part of public health nursing.

Within the local health department, public health nursing is generally organized as a service division, with a director of nursing and/or a supervisor for each eight or ten staff nurses. Each state health department has a division of public health nursing which acts as advisor to local units, as well as assisting them in planning nursing programs and in selecting and training personnel. In local communities, about one nurse per 5000 population is the recommended standard, or one per 2500 population, if bedside nursing is included as part of the service. Areas of particular concern in public health nursing include maternal and child health, communicable disease control, chronic illness and rehabilitation, psychiatric care, and nutritional education. The public health nurse may also provide instruction in public health matters to community groups, volunteer personnel, and professional nursing groups. Although there are specialized categories of public health nurses (e.g., tuberculosis nurses), "generalized" nursing is usually considered to be preferable particularly in connection with services to families. In "generalized" public health nursing, a nurse performs *all* public health nursing functions in the specified geographic area or district to which she is assigned.

LABORATORY SERVICES

Laboratories have an important role in the health services not only in the diagnosis and treatment of illness but also in the prevention and control of disease. The laboratories which perform these functions are found in several different kinds of settings. Hospitals constitute one of the principal settings and employ many thousands of laboratory personnel. In addition, an estimated 25,000 to 30,000 persons (other than nurses) perform some laboratory work in physicians' offices, and approximately 10,000 persons work in about 2000 private independent laboratories.[3] State and local health departments employ almost 4000 laboratory workers, as shown earlier in Table 15-3. Smaller numbers of personnel are estimated to be employed by industrial and independent research laboratories.

Most laboratories, aside from those under public health or research auspices, engage exclusively in the conduct of a wide variety of clinical tests to aid the physician in diagnosing illness. Public health laboratories also perform diagnostic tests but have numerous broader functions as well, particularly state health department laboratories and those in larger cities.[9] All states provide laboratory services for the diagnosis and control of communicable disease, and to a lesser but increasing degree they also provide services relating to certain noncommunicable diseases such as tissue examinations for cancer. Such services may be provided for physicians and hospitals as well as for public health workers. Public health laboratories also conduct chemical and bacteriologic examinations of food, milk, water, air, narcotics, drugs, and other substances. They distribute and sometimes manufacture biologicals, including serums, toxins, antitoxins, and vaccines. State public health laboratories may supervise the practices, procedures, personnel, and products of local and private laboratories through various methods such as inspections, licensing, and standard setting. A majority of state laboratories also conduct special research projects in addition to their routine activities.

Several different kinds of occupations are found in the field of laboratory services. An estimated 3500 or more professional *scientists* with graduate degrees in chemistry or the biologic sciences, such as microbiology, were employed in laboratory services in 1965.[3] *Medical technologists,* of whom there were about 32,000 in 1965, perform clinical, microscopic, bacteriologic, and other tests under the supervision of a pathologist or other physician. In addition, there are various clinical laboratory technicians and assistants who numbered in excess of 45,000 in 1965. These include, for example, *cytotechnologists* (or cytotechnicians), who specialize in screening slides for abnormalities that are warning signs of cancer, and *histologic technicians,* who specialize in cutting and staining body tissues for microscopic examination.

PHARMACOLOGIC SERVICES

Pharmacy is concerned with the discovery, standardization, manufacture, storage, distribution, and dispensing of medicinal products. Such products are used in the prevention, diagnosis, and treatment of disease. *Pharmacists* are specialists in the science of drugs. Of the 118,284 licensed, practicing pharmacists in the United States in 1965, a vast majority were practicing in retail community pharmacies.[3] Settings in which the remaining pharmacists were found included hospital pharmacies, pharmaceutical manufacturing and wholesale establishments, colleges of pharmacy, and government. Licensure to practice pharmacy requires graduation from an accredited pharmacy college, completion of a one-year internship (required in most states), and passing a state board examination. In 1965, there were 75 colleges of pharmacy in the United States and Puerto Rico, all but two of which were accredited by the American Council on Pharmaceutical Education.

The public health import of pharmaceuticals was, of course, recognized many years ago by the federal government and contributed to the establishment of the Food and Drug Administration. The Administration, within its broad responsibilities for drug protective services, is concerned with the purity, safety, and effectiveness of drugs. Drug laws are enforced by the Food and Drug Administration and by state and local official health agencies.

In local communities, retail pharmacists also have an important role in public health. Pharmacists are approached daily by patrons who ask for health-related information ranging from the causes of aches and pains to community health facilities for preventing and treating these ailments. Although the pharmacist does not give medical advice or treatment, he can inform such persons where to obtain the help they want, or he can make them aware of the fact that they need help. Thus, the community pharmacist makes a significant contribution to the promotion of well-being among people in his neighborhood, and his efforts can be further enhanced by active cooperation with physicians and with public and private agencies.

NUTRITIONAL AND DIETETIC SERVICES

Nutritional and dietetic services deal with the application of the scientific principles of nutrition to the consumption and utilization of food. Nutrition is recognized as a vital element in the promotion of health and the prevention of disease and in facilitating recovery and rehabilitation from many illnesses. Scientific research already has greatly expanded the knowledge of the relationship of nutrition to disease and to health. Nutritional factors in various diseases continue to be an important avenue of investigation, for example, the role of cholesterol (dietary fat) in atherosclerosis and of obesity in heart disease and diabetes. Today, nutrition is concerned not only with inadequacies in eating patterns, but also with the sources of possible food hazards such as fads and frauds, radiation, chemical fertilizers, and additives. Nutritional problems are complex because food habits are influenced not only by knowledge of nutrition, but also by many cultural, economic, psychological, and physiologic factors.

Nutritionists engage in investigating and solving problems of nutrition for the promotion of health. The *public health nutritionist* is responsible for the nutrition component of public health agency programs. She provides nutrition counseling to patients in the agency's clinics and serves as a consultant to other workers in health agencies and various community organizations. She provides current nutrition information to the public by teaching special classes, preparing informational material, and working with community leaders in planning nutrition programs. The *teaching nutritionist* conducts educational programs in nutrition for the preparation of professional workers as well as for the public. The *research nutritionist* is concerned with the interrelationship of nutrients in foods and the effects on health.[3]

Dietitians assume major responsibility for food selection, preparation, and management of food services. They plan and direct food service programs in hospitals, schools, restaurants, and other public and private institutions. Dietitians are employed as administrators of food-service programs, as therapeutic dietitians in hospitals, and as consultants. Some are also engaged in teaching and research.

SPECIAL THERAPEUTIC SERVICES

There are several special health services that are particularly concerned with the correction of impairments, restoration of function, and various aspects of rehabilitation. These include speech pathology and audiology, physical therapy, occupational therapy, and several specialized rehabilitation services including vocational rehabilitation counseling.

Speech Pathology and Audiology

Speech pathology and audiology are concerned with disorders in the production, reception, and perception of speech and language. *Speech pathologists* and *audiologists* help to identify persons who have such disorders and to determine the etiology, history, and severity of specific disorders through interviews and special tests. They facilitate optimal treatment and rehabilitation through speech, hearing, and language remedial or conservational procedures, counseling, and guidance. They also make appropriate referrals for medical or other professional attention.[3]

In 1965, there were about 14,000 speech pathologists and audiologists in active practice in the United States. A large proportion work in elementary or secondary schools, including schools and classes for the deaf. Others work in clinics in hospitals, rehabilitation centers, colleges, etc., and some are engaged in teaching and research. There were 240 schools in the United States which offered training programs in speech pathology and audiology in 1964. The American Speech and Hearing Association awards a "Certificate of Clinical Competence" in speech pathology and in audiology, each of which requires academic training at the master's degree level, one year of experience, and passing a national examination.

Physical Therapy

Physical therapy is concerned with the restoration of function and the prevention of disability following disease, injury, or loss of a bodily part. Upon referral by a physician, the *physical therapist* evaluates the needs of the patient and plans the program which will be most effective. Treatment may include exercises in warm baths or pools, other types of exercise, hot packs, special electrical currents to stimulate muscles, ultraviolet rays, or massage. Physical therapy services include instructing patients and their families on how to carry on prescribed treatment at home.

There were an estimated 12,000 physical therapists employed in the United States in 1965. A majority work in hospitals, while others are employed by rehabilitation centers, by schools or societies for crippled children, and by public health agencies. A license to practice physical therapy is required in 48 states and the District of Columbia. To obtain a license an applicant must have a degree or certificate from a school of physical therapy and pass a state board examination. In 1964, there were 42 colleges and universities offering training programs leading to professional qualification in physical therapy.

Occupational Therapy

Occupational therapy is the use of purposeful activity as treatment in the rehabilitation of persons with physical or emotional disability. The occupational therapist, as a vital member of the rehabilitation team, uses creative, educational, recreational, and prevocational activities in treatment programs that are geared to the individual needs of each patient. Through prevocational testing, the occupational therapist helps handicapped persons prepare for job training and employment or for possible changes in occupation.

Approximately 6000 occupational therapists were in active practice in the United States in 1965. About three fourths work in hospitals, with large numbers in federal installations. Others are employed in rehabilitation centers, nursing homes, homes for the aged, schools and camps for handicapped children, and teaching and research institutions. In 1965, there were 32 colleges and universities offering training programs in occupational therapy; these programs include supervised clinical experience. Graduates of approved schools of occupational therapy are eligible to take the national registration examination which is conducted by the American Occupational Therapy Association.

Specialized Rehabilitation Services

Rehabilitation is a complex process because many different services may be required to help people with physical or mental disabilities return to normal, or near normal, living. There are, however, two principal tasks in rehabilitation.[6] One task is concerned with repairing, or compensating for, the damage of illness or accident. There are several health services directed toward this phase of rehabilitation, two of which—physical therapy and occupational therapy—have just been described. In addition, there are several other kinds of therapists, each of whom has a particular, specialized skill in the rehabilitation of physically or mentally disabled persons. These include the *corrective therapist* (who utilizes physical exercises in treatment and may instruct patients in the use of orthopedic and prosthetic appliances), the *educational therapist*, the *manual arts therapist*, the *music therapist*, and the *recreational therapist*. Such occupations are relatively new and are concentrated in hospitals and rehabilitation centers (particularly those operated by the Veterans Administration) but are also found in certain schools that provide such programs.

The other principal task in rehabilitation is vocational guidance, training, and placement. Activities of this kind constitute the field of vocational rehabilitation counseling. The *vocational rehabilitation counselor* is concerned with evaluating the vocational potential of the individual. He tries to match the abilities of the client with a job when the time comes for starting work—either in the old job or the one for which job training or retraining becomes a part of rehabilitation. Counselors also engage in community activities to interest prospective employers, educators, and others in the problems of handicapped persons and the benefits of rehabilitation.[3] Most vocational rehabilitation counselors are employed in state rehabilitation programs which are financed jointly by federal and state funds. Others are employed in hospitals, in special schools, and by voluntary health agencies and other organizations with rehabilitation interests.

SOCIAL WORK IN THE HEALTH SERVICES

Of a total of 125,000 social workers in the United States in 1965, about 17,500 were in the health field.[3] Social work programs in the health field are designed to meet the special needs of persons who are ill, disabled, aged, or crippled. Two types of social work specialists are found in health work: *medical social workers* and *psychiatric social workers*. Both work directly with patients and their families, helping them to cope with problems related to severe or long illness, recovery, and rehabilitation. They also assess the significant social and emotional factors related to the patient's health problems and thus assist physicians and other health workers in the evaluation and treatment of the individual. They utilize community health agencies and other resources to assist the patient in adjustment to disability and to life in the community.[3]

The health settings in which social workers are employed include hospitals and their outpatient departments, clinics, voluntary organizations, and public health departments. Social workers in public health agencies may do family casework, serve as consultants to other health workers, or be involved in community organization, program planning, and research. They may have responsibilities in particular health department programs such as chronic disease, mental health, maternal and child health, alcoholism, or crippled children's services.

There were 60 graduate schools of social work in the United States in 1965 which were accredited by the Council on Social Work Education. In addition, at least 600 colleges and universities offer courses with social welfare content. More than half of the social workers employed in medical settings and three fourths of those in psychiatric settings have a masters degree.[3]

ENVIRONMENTAL HEALTH SPECIALTIES

The many different programs that constitute the field of environmental health, as described in Chapter 7, require numerous categories of personnel representing a wide variety of professional and technical skills. Those who have particularly central functions include sanitarians and environmental health engineers, specialists, and scientists. However, numerous practitioners and technologists in other health fields (e.g., physicians, epidemiologists, and veterinarians) may also have an important role in environmental health, as may several kinds of specialists outside the health field (e.g., urban planners, meteorologists, and automotive engineers).

Sanitarians and *sanitarian technicians* constitute the largest category of environmental health personnel, numbering 15,000 or more in 1965 in the United States. The sanitarian interprets and enforces city, state, federal, or other laws regarding sanitary standards in the various areas of environmental health. His responsibilities often include conferring with governmental and private groups for the purpose of interpreting and promoting environmental health programs. The professional sanitarian may be assisted by a sanitarian technician, aide, or sanitary inspector who investigates public and private establishments to determine compliance with or violation of public sanitation laws and regulations. The minimum educational qualification for a professional sanitarian is a bachelor's degree with specific training in a field relevant to environmental health; in addition, graduate training in environmental health sciences is desirable. At present, 29 states require registration or licensing of sanitarians.

Environmental health engineers hold engineering degrees and have specialized training or experience which enables them to plan and conduct programs for the prevention and control of environmental health hazards. Their job titles may reflect a special area of activity such as air pollution engineer, industrial hygiene engineer, or radiologic engineer, or they may have the more general designation of public health engineer or sanitary engineer.[3] There are also several kinds of *environmental health specialists,* notably industrial hygienists (who along with industrial hygiene engineers conduct health programs in industrial plants or similar installations to eliminate or control occupational health hazards and diseases) and radiologic health specialists (who have special training in the health aspects of radiation).

Environmental health scientists are concerned with the study and determination of the effects of environmental factors, singly and in the aggregate, on the health of human beings.[3] Their special capabilities are in the biologic, physical, and social sciences, and they are particularly concerned with the development of new knowledge and methods in the environmental health field.

TRAINING OPPORTUNITIES IN PUBLIC HEALTH

Preceding sections of this chapter have mentioned some of the many kinds of schools which offer training programs in the various health-service fields, and reference has been made to the fact that completion of a special academic program is a prerequisite for licensure or certification in a number of the health professions and occupations. The selected health fields described above have also illustrated the three-pronged nature of some of the fields, namely, direct service (which often requires a number of different occupational specialties), teaching, and research; each has its own particular training requirements.

For a few of the health occupations, of course, a high school general academic program is sufficient; for a few, specialized training offered by some high schools and vocational schools is needed; and for a few others, there are on-the-job training possibilities. However, many health professions and occupations now require from two to several years of academic training beyond high school. As health knowledge and technology advance, the need for formal training increases, and the new frontiers in science, medicine, and public health will no doubt continue to reinforce this trend.

The training of community health workers has for some time been recognized as the particular responsibility of schools of public health. Professional schools of public health were established in the United States early in the present century. In 1912, a formal program of instruction in biologic sciences and public health was organized by William Sedgwick at the Massachusetts Institute of Technology in cooperation with Harvard University. Subsequently, a conference of leaders of public health, medicine, and education set the pattern for the establishment of schools of public health by recommending that they be established as separate entities but affiliated with universities and their schools of medicine. In 1918, the Johns Hopkins University established a School of Hygiene and Public Health based on this principle. Professionalization of the field continued to develop thereafter, and in 1945, a system of accreditation of schools of public health was established by the American Public Health Association.

In 1964–1965, there were 15 schools of public health in North America, as shown in Table 15-4: 11 in continental United States, one each in Hawaii

TABLE 15-4   Location and Ownership of Schools of Public Health in North America: 1964–1965

Location	School	Ownership
California	University of California, Berkeley	Public
	University of California, Los Angeles	Public
Connecticut	Yale University, New Haven	Private
Louisiana	Tulane University, New Orleans	Private
Maryland	Johns Hopkins University, Baltimore	Private
Massachusetts	Harvard University, Boston	Private
Michigan	University of Michigan, Ann Arbor	Public
Minnesota	University of Minnesota, Minneapolis	Public
New York	Columbia University, New York	Private
North Carolina	University of North Carolina, Chapel Hill	Public
Pennsylvania	University of Pittsburgh, Pittsburgh	Private
Hawaii	University of Hawaii, Honolulu	Public
Puerto Rico	University of Puerto Rico, San Juan	Public
Canada	University of Montreal, Montreal	Private
	University of Toronto, Toronto	Public

Source: Adapted from U.S. Department of Health, Education, and Welfare, Public Health Service, National Center for Health Statistics. *Health Resources Statistics—Health Manpower, 1965,* p. 10.

and Puerto Rico, and two in Canada.* Of the schools in continental United States, four offered bachelors' degrees (the University of California at Berkeley and at Los Angeles, the University of Michigan, and the University of North Carolina), and all offered master's and doctor's degrees. Emphasis is on graduate education, and the schools are closing their undergraduate programs. Some students undertake master's or doctoral programs directly after they obtain a bachelor's degree with, perhaps, a major in public health. Many other students in the graduate-degree programs are already practitioners in various health fields, for example, in medicine, dentistry, nursing, veterinary medicine, engineering, environmental health, and numerous additional fields.

Curricula vary somewhat among schools of public health, of course, but in general the goal and content of a curriculum reflect the formulations of the Committee on Professional Education of the American Public Health Association, which is responsible for accrediting the schools. The general goal of training programs in schools of public health is considered to be the preparation of "competent, imaginative workers for careers in preventing disease and disability, and in analyzing, improving, promoting, and maintaining the health of the public." [10]

Several broad areas have been delineated in the curricula of schools of public health.[10] One of these has to do with the *health problems of the general population,* including the provision of comprehensive health care services, and several special considerations such as environmental hazards, infectious diseases, mental illness and retardation, and chronic diseases. A second broad area is concerned with the *health problems of special population groups,* such as mothers and children, occupational groups, and the aged. A third area consists of *special services for the general population or for special groups* and includes medical and hospital care, family planning, health education, nursing, nutrition, occupational health services, and rehabilitation. A fourth area pertains to *health resources and health economics,* and a fifth includes *technical and background subjects* such as epidemiology, biostatistics, demography, behavioral sciences, and research methodolgy.

In recent years, the training of students for professions in public health has been augmented significantly by federal legislation which provides funds for a variety of purposes, including student support, the development of programs of instruction, and the construction of teaching facilities. Through the Public Health Service, student support is provided either by training grants to the eligible institutions or through traineeships and fellowships awarded to individuals sponsored by the institution of their choice. The purpose of such support is to provide training opportunities for those interested in careers in research, teaching, and certain areas of clinical service.

* By 1967 two more schools of public health had been accredited by the American Public Health Association—those at the University of Oklahoma (Oklahoma City) and at Loma Linda University (Loma Linda, California).

REFERENCES

1. U.S. DEPARTMENT OF HEALTH, EDUCATION, AND WELFARE, Public Health Service. *Health Manpower Source Book,* Section 18. Manpower in the 1960's. U.S. Government Printing Office, Washington, D.C., 1964.

2. NATIONAL COMMISSION ON COMMUNITY HEALTH SERVICES, Task Force on Health Manpower. *Health Manpower—Action to Meet Community Needs.* Public Affairs Press, Washington, D.C., 1967.

3. U.S. DEPARTMENT OF HEALTH, EDUCATION, AND WELFARE, Public Health Service, National Center for Health Statistics. *Health Resources Statistics— Health Manpower, 1965.* U.S. Government Printing Office, Washington, D.C., 1966.

4. U.S. DEPARTMENT OF LABOR—U.S. Department of Health, Education, and Welfare. *Training Health Service Workers: The Critical Challenge.* Proceedings of the Conference on Job Development and Training for Workers in Health Services. U.S. Government Printing Office, Washington, D.C., 1966.

5. KEPPEL, FRANCIS. National responsibility for health manpower. In: U.S. Department of Labor—U.S. Department of Health, Education, and Welfare. *Training Health Service Workers: The Critical Challenge.* (Proceedings of the Conference on Job Development and Training for Workers in Health Services.) U.S. Government Printing Office, Washington, D.C., 1966.

6. U.S. DEPARTMENT OF LABOR, Bureau of Employment Security. *Health Careers Guidebook.* U.S. Government Printing Office, Washington, D.C., 1965.

7. BONNET, PHILIP D. Health manpower needs and requirements. In: U.S. Department of Labor—U.S. Department of Health, Education, and Welfare. *Training Health Service Workers: The Critical Challenge.* (Proceedings of the Conference on Job Development and Training for Workers in Health Services.) U.S. Government Printing Office, Washington, D.C., 1966.

8. YOUNG, W. O. Dental health. In: Commission on the Survey of Dentistry in the United States. *The Survey of Dentistry.* American Council on Education, Washington, D.C., 1961.

9. HANLON, JOHN J. *Principles of Public Health Administration,* 4th ed. The C. V. Mosby Company, St. Louis, 1964.

10. AMERICAN PUBLIC HEALTH ASSOCIATION, COMMITTEE ON PROFESSIONAL EDUCATION. Criteria and guidelines for accrediting schools of public health. *Amer J Public Health,* **56**:1308–18, August 1966.

INDEX

Illustrations are indicated by numbers in **boldface**.

SECRETARY

Under Secretary

| ASSISTANT SECRETARY (Education) | ASSISTANT SECRETARY (Community and Field Services) | ASSISTANT SECRETARY (Health and Scientific Affairs) Surgeon General Public Health Service | ASSISTANT SECRETARY (Legislation) |

American Printing House for Blind
Gallaudet College
Howard University

Office for Civil Rights
Center for Community Planning
Office of Consumer Services
Office of Field Coordination

PUBLIC HEALTH SERVICE

CONSUMER PROTECTION & ENVIRONMENTAL HEALTH SERVICE

Office of the Administrator

Environmental Control Administration

Food and Drug Administration

National Air Pollution Control Administration

HEALTH SERVICES & MENTAL HEALTH ADMINISTRATION

Office of the Administrator
National Center for Health Services Research and Development
National Center for Health Statistics
National Communicable Disease Center
National Institute of Mental Health
Health Facilities Planning and Construction Service
Community Health Service
Regional Medical Programs Service
Indian Health Service
Federal Health Programs Service

NATIONAL INSTITUTES OF HEALTH

Office of the Director
Bureau of Health Manpower
National Cancer Institute
National Heart Institute
National Institute of Allergy and Infectious Diseases
National Institute of Arthritis and Metabolic Diseases
National Institute of Child Health and Human Development
National Institute of Dental Research
National Institute of General Medical Sciences
National Institute of Neurological Diseases and Stroke
National Library of Medicine
Fogarty International Center

REGIONAL OFFICES

Regional Directors

| Regional Commissioners | Regional Health Directors |